Chronic Pain

Editors

JAMES P. ROBINSON
VIRTAJ SINGH

PHYSICAL MEDICINE AND REHABILITATION CLINICS OF NORTH AMERICA

www.pmr.theclinics.com

Consulting Editor
GREGORY T. CARTER

May 2015 • Volume 26 • Number 2

ELSEVIER

1600 John F. Kennedy Boulevard • Suite 1800 • Philadelphia, Pennsylvania, 19103-2899

http://www.theclinics.com

PHYSICAL MEDICINE AND REHABILITATION CLINICS OF NORTH AMERICA Volume 26, Number 2
May 2015 ISSN 1047-9651, ISBN 978-0-323-37615-0

Editor: Jennifer Flynn-Briggs
Developmental Editor: Don Mumford

Reprints. For copies of 100 or more of articles in this publication, please contact the Commercial Reprints Department, Elsevier Inc., 360 Park Avenue South, New York, NY 10010-1710. Tel.: 212-633-3874; Fax: 212-633-3820; E-mail: reprints@elsevier.com.

Physical Medicine and Rehabilitation Clinics of North America (ISSN 1047-9651) is published quarterly by Elsevier Inc., 360 Park Avenue South, New York, NY 10010-1710. Months of issue are February, May, August, and November. Business and Editorial Offices: 1600 John F. Kennedy Blvd., Suite 1800, Philadelphia, PA 19103-2899. Customer Service Office: 3251 Riverport Lane, Maryland Heights, MO 63043. Periodicals postage paid at New York, NY and additional mailing offices. Subscription price per year is $275.00 (US individuals), $486.00 (US institutions), $145.00 (US students), $335.00 (Canadian individuals), $640.00 (Canadian institutions), $210.00 (Canadian students), $415.00 (foreign individuals), $640.00 (foreign institutions), and $210.00 (foreign students). Foreign air speed delivery is included in all *Clinics* subscription prices. All prices are subject to change without notice. **POSTMASTER:** Send address changes to *Physical Medicine and Rehabilitation Clinics of North America*, Customer Service Office: Elsevier Health Sciences Division, Subscription Customer Service, 3251 Riverport Lane, Maryland Heights, MO 63043. **Customer Service: 1-800-654-2452 (US). From outside of the United States, call 314-447-8871. Fax: 314-447-8029. E-mail: JournalsCustomer Service-usa@elsevier.com (for print support); JournalsOnlineSupport-usa@elsevier.com (for online support).**

Physical Medicine and Rehabilitation Clinics of North America is indexed in *Excerpta Medica, MEDLINE/ PubMed (Index Medicus), Cinahl,* and *Cumulative Index to Nursing and Allied Health Literature.*

Contributors

CONSULTING EDITOR

GREGORY T. CARTER, MD, MS
Consulting Medical Editor, Medical Director, St Luke's Rehabilitation Institute, Spokane, Washington; University of Washington, School of Medicine, Seattle, Washington

EDITORS

JAMES P. ROBINSON, MD, PhD
Clinical Professor, Department of Rehabilitation Medicine, University of Washington, Seattle, Washington

VIRTAJ SINGH, MD
Clinical Faculty, Department of Rehabilitation Medicine, University of Washington; Medical Director, Seattle Spine and Sports Medicine, Seattle, Washington

AUTHORS

LARS ARENDT-NIELSEN, PhD, Dr Med Sci
Center for Sensory Motor Interaction, Department of Health Science and Technology, School of Medicine, University of Aalborg, Aalborg, Denmark

JANE C. BALLANTYNE, MD, FRCA
Professor, Department of Anesthesiology and Pain Medicine, University of Washington, Seattle, Washington

MICHELE CURATOLO, MD, PhD
Department of Anesthesiology and Pain Medicine, University of Washington, Seattle, Washington; Center for Sensory Motor Interaction, Department of Health Science and Technology, School of Medicine, University of Aalborg, Aalborg, Denmark

LINA FINE, MD, MPhil
Attending physician, Swedish Sleep Medicine, Swedish Neuroscience Institute, Swedish Medical Center, Seattle, Washington

ADRIELLE FRY, MD
Chief Resident, Department of Rehabilitation Medicine, University of Washington, Seattle, Washington

LEE S. GLASS, MD
Associate Medical Director, Department of Labor and Industries, Olympia, Washington

CATHERINE Q. HOWE, MD, PhD
Physical Medicine and Rehabilitation, University of Washington, Seattle, Washington

DANIEL KRASHIN, MD
Clinical Assistant Professor, Director of Chronic Fatigue Clinic UW, Department of Psychiatry, Anesthesiology and Pain Medicine, University of Washington, Seattle, Washington

HEATHER R. KROLL, MD
Medical Director, Rehabilitation Institute of Washington, PLLC; Clinical Assistant Professor, Department of Rehabilitation Medicine, University of Washington School of Medicine, Seattle, Washington

NIRIKSHA MALLADI, MD
Medical Director, Pacific Rehabilitation Centers, Bellevue, Washington

NATALIA MURINOVA, MD, MHA
Clinical Assistant Professor, Director, Headache Clinic, Department of Neurology, University of Washington, Seattle, Washington

ISUTA NISHIO, MD
Associate Professor, Department of Anesthesiology and Pain Medicine, University of Washington; Attending Physician, VA Puget Sound Health Care System, Seattle, Washington

JAMES P. ROBINSON, MD, PhD
Clinical Professor, Department of Rehabilitation Medicine, University of Washington, Seattle, Washington

RICHARD SEROUSSI, MD, MSc (Engin)
Clinical Courtesy Faculty, Department of Rehabilitation Medicine, University of Washington; Attending Physician, Seattle Spine and Sports Medicine, Seattle, Washington

CHARLES A. SIMPSON, DC, DABCO
Vice President, Clinical Affairs, The CHP Group, Beaverton, Oregon

VIRTAJ SINGH, MD
Clinical Faculty, Department of Rehabilitation Medicine, University of Washington; Medical Director, Seattle Spine and Sports Medicine, Seattle, Washington

MARK D. SULLIVAN, MD, PhD
Physical Medicine and Rehabilitation, University of Washington, Seattle, Washington

DAVID TAUBEN, MD, FACP
Chief, UW Division of Pain Medicine; Hughes M and Katherine G Blake Endowed Professor, Clinical Associate Professor, Departments of Medicine and Anesthesia and Pain Medicine, University of Washington, Seattle, Washington

HEATHER TICK, MD
Clinical Associate Professor, Department of Family Medicine; Gunn-Loke Endowed Professor of Integrative Pain Medicine; Clinical Associate Professor, Department of Anesthesiology and Pain Medicine, University of Washington, Seattle, Washington

ANDREA TRESCOT, MD
Medical Director, Pain and Headache Center, Wasilla, Alaska

Contents

Michele Curatolo and Lars Arendt-Nielsen

Clinical research has consistently detected alteration in central pain processing leading to hypersensitivity. Most methods used in humans are reliable and have face validity to detect widespread central hypersensitivity.
However, construct validity is difficult to investigate due to lack of gold
standards. Reference values in the pain-free population have been generated, but need replication. Research on pain biomarkers that reflect specific central hypersensitivity processes is warranted. Few studies have
analyzed the prognostic value of central hypersensitivity. Most medications acting at central level and some non-pharmacological approaches,
including psychological interventions, are likely to attenuate central
hypersensitivity.

Richard Seroussi

To be accurate with chronic pain assessment, the medical examiner
should be alert to specific diagnoses in addition to global markers of
decreased function associated with chronic pain, such as disability and
depression. The key to accurate assessment is to avoid making assumptions before doing a complete history and physical examination. This
article focuses on the history and examination and emphasizes pitfalls
associated with overreliance on medical technology.

Jane C. Ballantyne

Opioids remain the strongest and most effective analgesics available. The
downside is that they are addictive and potentially dangerous. Throughout
history, although recognizing the value of opioids in treating serious pain,
especially acute pain and pain at the end of life, there has been caution
about using opioids to treat chronic pain. This article presents how opioids
should be used to treat chronic pain considering recent concerns about
their efficacy and safety.

(CNS) amplification of pain and have a poor prognosis. In this context, specific pain generators from acute whiplash have been identified through clinical, biomechanical, and animal studies. This article gives a clinical perspective on current understanding of these pain generators, including the phenomenon of CNS sensitization.

Chronic daily headache (CDH) is a challenging condition to treat. CDH is often accompanied by significant comorbidities, such as chronic fatigue, depression, anxiety, and insomnia, which further complicate treatment. Unrealistic expectations of treatment goals can lead to patient frustration, and, as a result, decrease treatment adherence. Patients often desire headache-free status, but this outcome is not realistic for many patients with CDH. By contrast, an effective treatment goal starts with establishing the correct diagnosis and creating a multimodal treatment plan to improve function and well-being. With proper comprehensive treatment, the condition improves in most patients.

Physicians who treat injured workers with painful conditions face complex challenges that require skills beyond those of a clinician. To address these challenges effectively, physicians need to understand the logic of workers' compensation systems and the interests of the various participants in the systems. They must be prepared to interface constructively between their patients and the workers' compensation carrier and attend to a multitude of administrative issues. In the present article, the authors provide an extended case history with commentary to illustrate the challenges that physicians face and the ways they can respond to these challenges.

PHYSICAL MEDICINE AND REHABILITATION CLINICS OF NORTH AMERICA

VISIT THE CLINICS ONLINE!
Access your subscription at:
www.theclinics.com

DOWNLOAD
Free App!

Review Articles
THE CLINICS

NOW AVAILABLE FOR YOUR iPhone and iPad

Foreword

Chronic Pain

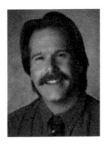

Gregory T. Carter, MD, MS
Consulting Editor

Much has happened in the field of chronic pain in the past few decades. Things continue to change, even in the way chronic pain is characterized, as well as in treatment strategies. In the field of chronic pain, the University of Washington has a longstanding history of excellence in both research and clinical care. Among the leaders here include my good friend and colleague, Dr Jim Robinson. Dr Robinson came immediately to mind when thinking of who could edit a *Physical Medicine and Rehabilitation Clinics of North America* issue on chronic pain. Thankfully, he was up for the challenge once again, as he has done this topic for the *Physical Medicine and Rehabilitation Clinics of North America* previously.

Along with coeditor, Dr Virtaj Singh, they have recruited leading clinicians and researchers to write articles ranging from basic science, through applications of assessment techniques, to practical treatments for chronic pain. This issue will be of immediate usefulness for practitioners, with innovative treatments to chronic pain discussed in great detail, and emphasizing their practical use.

I want to extend my personal gratitude to all of the esteemed authors, most of whom I consider good friends, for taking on this task and for producing such an excellent treatise on chronic pain.

Gregory T. Carter, MD, MS
St Luke's Rehabilitation Institute
711 South Cowley Street
Spokane, WA 99202, USA

E-mail address:
gtcarter@uw.edu

Phys Med Rehabil Clin N Am 26 (2015) xi
http://dx.doi.org/10.1016/j.pmr.2015.04.012
1047-9651/15/$ – see front matter © 2015 Published by Elsevier Inc.

Preface
Chronic Pain

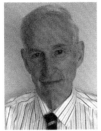 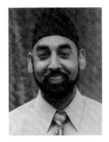

James P. Robinson, MD, PhD   Virtaj Singh, MD
Editors

This issue of the *Physical Medicine and Rehabilitation Clinics of North America* deals with strategies for evaluating and treating chronic pain. Physiatrists need skill in managing chronic pain because they encounter it frequently. Some physiatrists focus their clinical practices on patients who have pain as their major reason for seeking health care. These include physiatrists who work at pain centers, and ones who focus on the management of spinal disorders. Other physiatrists treat patients who are disabled by conditions that are not necessarily painful, such as spinal cord injury and stroke. For these physicians, pain might be construed as a secondary problem that complicates their attempts to rehabilitate patients. Unfortunately, it is a secondary problem that they are likely to encounter routinely, since epidemiologic research demonstrates a high prevalence of chronic pain in most of the patient populations that physiatrists treat.

APPROACHES TO PAIN

Physicians usually provide an eclectic mixture of therapies when they treat patients with chronic pain. Some of the therapies defy any simple classification scheme. For purposes of exposition, though, it is possible to classify most of them into 3 broad groups: curative/disease modifying, rehabilitative, and palliative.

The curative approach is the simplest to understand and the preferred one when it is applicable. From this perspective, pain is a symptom that, in combination with other symptoms and signs, helps the physician identify a pathophysiologic process that becomes the target of treatment. In an ideal situation, once the underlying biological disturbance has been identified and reversed, the patient's symptoms resolve without any additional treatments. Common examples of pain treatment based on the curative perspective include internal fixation and casting for a patient who presents with a painful wrist fracture, appendectomy for a patient who presents with right lower quadrant pain secondary to appendicitis, and angioplasty for a patient who presents with chest pain secondary to cardiac ischemia.

Phys Med Rehabil Clin N Am 26 (2015) xiii–xvii
http://dx.doi.org/10.1016/j.pmr.2015.01.006
1047-9651/15/$ – see front matter © 2015 Published by Elsevier Inc.

pmr.theclinics.com

Unfortunately, attempts to relieve pain by curing an "upstream" pathophysiologic process sometimes fail. The reasons for such failure are multiple. An obvious one is that physicians sometimes have difficulty identifying the offending pathophysiologic process. This situation frequently occurs when physicians attempt to help patients with chronic pain, perhaps because the underlying problem in these patients is often an alteration in the manner in which their nervous systems encode and process sensory information, rather than ongoing nociception from tissue injury.

A rehabilitative model to pain management is most appropriate when 2 conditions apply: the curative model is not appropriate, and a major goal of the pain management program is to improve a patient's ability to function. Most of the articles in this issue of the *Physical Medicine and Rehabilitation Clinics of North America* incorporate a rehabilitative model.

In a general way, pain rehabilitation is similar to rehabilitation of any medical condition—its goal is to optimize functioning through a combination of physical conditioning, skills training, education, and mobilization of patients' psychological resources. Many of the patients treated by physiatrists undergo rehabilitative treatment for disorders (eg, spinal cord injury) that may be associated with pain, but invariably involve numerous functional deficits unrelated to pain. For these patients, pain rehabilitation becomes a component of the overall rehabilitation program. Thus, for example, a paraplegic who reports shoulder pain as he transfers or uses his wheelchair might experience pain resolution as a result of conditioning to improve his upper body strength and training to improve his transfer techniques. In other settings, pain is the focus of rehabilitative treatment. The best example of this is multidisciplinary pain rehabilitation.

Although rehabilitative therapies influence pain indirectly by addressing secondary effects of the pain (eg, deconditioning) and improving patients' coping skills, palliative therapies focus directly on the pain experience itself. For example, opiates can blunt the experience of pain, without requiring patients to do the kind of work that is demanded by rehabilitative therapies.

In practical situations, physicians typically manage chronic pain by some combination of rehabilitative and palliative strategies. For example, they will frequently prescribe medications to ease the pain experiences of patients, and at the same time, refer the patients to physical therapy in order to improve their functional capabilities.

PREVIEW

The present issue of the *Physical Medicine and Rehabilitaion Clinics of North America* starts with an article on altered nervous system functioning in chronic pain. Most pain specialists believe that such altered functioning plays a key role in many chronic pain conditions and, to a large extent, explains why these conditions are difficult to treat. However, unless physicians have reliable methods to determine whether the altered functioning is occurring in individual patients, the hypothesis that chronic pain is often governed by altered nervous system functioning (rather than ongoing nociception from damaged tissues) is tenuous. The authors of this article have done extensive research on methods to assess altered nervous system functioning among pain patients and summarize their findings in the article.

The article by Seroussi addresses the crucial practical issue of assessment of chronic pain. Early on in medical school, students are taught the importance of taking a thorough history and conducting a comprehensive physical examination. This in-depth assessment is of particular importance when treating patients with chronic pain. Although physiatrists are typically well trained in the performance of thorough neuromuscular examinations, accurate assessment in patients with chronic pain also requires the ability to identify comorbid factors, such as depression, deconditioning, disability, substance abuse, and so forth. This article discusses how to perform a thorough biopsychosocial assessment in the setting of chronic pain.

Broadly speaking, nine articles address treatment options for patients with chronic pain and various issues that physicians should consider when developing treatment plans.

More specifically, 2 articles address pharmacologic management of chronic pain. The article by Ballantyne is devoted entirely to a discussion of opioid therapy. This subject is crucial in large part because of the enormous changes that have occurred over the past 20 years in our understanding of the pros and cons of such therapy. The article by Tauben discusses a wide range of pharmacologic agents other than opioids that can be prescribed for patients with various chronic pain problems. These agents include acetaminophen, nonsteroidal anti-inflammatory medications, steroids, antidepressants, anticonvulsants, benzodiazepines, and less widely used agents (eg, ketamine).

The article by Singh describes injection therapies that can be used in the treatment of chronic pain. It is important to note that some injections may be of limited utility by the time pain becomes chronic. However, there is sometimes a limited role for injections to help clarify potential sources of pain ("pain generators") and facilitate participation in a more active rehabilitation program. There is extant literature (including prior issues of the *Physical Medicine and Rehabilitation Clinics of North America*) that addresses the use of epidural steroid injections and facet injections for the treatment of spinal pain, both axial and radicular. As such, these topics will not be covered in this article. Instead, less well-covered topics are the focus, including trigger point injections, prolotherapy and other regenerative injections, and botulinum toxin injections.

The article by Kroll discusses exercise therapy for chronic pain. The material in this article is particularly important for 2 reasons. First, exercise is the most direct form of rehabilitative treatment—it directly addresses and attempts to reverse functional limitations that patients have because of their pain. Second, physiatrists have more expertise in exercise therapy than physicians with other kinds of training. As a result, they are in an optimal position to supervise exercise programs.

Many patients with chronic pain have coexisting emotional dysfunction. Physiatrists who treat these patients need to have a high index of suspicion for the emotional problems that are likely to plague their patients, and they need to understand the perspectives and treatment approaches of the psychiatrists and clinical psychologists who are often called on to intervene. The article by Howe and colleagues addresses psychiatric and psychological problems that are commonly seen in patients with chronic pain. It is written from the perspectives of psychiatrists (Howe and Sullivan) and a psychologist (Robinson).

Two articles address issues that are crucially important in the management of chronic pain, but are often not emphasized in traditional medical training. In particular, sleep, the focus of the article by Fine, has emerged as an area that demands attention. The reason for this is that patients with chronic pain often find themselves in a vicious circle. Their pain and accompanying emotional distress make it difficult to sleep, and their inadequate sleep leaves them exhausted and less ready to cope with pain. Tick's article addresses the role of nutrition in chronic pain and outlines several practical strategies that physicians can follow to assess and remediate nutritional deficiencies in their patients with chronic pain.

The article by Simpson addresses another arena that typically receives little attention in traditional medical training—complementary and alternative therapies (CAM).

As Simpson makes clear, a high proportion of patients with chronic pain avails themselves of CAM therapies, and evidence for the effectiveness of many CAM therapies is as good as evidence for allopathic therapies. Brief descriptions are included of the rationales for several common CAM therapies and of the evidence supporting their effectiveness.

The article by Malladi addresses multidisciplinary pain rehabilitation. There are at least 2 reasons physiatrists should be familiar with this approach to chronic pain. One reason is that multidisciplinary treatment of some kind is recommended by virtually every expert panel that provides guidelines for treating various chronic pain problems. A major reason for this is that chronic pain has multifactorial roots. It is typical for patients to suffer from deconditioning, emotional dysfunction, sleep deprivation, various nutritional deficiencies, and work disability. It is virtually impossible for a single physician to address all these domains during office visits with a patient. Second, the structure and organization of multidisciplinary pain rehabilitation programs are similar in many ways to the rehabilitation programs used for common rehabilitation problems such as stroke or spinal cord injury. In fact, the architect of the original multidisciplinary pain rehabilitation program, which was started at the University of Washington (UW) in the late 1960s, was a psychologist in the Department of Rehabilitation Medicine at UW.

The articles by Seroussi and colleagues and Murinova and Krashin describe how concepts developed in the earlier articles of the issue can be applied to 2 populations of patients with chronic pain: those with whiplash injuries, and those with chronic headaches. These 2 chronic pain populations frequently present in a physiatric practice.

Finally, the article by Robinson and Glass addresses the management of pain in patients with workers' compensation claims. The discussion emphasizes the fact that a physician who treats pain in an injured worker must do much more than provide effective medical care for the patient. In particular, such a physician must be prepared to interact with several different interested parties and to address complex issues regarding the patient's disability.

A FINAL WORD

Many physicians find chronic pain difficult and emotionally challenging to treat. Their reticence reflects 3 basic facts about chronic pain. First, pain is a personal experience that cannot be fully confirmed by a physician or any other third party. Thus, a treating physician will frequently experience uncertainty about how to interpret a patient's pain complaints. This ambiguity becomes especially challenging if the patient demands high doses of opiates to control pain or reports a degree of incapacitation that appears to be excessive relative to the severity of the medical condition. Second, chronic pain reflects the combined influence of a wide range of biological, psychological, and social factors. Thus, a physician who tries to understand the factors underlying a patient's pain complaints must have expertise in areas other than just the pathophysiology of injuries and diseases. Third, many of the commonly used treatments for chronic pain have not been validated in well-designed studies, and the treatments that have been validated generally demonstrate only modestly beneficial effects. As a result, a physician who treats chronic pain usually cannot practice evidence-based medicine and must be prepared to encounter frequent failures.

The articles in this issue of the *Physical Medicine and Rehabilitation Clinics of North America* do not eliminate the above challenges. In particular, since the various therapeutic approaches described in the issue have essentially never been subjected to head-to-head comparisons, the material in this issue does not provide anything like a simple algorithm to follow when treating pain patients. But we do believe that the articles will provide physiatrists with an appreciation of the complexities of chronic pain and also with a set of practical strategies that they can use when they agree to manage patients with chronic pain.

ACKNOWLEDGMENTS

We would like to express our appreciation to the authors of this issue of the *Physical Medicine and Rehabilitation Clinics of North America*. They are all very busy clinicians and scholars. It is impressive that they were willing to take the time to write their articles. We believe that their cumulative efforts have resulted in an issue that provides both conceptual clarity and practical tools for physiatrists.

James P. Robinson, MD, PhD
Department of Rehabilitation Medicine
University of Washington
4225 Roosevelt Way NE, 4th floor
Seattle, WA 98105, USA

Virtaj Singh, MD
Department of Rehabilitation Medicine
University of Washington
Seattle Spine & Sports Medicine
3213 Eastlake Avenue E, Suite A
Seattle, WA, 98102, USA

E-mail addresses:
jimrob@uw.edu (J.P. Robinson)
vsingh@seattlespine.com (V. Singh)

Erratum

Please note that Dr. Reina Nakamura's last name was misspelled as "Nakamurra" in the November 2014 issue of *Physical Medicine and Rehabilitation Clinics* (Volume 25, Issue 4).

Phys Med Rehabil Clin N Am 26 (2015) xix
http://dx.doi.org/10.1016/j.pmr.2015.03.001
1047-9651/15/$ – see front matter © 2015 Elsevier Inc. All rights reserved.

pmr.theclinics.com

Central Hypersensitivity in Chronic Musculoskeletal Pain

Michele Curatolo, MD, PhD[a,b,*], Lars Arendt-Nielsen, PhD, Dr Med Sci[b]

KEYWORDS

- Chronic pain • Central sensitization • Hyperalgesia • Quantitative sensory tests

KEY POINTS

- Pain states may be associated with enhanced sensitivity of peripheral and central nociceptive pathways, potentially leading to pain amplification and increased disability.
- Hypersensitivity can be evaluated in patients by quantitative sensory tests (QSTs).
- Widespread hyperalgesia may be caused by central sensitization.
- Evidence on clinical applicability of QSTs has improved with recent research on reliability and reference values.
- Further research is needed to identify more mechanistic biomarkers and link the measurements with clinically relevant outcomes.

INTRODUCTION

Injuries and inflammatory processes of peripheral tissues and nerves are associated with profound changes in peripheral and central nociceptive pathways: receptors become hyperexcitable, neural structures involved in the transmission of sensory input become hypersensitive, and endogenous pain-inhibiting mechanisms are less functional.[1] As a result, nociceptive stimuli of low intensity and even innocuous stimuli lead to enhanced pain responses and spread of pain to noninjured areas (**Fig. 1**).

It is widely accepted that the intensity of a primary nociceptive stimulus is not necessarily the only or main determinant of pain and disability. Pain syndromes are

Disclosure: The authors do not have any conflict of interest.
[a] Department of Anesthesiology and Pain Medicine, University of Washington, 1959 Northeast Pacific Street, Seattle, WA 98195, USA; [b] Center for Sensory Motor Interaction, Department of Health Science and Technology, School of Medicine, University of Aalborg, Fredrik Bajers Vej 7, Bld. D3, Aalborg 9220, Denmark
* Corresponding author. Department of Anesthesiology and Pain Medicine, University of Washington, 1959 Northeast Pacific Street, Seattle, WA 98195.
E-mail address: curatolo@uw.edu

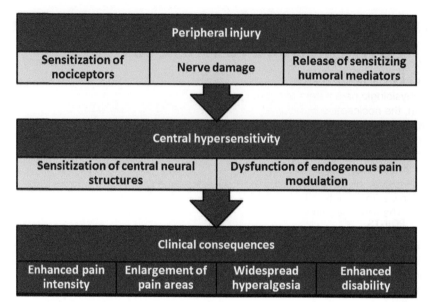

Fig. 1. Path between peripheral lesion, central hypersensitivity, and a selection of possible clinical consequences.

indeed often characterized by a discrepancy between the magnitude of tissue damage and symptoms. It is conceivable that part of this discrepancy is explained by hypersensitivity of central pain pathways.

This article focuses on the current status of translational research in central hypersensitivity. The article discusses the currently available methods to detect hypersensitivity in patients, examines the evidence for the presence of this phenomenon in human chronic pain, and highlights actual and potential bedside applications of measures of central hypersensitivity. The scope of the article is limited to human chronic musculoskeletal pain conditions; only methods that can be used clinically or have potential clinical application are discussed.

METHODS TO DETECT CENTRAL HYPERSENSITIVITY

The current knowledge on the presence and mechanisms of central hypersensitivity stems mostly from basic research. Clinical research has had an obvious constraint: the very limited accessibility of nociceptive pathways in humans. Most of the evidence on central hypersensitivity in human pain is therefore based on indirect measures.

Psychophysical Assessments

The most widely used paradigm to assess central hypersensitivity consists in the application of a standardized stimulus to a peripheral tissue and the recording of a subject's response.[2] These measurements are known as quantitative sensory tests (QSTs). However, if such tests stand alone it is difficult to conclude if a detected hypersensitivity is caused by a peripheral mechanism, central mechanisms, or a combination of the two. Examples of responses to the stimulus are pain intensity and pain threshold. The paradigm relies on the assumption that a nonpainful stimulus, when applied to a noninjured tissue, can evoke pain only if central nociceptive pathways are hypersensitive. Similarly, a low-input noxious stimulus applied to a noninjured tissue would produce exaggerated pain in the presence of hypersensitive central pain pathways (hyperalgesia and/or allodynia).

Objective Assessments

The aforementioned methods rely on subjective pain reports. Different objective electrophysiologic parameters of central hypersensitivity have been investigated. Among them, the nociceptive withdrawal reflex (NWR) has potential for clinical applications, because it consumes little time and requires relatively simple equipment. The NWR is typically measured by applying percutaneously an electrical stimulus to a sensory nerve of the lower extremity, such as the sural nerve at the foot, and registering the electromyography response during leg withdrawal.[3] It is considered as a measure of sensitivity of spinal nociceptive pathways. For instance, if the reflex is elicited with low stimulus intensities, it can be inferred that these spinal pathways are sensitized. The NWR has also been used as response for the assessment of endogenous pain modulation[4] and temporal summation (discussed later).[5]

Spread of Pain and Referred Pain Areas

Spread of pain areas from the site of primary injury to noninjured body areas is a commonly observed clinical phenomenon. Extensive basic research has revealed structural changes in the central nervous system that account for spread of pain areas.[1] Several experimental studies have described this phenomenon in humans. For instance, pain after the injection of hypertonic saline into a muscle is perceived at a much wider body area in chronic pain patients, compared with pain-free subjects.[6] The combined findings of basic and clinical research indicate that neuroplastic changes at least contribute to, and are likely the main determinants for, spreading of pain areas outside the primary site of injury.

Therefore, measuring the area of pain in general and referred pain in particular may be simple methods to assess central hypersensitivity. For this parameter, there are no normative values or guidelines. Nevertheless, whenever the pain area significantly spreads outside the primary site of lesion, the clinician may suspect that sensitization processes are relevant components of the patient's complaints.

Measurement of Endogenous Modulation

Central hypersensitivity may also be the result of inefficient endogenous pain modulation (balance between descending inhibition and facilitation). In humans, the most established paradigm to measure this phenomenon is conditioned pain modulation, which mirrors diffuse noxious inhibitory control tested in animal models.[7] Conditioned pain modulation assessment consists of applying two concomitant painful stimuli at two distant body areas: a conditioning and a test stimulus. If endogenous pain modulation is efficient, the conditioning stimulus is expected to attenuate the pain (increase the pain threshold or decrease the pain intensity to a given stimulus) elicited by the test stimulus.[8] For instance, pressure pain threshold to stimulation of the lower extremity increases when immersing the hand into ice water (cold pressor test).[9]

Measurement of Temporal Summation

Temporal summation occurs when a stimulus, delivered at constant intensity, evokes increased pain reactions.[10] For instance, repeating an electrical stimulus every 0.5 seconds leads to increased pain sensation during the stimulation, although the intensity of the stimuli is constant.[11] This phenomenon can also be analyzed by electromyography, whereby a withdrawal spinal reflex is evoked only by the last one or two of a train of five stimuli.[11]

Temporal summation is thought to reflect facilitatory mechanisms within the central nervous system. Several investigations have found a facilitation of temporal summation in pain patients.[12–14]

CLINICAL APPLICABILITY
Evidence for Central Hypersensitivity in Musculoskeletal Pain

The issue of central hypersensitivity has been extensively investigated in humans. The typical study design has involved the comparison between a group of patients and a control group of pain-free subjects. Different QST methods have been used to profile the two groups. These studies have applied stimuli of different nature to different body areas. Despite heterogeneity, they have consistently shown enhanced pain responses in patients compared with control subjects. Hypersensitivity has been found in a variety of pain conditions, including low back,[15] neck,[16,17] temporomandibular joint,[18] elbow,[19] and knee pain[20]; tension-type headache[21]; endometriosis[22]; and fibromyalgia.[12] More details are available in previous reviews.[2,6,23] A first epidemiologic study on a large patient population in a university pain clinic used pressure algometry at the toe to determine the prevalence of widespread hypersensitivity; depending on the percentile of normative values considered, generalized central hypersensitivity affected 17.5% to 35.3% of patients.[9]

These studies have provided a better understanding of phenomena that had been poorly recognized. Exaggerated pain and expansion of pain areas can occur after limited tissue damage. This can be the result of enhanced nociceptive processes within the central nervous system. Clinicians should be aware of this pathophysiology and should explain it to their patients as one of the possible determinants of their symptoms. Noticeably, one of the primary expectations of patients in a pain clinic is to gain a better understanding of their problems.[24]

Limitations

Several limitations apply to these kinds of studies. QST is a measure of pain sensitivity and does not allow conclusions on the causes and mechanisms underlying hypersensitivity. When the stimulus is applied to tissues that cannot be a primary source of nociception, such as the lower limb in neck pain, it is reasonable to infer that some site of the central nervous system is sensitized. Unfortunately, we cannot say much more. For instance, clinicians are still unable to say whether or to what extent pain hypersensitivity is the result of psychosocial factors. Cognitive and affective components may be determinants of hypersensitivity at brain level, or at the level of descending pathways that facilitate pain transmission at the spinal cord.[25]

Some models may allow more mechanistic inferences. For instance, facilitated NWR is likely the result of sensitization of spinal pathways. Enlargement of nociceptive reflex receptive fields after electrical stimulation is suggestive for the presence of sensitization of spinal neurons not directly connected to the site of primary stimulation.[15,22]

Importantly, QST may allow detection of only widespread central hypersensitivity. The sensitivity of central nociceptive pathways connected to the site of primary nociceptive input cannot be tested with QST, because these tests do not differentiate central from peripheral sensitization. For example, a low pain threshold detected with pressure stimulation of the knee in patients with knee pain does not tell whether sensitization of injured tissues of the knee, sensitization of central pathways, or both are being detected.[20]

Reliability

One of the requirements for clinical applicability of any test is reliability. It can be defined as the degree to which a test measures the same way each time it is used under the same condition with the same subjects. Ideally, the results of a test on a subject should be the same even if different examiners are involved and the assessment is made at different time-points.

Several studies have investigated the reliability of QSTs. Collectively, the data show that the reliability of most QSTs is at least acceptable.[26–30] Most studies have been conducted on pain-free subjects, but studies on patients have been recently published. Most of them have confirmed the encouraging results obtained with healthy volunteers.[26,30,31]

Reference Values

For research purposes, mean scores of patient groups are typically compared with those of groups of pain-free subjects. This approach is obviously not applicable if abnormalities are to be detected in individual patients. For this purpose, the availability of reference values in the pain-free population is essential. In recent years, some large studies that aimed to determine reference values of QSTs have been published. Some of them are suitable for profiling patients with neuropathic pain[32,33]; others have been designed for painful musculoskeletal conditions.[34–36]

Such studies are demanding because they require large sample sizes and the control of several factors that may influence the measurements, such as demographic or psychosocial variables. The available investigations are important steps toward the clinical application of QSTs. However, they require replication to ensure generalizability. Furthermore, the reference values depend on the body site where the stimuli are applied. Thus, the available data have to be taken with caution when applied to clinical practice.

Validity

The use of QSTs for the assessment of central hypersensitivity is largely based on face validity. Face validity can be defined as the extent to which a test seems "on its face" to sample what it was intended to measure. For example, an innocuous stimulus applied to the lower extremity may be perceived as painful by patients with neck pain.[17] Because there is no pathology at the lower extremity, it can be inferred that the pain evoked in these patients is the result of sensitization processes in the central nervous system. This assumption, although reasonable, does not provide firm evidence for central hypersensitivity. Ideally, clinicians need to ensure that tests are measuring the construct they claim to be measuring (ie, they need to demonstrate construct validity). In the case of central hypersensitivity, construct validity could be studied by comparing the results of a QST with the results of a reference method (gold standard) that directly measures sensitization of central nociceptive pathways. This would allow the calculation of sensitivity, specificity, and likelihood ratios of the QST, and ultimately the estimation of their diagnostic value. Because of the lack of an established gold standard for central hypersensitivity in humans, construct validity of QST cannot be assessed.

Therapeutic Options

Central hypersensitivity is at least initiated by a nociceptive input arising from the injured area. It is therefore possible that any treatment that reduces or abolishes the transmission of the nociceptive flow to the spinal cord can attenuate or reverse central hypersensitivity.

A recent study in an animal model of cervical facet joint injury found that intra-articular bupivacaine, administered immediately after injury, significantly attenuated hyperalgesia, neuronal hyperexcitability, and dysregulation of excitatory signaling proteins; however, bupivacaine at Day 4 had no effect on these outcomes.[37] These data suggest that reversion of central plasticity changes may not be achieved by late interventions at the primary site of injury.

However, clinical studies have shown that after hip or knee replacement pain relief was associated with attenuation of central hypersensitivity.[38,39] Similarly, a study in chronic neck pain after whiplash injury found that medial branch radiofrequency neurotomy reduced indicators of augmented central pain processing.[40] These findings suggest that central augmentation processes are maintained by peripheral nociceptive input and can therefore be reversed also in the chronic phase. The issue of peripheral modulation of central hypersensitivity remains an important field of future research.

Virtually all centrally acting medications have the potential to provide pain relief by acting, at least partly, on central hypersensitivity. Some of them can do so nonspecifically by reducing the amount of nociceptive flow within the central nervous system. Others can more specifically target mechanisms of neuronal hyperexcitability. N-methyl-D-aspartate antagonists (NMDA) are among medications that act specifically on central hypersensitivity, given the involvement of the N-methyl-D-aspartate receptor in the generation of neuronal hyperexcitability.[41] Ketamine is the most effective drug of this class, but its use in chronic pain is limited by an unfavorable side effect profile, concerns regarding potential drug abuse, lack of long-term clinical data, and limited bioavailability after oral administration.[42]

Inflammatory and neuropathic conditions are associated with a reduction in inhibitory glycinergic and GABAergic control of dorsal horn neurons; this reduction in γ-aminobutyric acid (GABA)–mediated endogenous inhibitory control leads to exaggerated pain and hyperalgesia.[43] Potentiation of $GABA_A$ receptor–mediated synaptic inhibition by benzodiazepines reverses hypersensitivity in animal studies.[44,45] A preliminary experimental human study suggested that benzodiazepines may be antihyperalgesic.[46] However, these compounds produce sedation and tolerance, which severely limit dose escalation and clinical applicability. Subtype-selective compounds targeting the α_2 and/or α_3 subunit of the $GABA_A$ receptor produce antihyperalgesia in mice and rats, without causing sedation or tolerance.[47] These findings, if confirmed in human studies, may open new perspectives for a more selective targeting of hypersensitivity with GABAergic drugs. Gabapentin[48] and pregabalin[49] may attenuate central sensitization presumably by acting at the calcium channel alpha-2-delta-1 subunit that is upregulated in hypersensitivity states.

Pharmacologic inhibition of central sensitization can be achieved by opioids and antidepressants, via descending opioidergic,[50] serotoninergic,[51] and noradrenergic[51] pathways. However, opioids can also enhance pain sensitivity[52] and severe concerns regarding their use in chronic pain have been raised in recent years.[53]

Inhibitors of the 5-HT3 receptors, such as tropisetron and ondansetron, may attenuate generalized central hypersensitivity because of the role of mechanisms involving these receptors in hypersensitivity states.[54] Clinical studies have shown an effect of inhibitors of the 5-HT3 receptors on fibromyalgia[55] and neuropathic pain.[56] However, a more recent study on low back pain yielded negative results on intensity of low back pain and parameters of central hypersensitivity.[57]

It is conceivable that psychological treatments attenuate central hypersensitivity by acting at modulatory mechanisms within the brain and descending inhibitory pathways. The authors are not aware of investigations that have addressed this issue.

SUMMARY

There is established evidence that many pain states are associated with enhanced sensitivity of central nociceptive pathways, potentially leading to pain amplification and increased disability in human chronic pain. Central hypersensitivity can be evaluated in patients by QSTs. Evidence of the clinical applicability of these tests has improved with recent research on reliability and reference values. Further research is needed to identify more mechanistic biomarkers. Furthermore, future research is expected to clarify the links between bedside measurements of central hypersensitivity and clinically relevant outcomes.

REFERENCES

1. Woolf CJ, Salter MW. Neuronal plasticity: increasing the gain in pain. Science 2000;288:1765–9.
2. Arendt-Nielsen L, Curatolo M. Mechanistic, translational, quantitative pain assessment tools in profiling of pain patients and for development of new analgesic compounds. Scand J Pain 2013;4(4):226–30.
3. Sandrini G, Serrao M, Rossi P, et al. The lower limb flexion reflex in humans. Prog Neurobiol 2005;77(6):353–95.
4. Biurrun Manresa JA, Fritsche R, Vuilleumier PH, et al. Is the conditioned pain modulation paradigm reliable? A test-retest assessment using the nociceptive withdrawal reflex. PLoS One 2014;9(6):e100241.
5. Rhudy JL, Martin SL, Terry EL, et al. Pain catastrophizing is related to temporal summation of pain but not temporal summation of the nociceptive flexion reflex. Pain 2011;152(4):794–801.
6. Graven-Nielsen T, Curatolo M, Mense S. Central sensitization, referred pain, and deep tissue hyperalgesia in musculoskeletal pain. In: Flor H, Kalso E, Dostrovsky JO, editors. Proceedings of the 11th world congress on pain. Seattle (WA): IASP Press; 2006. p. 217–30.
7. Yarnitsky D, Arendt-Nielsen L, Bouhassira D, et al. Recommendations on terminology and practice of psychophysical DNIC testing. Eur J Pain 2010;14(4):339.
8. Pud D, Granovsky Y, Yarnitsky D. The methodology of experimentally induced diffuse noxious inhibitory control (DNIC)-like effect in humans. Pain 2009; 144(1–2):16–9.
9. Schliessbach J, Siegenthaler A, Streitberger K, et al. The prevalence of widespread central hypersensitivity in chronic pain patients. Eur J Pain 2013;17(10): 1502–10.
10. Price DD. Characteristics of second pain and flexion reflexes indicative of prolonged central summation. Exp Neurol 1972;37:371–87.
11. Arendt-Nielsen L, Brennum J, Sindrup S, et al. Electrophysiological and psychophysical quantification of central temporal summation of the human nociceptive system. Eur J Appl Physiol Occup Physiol 1994;68:266–73.
12. Banic B, Petersen-Felix S, Andersen OK, et al. Evidence for spinal cord hypersensitivity in chronic pain after whiplash injury and in fibromyalgia. Pain 2004; 107:7–15.
13. Maixner W, Fillingim R, Sigurdsson A, et al. Sensitivity of patients with painful temporomandibular disorders to experimentally evoked pain: evidence for altered temporal summation of pain. Pain 1998;76:71–81.
14. Staud R, Vierck CJ, Cannon RL, et al. Abnormal sensitization and temporal summation of second pain (wind-up) in patients with fibromyalgia syndrome. Pain 2001;91:165–75.

15. Biurrun Manresa JA, Neziri AY, Curatolo M, et al. Reflex receptive fields are enlarged in patients with musculoskeletal low back and neck pain. Pain 2013; 154(8):1318–24.
16. Sterling M, Jull G, Vicenzino B, et al. Sensory hypersensitivity occurs soon after whiplash injury and is associated with poor recovery. Pain 2003;104:509–17.
17. Curatolo M, Petersen-Felix S, Arendt-Nielsen L, et al. Central hypersensitivity in chronic pain after whiplash injury. Clin J Pain 2001;17:306–15.
18. Sarlani E, Greenspan JD. Evidence for generalized hyperalgesia in temporomandibular disorders patients. Pain 2003;102:221–6.
19. Slater H, Arendt-Nielsen L, Wright A, et al. Sensory and motor effects of experimental muscle pain in patients with lateral epicondylalgia and controls with delayed onset muscle soreness. Pain 2005;114(1–2):118–30.
20. Skou ST, Graven-Nielsen T, Rasmussen S, et al. Facilitation of pain sensitization in knee osteoarthritis and persistent post-operative pain: a cross-sectional study. Eur J Pain 2014;18(7):1024–31.
21. Bendtsen L, Jensen R, Olesen J. Decreased pain detection and tolerance thresholds in chronic tension-type headache. Arch Neurol 1996;53:373–6.
22. Neziri AY, Haesler S, Petersen-Felix S, et al. Generalized expansion of nociceptive reflex receptive fields in chronic pain patients. Pain 2010;151:798–805.
23. Curatolo M, Arendt-Nielsen L, Petersen-Felix S. Central hypersensitivity in chronic pain: mechanisms and clinical implications. Phys Med Rehabil Clin N Am 2006; 17(2):287–302.
24. Petrie KJ, Frampton T, Large RG, et al. What do patients expect from their first visit to a pain clinic? Clin J Pain 2005;21(4):297–301.
25. Sterling M, Hodkinson E, Pettiford C, et al. Psychologic factors are related to some sensory pain thresholds but not nociceptive flexion reflex threshold in chronic whiplash. Clin J Pain 2008;24(2):124–30.
26. Biurrun Manresa JA, Neziri AY, Curatolo M, et al. Test-retest reliability of the nociceptive withdrawal reflex and electrical pain thresholds in chronic pain patients. Eur J Appl Physiol 2011;111:83–92.
27. Chesterton LS, Sim J, Wright CC, et al. Interrater reliability of algometry in measuring pressure pain thresholds in healthy humans, using multiple raters. Clin J Pain 2007;23(9):760–6.
28. Geber C, Klein T, Azad S, et al. Test-retest and interobserver reliability of quantitative sensory testing according to the protocol of the German Research Network on Neuropathic Pain (DFNS): a multi-centre study. Pain 2011;152(3):548–56.
29. Jones DH, Kilgour RD, Comtois AS. Test-retest reliability of pressure pain threshold measurements of the upper limb and torso in young healthy women. J Pain 2007;8(8):650–6.
30. Prushansky T, Handelzalts S, Pevzner E. Reproducibility of pressure pain threshold and visual analog scale findings in chronic whiplash patients. Clin J Pain 2007;23(4):339–45.
31. Agostinho CM, Scherens A, Richter H, et al. Habituation and short-term repeatability of thermal testing in healthy human subjects and patients with chronic non-neuropathic pain. Eur J Pain 2009;13(8):779–85.
32. Magerl W, Krumova EK, Baron R, et al. Reference data for quantitative sensory testing (QST): refined stratification for age and a novel method for statistical comparison of group data. Pain 2010;151(3):598–605.
33. Rolke R, Baron R, Maier C, et al. Quantitative sensory testing in the German Research Network on Neuropathic Pain (DFNS): standardized protocol and reference values. Pain 2006;123:231–43.

34. Neziri AY, Andersen OK, Petersen-Felix S, et al. The nociceptive withdrawal reflex: normative values of thresholds and reflex receptive fields. Eur J Pain 2010;14:134–41.
35. Neziri AY, Scaramozzino P, Andersen OK, et al. Reference values of mechanical and thermal pain tests in a pain-free population. Eur J Pain 2011;15:376–83.
36. Scaramozzino P, Neziri AY, Andersen OK, et al. Percentile normative values of parameters of electrical pain and reflex thresholds. Scand J Pain 2013;4:120–4.
37. Crosby ND, Gilliland TM, Winkelstein BA. Early afferent activity from the facet joint after painful trauma to its capsule potentiates neuronal excitability and glutamate signaling in the spinal cord. Pain 2014;155(9):1878–87.
38. Kosek E, Ordeberg G. Abnormalities of somatosensory perception in patients with painful osteoarthritis normalize following successful treatment. Eur J Pain 2000;4:229–38.
39. Graven-Nielsen T, Wodehouse T, Langford RM, et al. Normalization of widespread hyperesthesia and facilitated spatial summation of deep-tissue pain in knee osteoarthritis patients after knee replacement. Arthritis Rheum 2012;64(9): 2907–16.
40. Smith AD, Jull G, Schneider G, et al. Cervical radiofrequency neurotomy reduces central hyperexcitability and improves neck movement in individuals with chronic whiplash. Pain Med 2013;15:128–41.
41. Dickenson AH, Sullivan AF. Evidence for a role of the NMDA receptor in the frequency dependent potentiation of deep rat dorsal horn nociceptive neurones following C fibre stimulation. Neuropharmacology 1987;26:1235–8.
42. Yanagihara Y, Ohtani M, Kariya S, et al. Plasma concentration profiles of ketamine and norketamine after administration of various ketamine preparations to healthy Japanese volunteers. Biopharm Drug Dispos 2003;24:37–43.
43. Zeilhofer HU. The glycinergic control of spinal pain processing. Cell Mol Life Sci 2005;62(18):2027–35.
44. Knabl J, Zeilhofer UB, Crestani F, et al. Genuine antihyperalgesia by systemic diazepam revealed by experiments in GABAA receptor point-mutated mice. Pain 2009;141(3):233–8.
45. Reichl S, Augustin M, Zahn PK, et al. Peripheral and spinal GABAergic regulation of incisional pain in rats. Pain 2012;153(1):129–41.
46. Vuilleumier PH, Besson M, Desmeules J, et al. Evaluation of anti-hyperalgesic and analgesic effects of two benzodiazepines in human experimental pain: a randomized placebo-controlled study. PLoS One 2013;8(3):e43896.
47. Knabl J, Witschi R, Hosl K, et al. Reversal of pathological pain through specific spinal GABAA receptor subtypes. Nature 2008;451(7176):330–4.
48. Luo ZD, Calcutt NA, Higuera ES, et al. Injury type-specific calcium channel alpha 2 delta-1 subunit up-regulation in rat neuropathic pain models correlates with antiallodynic effects of gabapentin. J Pharmacol Exp Ther 2002;303(3):1199–205.
49. Fink K, Dooley DJ, Meder WP, et al. Inhibition of neuronal Ca(2+) influx by gabapentin and pregabalin in the human neocortex. Neuropharmacology 2002;42(2): 229–36.
50. Yu XM, Hua M, Mense S. The effects of intracerebroventricular injection of naloxone, phentolamine and methysergide on the transmission of nociceptive signals in rat dorsal horn neurons with convergent cutaneous-deep input. Neuroscience 1991;44:715–23.
51. Li P, Zhuo M. Cholinergic, noradrenergic, and serotonergic inhibition of fast synaptic transmission in spinal lumbar dorsal horn of rat. Brain Res Bull 2001;54: 639–47.

52. Angst MS, Clark JD. Opioid-induced hyperalgesia: a qualitative systematic review. Anesthesiology 2006;104(3):570–87.
53. Ballantyne JC, Shin NS. Efficacy of opioids for chronic pain: a review of the evidence. Clin J Pain 2008;24(6):469–78.
54. Suzuki R, Morcuende S, Webber M, et al. Superficial NK1-expressing neurons control spinal excitability through activation of descending pathways. Nat Neurosci 2002;5:1319–26.
55. Farber L, Stratz TH, Bruckle W, et al. Short-term treatment of primary fibromyalgia with the 5-HT3-receptor antagonist tropisetron. Results of a randomized, double-blind, placebo-controlled multicenter trial in 418 patients. Int J Clin Pharmacol Res 2001;21:1–13.
56. McCleane GJ, Suzuki R, Dickenson AH. Does a single intravenous injection of the 5HT3 receptor antagonist ondansetron have an analgesic effect in neuropathic pain? A double-blinded, placebo-controlled cross-over study. Anesth Analg 2003;97:1474–8.
57. Neziri AY, Dickenmann M, Scaramozzino P, et al. Effect of intravenous tropisetron on modulation of pain and central hypersensitivity in chronic low back pain patients. Pain 2012;153(2):311–8.

Chronic Pain Assessment

Richard Seroussi, MD, MSc (Engin)

KEYWORDS

- Chronic pain • Assessment • Review • Musculoskeletal • Neurologic • Physiatry

KEY POINTS

- Although physiatrists are ideally suited to assess chronic pain, they need to perform a careful history and physical examination for accurate assessment.
- Specific attention should be given to comorbid factors, such as depression, disability, and deconditioning, at the same time searching for a treatable nociceptive focus driving the patient's chronic pain.
- The examiner should avoid overreliance on medical technology in making their assessment because this approach is fraught with false-positive and false-negative pitfalls that may be harmful to the patient.

INTRODUCTION

In contrast to acute nociceptive pain, the paradox of chronic pain is that many who suffer with this condition experience amplified rather than decreased pain over time. Chronic pain is often associated with widespread functional deficits such as sleep disruption, muscle stiffness, and the loss of ability to perform activities of daily living (ADL). Functional loss is often associated with higher level ADL, such as grocery shopping and housecleaning, but can involve more basic ADL in the setting of more severe injuries.

To put this information into context, up to 100 million Americans may suffer with chronic pain and a recent study estimated the annual burden of chronic pain, including work loss, to be more than $500 billion.[1] Physiatrists are often first-line specialists for patients with chronic pain. This article describes a clinician's approach to the assessment of chronic pain. The literature is replete with more theoretic discussions on the nature of chronic pain. This discussion will be more practical and grows out of years of experience as a practicing clinician.

CLINICAL PRESENTATION: HISTORY

Patients who have chronic pain can be identified by several factors. Foremost, patients typically have pain of at least 3 to 6 months' duration (and often much longer

Seattle Spine & Sports Medicine, 3213 Eastlake Avenue East, Suite A, Seattle, WA 98102, USA
E-mail address: res@seattlespine.com

Phys Med Rehabil Clin N Am 26 (2015) 185–199
http://dx.doi.org/10.1016/j.pmr.2014.12.009
pmr.theclinics.com
1047-9651/15/$ – see front matter © 2015 Elsevier Inc. All rights reserved.

duration). Pain-body diagrams may illustrate a diffuse pain pattern, with fairly high baseline levels of visual analog scale pain. **Fig. 1** illustrates a typical example for a clinic patient with severe chronic spinal pain.

The distribution of pain on the pain-body diagram may not follow any clear-cut, focal anatomic pattern. Practitioners may suspect a chronic pain syndrome for a new patient by simply scanning their pain-body diagram before entering the examination room.

Another feature of chronic pain is a significant loss of function. This loss of function can be assessed and tracked with the use of a functional index. Note, however, that simply tallying the total items of impaired function, for example with the Roland-Morris Disability Questionnaire,[2] should not be considered diagnostic for identifying a patient with a generalized chronic pain syndrome. **Fig. 2** illustrates such a scale for a patient who has chronic and severe, but focal, lower back pain from a specific injury. Although this impressive list of impaired function might imply a more generalized disorder such as fibromyalgia syndrome, this patient had a nociceptive focus as the source of his global decrease in function.

The Dreaded Ds

In practice, it may be helpful to collate and track the so-called dreaded Ds in assessing a patient with chronic pain. If patients have 3 or more of these features, their chronic pain often affects their daily function, their ability to work, and their quality of life. For

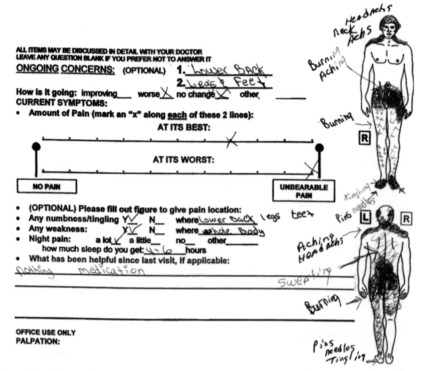

Fig. 1. Sample pain body diagram and symptom report from a patient with severe chronic pain.

CURRENT FUNCTION:
When your back / neck / joint hurts, you may find it difficult to do some of the things you normally do. This list contains some sentences that people have used to describe themselves when they have back / neck / joint pain. When you read them, you may find that some stand out because they describe you TODAY. As you read the list, think of yourself TODAY. When you read a sentence that describes you TODAY, put an "X" next to it. If the sentence does not describe you; then leave the space blank and go on to the next one. Remember, only "X" the sentence if you are sure that it describes you TODAY.

____ 1) I stay at home most of the time because of my back / neck / joint.
X 2) I change position frequently to try and get my back / neck / joint comfortable.
X 3) I walk more slowly than usual because of my back / neck / joint.
X 4) Because of my back / neck / joint, I am not doing any of the jobs that I usually do around the house.
X 5) Because of my back / neck / joint, I use a handrail to get up stairs.
X 6) Because of my back / neck / joint, I lie down to rest more often.
X 7) Because of my back / neck / joint, I have to hold on to something to get out of an easy chair.
X 8) Because of my back / neck / joint, I try to get other people to do things for me.
X 9) I get dressed more slowly than usual because of my back / neck / joint. Can't lift knee up to dre
X 10) I only stand for short periods of time because of my back / neck / joint.
X 11) Because of my back / neck / joint, I try not to bend or kneel down. I do every day but less than
____ 12) I find it difficult to get out of a chair because of my back / neck / joint. sometimes   normal
X 13) My back / neck / joint is painful almost all the time.
X 14) I find it difficult to turn over in bed because of my back / neck / joint pain.
____ 15) My appetite is not very good because of my back / neck / joint pain.
X 16) I have trouble putting on my socks (or stockings) because of the pain in my back / neck / joint.
____ 17) I only walk short distances because of my back / neck / joint.
X 18) I sleep less well because of my back / neck / joint.
____ 19) Because of my back / neck / joint pain, I get dressed with help from someone else.
____ 20) I sit down for most of the day because of my back / neck / joint.
X 21) I avoid heavy jobs around the house because of my back / neck / joint.
X 22) Because of my back / neck / joint pain, I am more irritable and bad tempered with people than usual.
X 23) Because of my back / neck / joint, I go up stairs more slowly than usual.
____ 24) I stay in bed most of the time because of my back / neck / joint.

Fig. 2. Sample Roland-Morris Disability Questionnaire for a patient with severe chronic pain with nociceptive focus in the lumbar region. Note that items 17/24 are positive, which might indicate a patient with generalized centrally mediated pain, which was not the case for this patient.

these patients, I recommend physiatry referral, sooner rather than later. The dreaded Ds are as follows:

1. Disability
2. Depression
3. Deconditioning
4. Dependence on opioids
5. Dysfunctional relationships, including divorce as a result of the patient's loss of function and chronic pain
6. Drinking and other substance abuse.

I cannot provide simple weighted averages to the various dreaded Ds. However, in my experience, vocational disability is often one of the most important factors to complicate a patient's course of care. Patients who are unable to return to gainful employment generally do not have as good a prognosis as those who continue to work. There are no value judgments here. Rather, I offer my dispassionate view of outcomes from treating patients with traumatic injuries, mostly in the setting of personal injury and/or workers' compensation.

Some of the dreaded Ds are likely not independent. For example, many injured patients will develop depression as a result of their loss of function. For some patients, if their function can be restored or their pain relieved, their depression will often melt away. For example, Barbara Wallis and colleagues[3] conducted an elegant study showing resolution of depression and anxiety symptoms among patients with chronic whiplash injuries whose pain was successfully treated with facet joint neurotomy for chronic neck pain.

There are other patients who have a more complex relationship between their emotional state and their physical disability, evidenced within my clinical practice and in the literature on chronic whiplash.[4-7] For example, patients who have a history of posttraumatic stress disorder (PTSD) may have this condition reactivated by a motor vehicle crash. In this setting, these patients often do poorly unless psychological factors can be addressed in addition to their physical pain. By contrast, others have a much more straightforward relationship between their chronic pain and their emotional state and resolve their dysphoria lock-step with improvement in pain and physical function.

Integrative Approach to the Complex Patient with Chronic Pain

In my experience, if a patient has at least 3 of the above 6 factors, usually a specialist with a physiatry approach to injury is required. In other words, if an orthopedic surgeon, for example, works with a patient who has had focal joint injuries but also more widespread problems with the dreaded Ds, the patient may well have relief of their focal joint pain from the orthopedic treatment but they are not likely to improve their functional status to the point of return to work and other functional gains.

Similarly, a chiropractor may do well to treat the patient's spinal pain and help them avoid dependence on opioid-based pain medications. However, in my experience, they generally do not have enough scope of practice to address many of these other issues, such as disability, deconditioning, and depression. It has been my experience that the well-trained physiatrist, who is attuned to these multiple nonphysical issues, is ideally suited to treat the complex patient with chronic pain. Having physiatry training alone does not guarantee an ability to treat these larger issues. One needs to have a propensity and level of patience to identify the dreaded Ds and to formulate an integrative treatment plan.

One of the classic pitfalls I see in my clinical practice and work as an expert witness, is that patients who have experienced multiple complex injuries from major trauma are often passed from one orthopedic specialist to the next. There is no single specialist taking an overall view of the patient's injuries and loss of function. Thus, they may get a focal shoulder consultation with surgery, then knee surgery, then foot and ankle assessment, and perhaps even physiatry spinal assessment with spinal injections given for diagnostic purposes. This barrage of specialty treatment is provided without any single provider giving an overall view of the patient's functional status and the nonphysical barriers to rehabilitation. This pattern represents a major danger associated with the current specialized form of treatment and is one that, as physiatrists, we are naturally equipped to help prevent.

Special Case of Workers' Compensation

In the workers' compensation setting, I have found that the following additional dreaded Ds are relevant:

1. Decision to litigate.
2. Disagreement with employer.

Decision to litigate

The treating provider should not blame either the patient or the workers' compensation claim company or employer for the presence of litigation. However, patients who decide to have legal representation in the workers' compensation setting generally have claims that are more complex and almost always associated with chronic disability.

This association may not be coincidental because workers' compensation attorneys generally are not paid unless the patient is on time loss. Thus, patients who are not on time loss may not find it either worthwhile or feasible to obtain legal representation in the workers' compensation setting. In the personal injury setting, it is controversial whether litigation per se leads to a worsened outcome.[4,8–12] Specifically, legal representation in the personal injury setting may represent the response to, rather than the cause of, worsening prognosis after chronic whiplash injuries. In other words, many patients do not bother with legal representation for the first few months after injury. However, they may seek an attorney if their injuries become more chronic.

Disagreement with employer

Again, the examiner should not take sides and decide whether the employer or the employee is to blame for a litigious or contentious claim. In my experience, if the employer and the injured worker have a mutual level of suspicion, the outcome of the claim will generally sour. For example, injured workers may be fearful that the employer will seek retaliation. Specifically, if the employer states that they are willing to have the patient return to work in a lighter duty capacity, given functional loss from a spinal injury, the worker may be concerned that they will be laid off shortly after the claim is closed. For their part, the employer may expedite claim closure by returning the patient to lighter duty employment, avoiding the expense for vocational consultation or retraining. Their offer for employment may be either in good faith or disingenuous. This uncertainty is a major source of concern for some injured workers, especially in industries in which there is no light duty, such as construction and other building trades. Because of this fear of being laid off once the claim is resolved, injured workers who are suspicious of their employers are often wary of accepting lighter duty work options. They assume, sometimes based on the experiences of their fellow injured workers, that the employer will terminate them once the claim is closed. In my experience, this problem of disagreement with employer is often one of the most important factors predicting outcome in a workers' compensation setting. If the injured worker and the employer have a relationship of mutual respect, lighter duty work options or reasonable accommodations often emerge, and the claim may resolve successfully.

Again, the physician should try not to judge the employer or the injured worker. Instead, they should give a dispassionate rendering of medical treatment, at the same time acknowledging that the level of trust between injured worker and their employer is an important factor in the success of a claim. Although this factor may not have a direct bearing on the experience of chronic pain, the distinction between chronic pain and workers' compensation claim-related factors can become blurred.

As an example, imagine a patient who is a pipefitter making approximately 4 times the minimum wage plus overtime and other benefits. If the pipefitter sustains a low back injury and is unable to return to their profession, he or she may be found eligible for permanent lighter duty work. In Washington State, there is no need to match patients to their previous level of earnings. This injured pipefitter might be found eligible to become a security guard, making slightly more than minimum wage. In my experience, most injured pipefitters remain reluctant to accept the career switch to security guard. Whether the patient is actually malingering or whether their behavior needs to be understood from a biopsychosocial approach to chronic pain should be addressed on a case-by-case basis.

Keep in mind that the choices for the injured pipefitter are (1) to receive 60% to 80% of their baseline wage on time loss, or more than twice the minimum wage, and remain resting at home, or (2) return to work as a security guard, with increased chances for aggravating their low back pain with return to physical activity and a significant pay cut going from time loss to working full-time. It may not be surprising from a cognitive-behavioral viewpoint, without considerations of malingering, that this injured worker may naturally feel entrenched with chronic spinal pain.

The employer may believe that the injured worker is malingering or overly invested in their disability. They may perform secret surveillance on the patient, with the goal of determining whether the patient is voluntarily underperforming or malingering. In some cases, the suspicion of excessive pain behavior with underperformance or malingering is verified, either through a functional capacity evaluation or video surveillance.

CLINICAL PRESENTATION: PHYSICAL EXAMINATION

Regarding physical examination, I note that chronic pain patients often have fairly globally reduced spinal range of motion. Lateral bending of the spine often causes contralateral paraspinal pain. For example, if patients undergo left lateral bending of the neck, they may develop right upper trapezius pain. This may be the manifestation of stiff and tightened muscles. For the cervical spine, in the setting of chronic whiplash, I often use quantitative cervical spine range of motion measurements to help track response to treatment.[13] However, lumbar range of motion as a measure of impairment is more controversial and may not yield meaningful results.[14]

There may be further loss of range of motion in the extremities, although generally this is limited to proximal joints, such as the shoulders and hips. In these more proximal joints, pain with range of motion is usually not localizable to an intra-articular joint problem. For example, although shoulder overhead range of motion may be limited, the resultant pain is often in the upper trapezius area, rather than in the lateral humeral area, which indicates a nociceptive focus within the shoulder joint, such as a rotator cuff tendinitis. Another example is the straight leg raise maneuver, which will often cause low back or buttock pain but not the lower extremity pain classic of lumbar radiculopathy. In fairness, the back and buttock pain may reflect a nociceptive focus, such as a discogenic pain generator, rather than a myofascial phenomenon of a painful muscle stretch.

The astute examiner should be alert to the coexistence of chronic centrally mediated pain and a focal nociceptive source of pain.[15–17] For example, it is reasonable to assume that patients with chronic cervical facet-mediated pain after whiplash injuries have concomitant centrally mediated pain.[18–20] Thus, a nociceptive focus can be thought of as driving a more generalized centrally mediated pain syndrome. As stated in one review on chronic whiplash pain, "The initial tissue damage and ensuing nociception may induce central hyperexcitability...This could be maintained by ongoing peripheral nociception or due to central changes that remain after resolution of the tissue injury."[21]

In my practice, I use simple bedside maneuvers to help me gauge whether there is centrally mediated pain or pain from peripheral sensitization from an original nociceptive focus. For example, with the patient prone, the examiner may do a test by rolling the skin over the area that has been painful, as illustrated in **Fig. 3**. I believe exquisite segmental discomfort in response to this test is an indicator of centrally mediated pain or peripheral sensitization.

Alternatively, or additionally, the practitioner could perform what I call the skin scratch test in which the end of a paperclip is run along the paraspinal region with the patient prone and the examiner tries to identify a segment or set of segments causing focal pain for the patient (illustrated in **Fig. 4**).

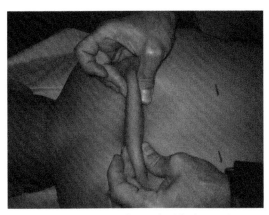

Fig. 3. Illustration of the skin roll test, performed with the patient prone. This test helps identify hypersensitive regions of spinal pain, usually over several segmental levels. Patients are often surprised to find repeatable evidence of pain with rolling of the skin.

This finding is often repeatable and surprising to the patient. Although I do not have peer-reviewed literature that describes the clinical significance of these findings, I find that the skin roll and skin scratch tests often identify patients who have experienced sleep disruption and other features of chronic pain syndrome. These tests also help me localize areas to perform trigger point therapy for patients suffering with chronic pain. They can also be used as serial gauges of recovery from injury.

In summary, history and physical examination are critical for identifying chronic pain syndromes. However, the astute clinician needs to understand that a nociceptive focus, such as a cervical facet joint injury after whiplash, may perpetuate the state of chronic centrally mediated pain. Thus, unless a nociceptive focus can be more durably treated, for example, with radiofrequency neurotomy of the facet joint nerves, it can be assumed that the nociceptive focus will drive the state of chronic centrally mediated pain.

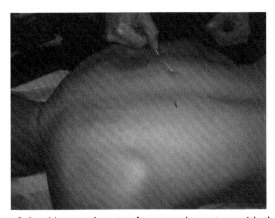

Fig. 4. Illustration of the skin scratch test, often complementary with the skin roll test. A ballpoint pen should be used to mark the region of hypersensitivity for the right and left sides separately. The test should be repeated for reliability, which is generally seen within one segment level.

PITFALLS WITH ASSESSMENT

The history and physical examination are critical in terms of establishing an overall diagnostic impression. However, in my experience, if the patient does not have repeatable physical examination findings, they will not benefit from treatments directed at a focal anatomic problem. Consider a patient who has tenderness of the right upper cervical facet joint area on initial examination but, on another date, has tenderness of the lower cervical facet joint area with resolution of the right upper cervical facet joint tenderness. This type of patient generally will not benefit from anatomically oriented focal treatments, such as diagnostic cervical facet joint injections with the goal of providing radiofrequency neurotomy treatment of longer term pain relief.

This is not to say that patients who have inconsistent examination findings are malingering. There are many reasons for physical examination findings to vary from visit to visit. Some variability arises from the shortcomings of biological measurement during physical examination. There is probably a larger fraction of inconsistencies due to patients experiencing variable physical states from one visit to the next. Finally, there is the possibility that patients may be voluntarily underperforming, or malingering, which is actually fairly rare. In any event, in my experience, if there is a wide variability in physical examination findings from one date to the next, patients generally do not benefit from focal anatomically directed treatments for chronic pain. They may benefit from a multidisciplinary pain management program.

In addition, the careful examiner should understand the importance of teasing out focal anatomic deficits from more generalized physical symptoms and examination findings. I am fond of saying that fibromyalgia syndrome is not Latin for "doctor doesn't know." In other words, if a physician fails to render an accurate history and physical examination for the patient, she or he may miss an underlying medical diagnosis amenable to focal anatomically directed treatment. In my clinical career, I have had a few patients labeled as having fibromyalgia syndrome but who actually had lumbar spinal stenosis. One of the key physical examination findings for these patients is weakness of extensor hallucis longus (EHL), a key painless muscle to test for radiculopathy.[22] EHL testing is increasingly ignored in the current medical milieu, which emphasizes advanced imaging and other diagnostic studies. Despite this trend toward high-tech medicine, I often label EHL as the poor man's MRI scan to my patients, given its exquisite ability to discriminate the presence of lumbar radiculopathy. The presence of radiculopathy is often then confirmed with the patient prone, with detailed testing of the knee flexor (hamstring) muscles. Careful technique for assessing the strength of both of these muscles is critical. I have found that these proficiencies are sometimes lacking when I review the examination skills of physiatry residents who have rotated through my clinic.

In my career, I have also seen a patient labeled with myofascial pain syndrome who actually had suprascapular nerve palsy. Further, I have had patients who were labeled as suffering from disc herniations based on MRI scan results but who did not have clinical features of lumbosacral radiculopathy. Finally, I have had patients thought to have spinal stenosis who actually had hip claudication from vascular disease. Although there is no guarantee that careful physical examination will prevent these diagnostic mishaps, all of these patients could have been correctly diagnosed with careful physical examination. Thus, the inability to perform a careful history and physical examination not only creates inaccurate diagnoses but can also lead to labeling patients with diagnoses based on advanced imaging findings or electrodiagnostic studies without sufficient clinical correlation.

As a final extreme example, I have had a few patients who have come to my office with the scars of anterior cervical decompression and fusion who actually had thoracic outlet syndrome (TOS). Typically, these patients had a disc protrusion on cervical MRI with tingling into the arm. The treating physicians had not recognized that the patients had TOS. Fusion surgery was performed for the visible abnormality (eg, the disc herniation at C5-6 visualized on MRI scan) and yet the patients did not improve. For these patients, careful examination often reveals focal tenderness in the scalene muscles, intolerance to overhead activities, and focal upper extremity weakness limited to the hand intrinsic muscles, a constellation of physical examination findings more consistent with TOS than most forms of cervical radiculopathy.

In summary, patients may have nociceptive pain without imaging abnormalities, including MRI, demonstrating the structural lesion. For example, cervical MRI scans in the setting of nonradicular whiplash injuries, the most common type of neck pain after a motor vehicle crash, often show degenerative changes at C5-6 and C6-7. However, as illustrated in **Fig. 5**, carefully controlled image-guided anesthetic blocks directed at the facet joints or the sensory nerves supplying the facet joints, the so-called medial branch nerves, are the gold standard for diagnosing facet joint injuries. Carefully controlled studies have revealed that the C2-3 facet joint level is the most common cause of chronic pain after a whiplash injury.[23,24] Paradoxically, MRI scanning is almost always normal at the C2-3 level, supporting the view that MRI scanning in the setting of axial neck pain generally has very little, if any, diagnostic yield.[25,26] I often discuss with patients that MRI scans will show the facet joints but not pain from or injury to these joints.

It is important for the examiner to remember that there are type 2 errors in our age of medical technology. As an example, before MRI became available, if we assumed radiographs should show disc herniations, we would have failed to detect the most actual disc herniations. Analogously, although MRI scanning has been quite helpful in detecting disc herniations, it is fairly useless for diagnosing facet joint injuries. In

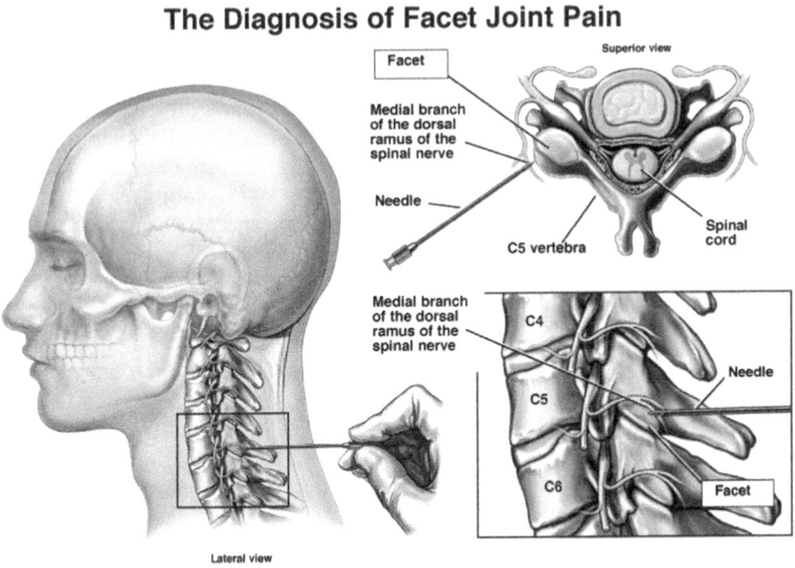

The Diagnosis of Facet Joint Pain

Fig. 5. Medical illustration showing anesthetic block of the medial branch of the dorsal ramus of the spinal nerve root for the diagnosis of cervical facet-mediated pain. (*Courtesy of* Nucleus Medical Media, Kennesaw, GA; with permission. Images © 2002 Nucleus Communications. Available at: www.nucleusinc.com.)

other words, disc herniations are to radiographs as facet joint injuries are to MRI scans: just as an occasional radiograph may show a calcified disc herniation, so too may a rare lumbar or cervical MRI scan show a facet joint injury. However, this is an exception and not a rule. In the most cases, MRI scanning is subject to type 2 error with respect to facet joint injuries (ie, it will yield normal results in the setting of an actual facet joint injury). The injury may instead be confirmed more accurately with history, careful repeated physical examinations on different clinic visits, and image-guided diagnostic injections directed at detecting facet joint injury.

Putting imaging and other diagnostic studies before a clear and accurate history and physical examination of the patient may be associated with additional problems, because this

1. Leads to over-testing, over-treating, and inaccurate care of the patient
2. Causes possible injury to the patient, including the injury associated with delay in diagnosis
3. Degrades the quality of the practitioner, who may ultimately become more focused on reviewing diagnostic studies rather than maintaining focus on the patient's history and physical examination.

In my clinical experience, this excessive focus on diagnostic studies, sometimes accompanied by normal physical examination templates in an electronic medical record (EMR), may lead to a range of poor outcomes. At the most benign end of the spectrum, I have encountered EMR errors from the casual use of normal physical examination templates. For example, one patient with a C2 potentially unstable cervical fracture was documented to have a neck examination that found the neck was supple and without lymphadenopathy. Despite this glaring error in the EMR, this patient received excellent neurosurgical assessment and treatment. Although this paper error might be seen as something almost humorous in retrospect, it degrades the integrity of the entire medical record.

At a much more severe level, focus on diagnostic studies without an accurate foundation of thorough history and physical examination can lead to disastrous consequences in the delay of diagnosis. In my clinical career, this has included the inability to detect cervical myelopathy and cauda equina syndrome with grossly inadequate neurologic examinations; the inability to detect a proximal median nerve injury in an anticoagulated patient, which resulted in pseudoaneurysm of the brachial artery; and Parsonage-Turner syndrome affecting the anterior interosseous nerve in a patient who underwent exploratory surgeries of her finger and thumb flexor tendons. All of these examples could have been prevented if a careful history and physical examination had been conducted on the patient.

In my clinic, the physicians are fond of saying, "Treat the patient, not the picture," referring to the importance of evaluating a patient by history and physical examination before reviewing their MRI studies. When I walk into the examination room, several patients are desperate to know if I reviewed their imaging studies. I often need to remind them that the most important clinical data comes from my listening to their story and doing a careful physical examination.

Examples of key pieces of history include whether the patient relies on a grocery cart when shopping in the mall and whether they can lie on their side if they are complaining of hip pain. The former is exquisitely sensitive and specific, in my experience, for detecting patients with spinal stenosis. The latter often goes with trochanteric bursitis, in the setting of other factors such as female gender, middle age, and increased body mass index. These are but a few of the pieces of history one should obtain when narrowing the differential diagnosis while interviewing a patient.

For the electrodiagnostic consultant, a corollary to treating the patient and not the picture is treat the numbness, not the numbers. For example, in my experience, many patients will have some measure of median neuropathy at the wrist by electrodiagnostic studies. This result may correlate clinically to the presence of carpal tunnel syndrome but not in all cases. Many patients who are in the building trades may have median neuropathy at the wrists without clinical evidence of carpal tunnel syndrome. Competing diagnoses may be present, such as radiculopathy without electrodiagnostic abnormalities or TOS. If the examiner is not astute and accurate, unnecessary treatments, including surgeries, may occur, resulting in scarring, increased expenses, and no clear resolution of the problem for the patient.

Psychological disorders, such as depression and anxiety, should be similarly treated as diagnoses of exclusion. This situation is analogous to the elderly patient who may present with weight loss. Although it is true that depression in the elderly can cause weight loss, more serious structural abnormalities, such as cancer, need to be addressed initially. Similarly, many patients have depression and anxiety in the setting of chronic pain. The astute examiner should ensure that they have ruled out physical conditions before attributing the patient's loss of function to a primary psychological condition. Even if the examiner has a strong suspicion that psychological problems are affecting the patient's physical functioning, they should not cut corners in terms of performing a rigorous neurologic and musculoskeletal evaluation.

As a final example, I have had a patient who was hospitalized with ataxia and diagnosed with conversion disorder. This diagnosis was augmented by input from a clinical psychologist during the patient's hospital admission. The patient actually had an atypical form of Guillain-Barré syndrome, causing sensory ataxia with normal motor strength. The patient was not promptly treated and was labeled as being hysterical with conversion disorder. The patient underwent several MRI scans but she did not have the key studies that would have made her diagnosis: nerve conduction studies and electromyography. Again, if the practitioner is not sufficiently astute to form a cogent differential diagnosis of neurologic and musculoskeletal findings, any amount of fishing, such as collecting MRI scans across the spine, will not lead to an accurate diagnosis.

A final note about biopsychosocial influences on the patient's clinical presentation, including the history and physical examination, is that an experienced practitioner can often detect malingering or exaggeration in the setting of the patient's history, even before performing physical examination. However, it should be remembered that malingering and conversion disorder are generally fairly rare and more organic diagnoses should be initially addressed.

CLINICAL SHINY-ROUND-OBJECTS-SOMETIMES-FOUND-IN-OYSTERS

As a final note, I have developed many observations based on a clinical career spanning almost 20 years since my residency.

Influence of Social Security Disability

In my clinical experience, if a patient is actively applying for Social Security disability benefits at the time of their initial evaluation with you, they generally will not benefit from your treatment. Even if the patient is not explicitly coming to you for endorsement of their disability status, my experience is that patients have often already thrown in the towel by the time they apply for Social Security disability. In this setting, they may be going to a physiatrist to help reassure themselves that they have done the utmost possible to improve their underlying functional status. However, the application to

Social Security disability is often a signature of a patient's hopelessness with regard to future employability.

Patients with Chronic Widespread Pain

If patients with this condition are not improving within a few months of physiatry treatment, they likely will not benefit from any further focal treatment within a single provider's medical clinic. They may benefit from a multidisciplinary pain management program. The practitioner should remain alert to the patient's compliance with treatment, the provider's sense that the patient wants to get on with their life, and the patient's actions regarding avoiding long-term disability.

Restorative Sleep

For patients with chronic pain, if they cannot establish a restorative sleep pattern, usually they will not make any further progress in their physical or functional rehab program. High-quality sleep should be considered as the first order of recovery. At times, patients will state that they feel they sleep fairly well but the practitioner should inquire whether they feel rested when they wake up. If this is not the case, sleep disruption is still present unless proven otherwise.

Although this article is not about treatment, patients with chronic pain may benefit from a sleep study if simple pharmacologic measures are not effective. For example, among traumatic brain injury and whiplash patients, sleep disruption is a common symptom[27,28] and should be aggressively treated by the practitioner. Even patients with fairly focal and milder pain symptoms benefit from simple interventions for sleep disruption. For example, in my practice, many patients referred by chiropractors are resistant to medication. However, if they have sleep disruption, I often can help them with their function and pain levels by an initial prescription of 5 mg of cyclobenzaprine at night. On follow-up, they are often surprised that the improvement in their sleep has given them global benefit.

Influence of Posttraumatic Stress

This condition is much less common than sleep disruption, and can have a spectrum of presentation. For example, patients who have been in a motor vehicle crash may have some crash-related anxiety for several months after the crash. Unless they are having frequent flashbacks and nightmares, they may not meet criteria for PTSD but may still need treatment of crash-related anxiety in conjunction with physical rehabilitation.

In my experience, if these emotional issues are not adequately treated, patients will never recover from their physical injuries. I am not sure of the neurobiology of this condition; however, I know this to be true based on my clinical experience. I suspect it has something to do with patients no longer feeling like perpetual victims once they are able to recognize and control the emotional trauma associated with their physical injuries. This may have some corollary to patients moving toward a higher-level of cognitive processing regarding their injury, as opposed to a fight-or-flight response associated with chronic PTSD. In any event, if patients continue to have intrusive posttraumatic emotional symptoms after a set of physical injuries, I recommend these symptoms be addressed as part of an overall treatment plan.

Patients with Low Back Pain and Falling

In my experience, patients with lower back pain generally do not fall because of their low back pain. This is to say that if you understand from a patient that they have fallen as a result of lower back pain, you should be alert to a possible more serious underlying cause or nonphysical cause for the falling. In the former case, I have seen instances of cauda equina syndrome, massive lower thoracic disc herniation, and spinal arteriovenous malformation that caused falling with lower back pain. All of these are extremely rare conditions but they should not be missed. Alternatively, the patient may be fabricating their injury and deliberately pretending to fall as a result of lower back pain. They may also have comorbid conditions having nothing to do with their lower back pain, such as peripheral neuropathy or stroke. All these possibilities should all be taken into account with clinical assessment.

Consistency of Clinical Examination Findings

This topic is touched on in the previous sections. Put concisely, if a patient does not exhibit fairly repeatable findings, accounting for biologic variability from day to day interactions with the patient, they generally will not be helped by focal anatomic treatments. This is not to say that the patient is necessarily malingering. However, focal anatomic treatments should flow from focal anatomic findings. For example, if a patient does not have fairly focal tenderness of one or more spinal facet joints on repeated clinic visits, I do not pursue an extensive set of diagnostic spinal injections to identify an injured facet joint. By contrast, if consistent clinical findings are occult from advanced imaging such as MRI scanning, patients may still benefit from focal treatment. For example, radiofrequency neurotomy procedure for facet-mediated pain of the neck after whiplash is a focal treatment given to patients without visible structural abnormalities.

Avoid Medicalizing Patients

In my opinion, this medicalizing tends to occur more in other specialties. For example, the polytrauma patient may have multiple injured joints addressed by different orthopedic specialists, who may even be colleagues within the same clinic. There is nothing necessarily wrong with this treatment but there should be an overarching overseer of treatment. A physiatrist is ideally suited to fill this role and to help guide the patient toward an optimal number of interventions without excessive treatment.

A physiatrist can also screen for multiple other factors, including several the dreaded Ds cited previously. In my experience, more specialized neurologic and musculoskeletal practitioners, such as neurologists and orthopedists, may not orient themselves to the patient's overall functional status and instead focus on focal anatomic deficits. It may be my bias, but I believe physiatry is ideally suited for treating patients in this setting.

With patients who have complex sets of injuries, I often explain to them that we will take a stepwise approach to their care. If the patient has fairly acute injuries, such as soon after motor vehicle crash, I will err on the side of documenting all of the diagnoses that may be possible or probable but avoid working up many of these diagnoses unless symptoms become more problematic with time. In a sense, I am triaging from day one while trying to be astute without missing diagnoses that may not resolve with time.

Avoid Excessive Advanced Imaging Studies

I generally avoid advanced imaging of the spine, such as MRI scanning, unless patients present with radicular findings specifically on physical examination. Even with radiculopathy, if we have the luxury of time, for example in the several weeks after an acute injury, I often hold off on advanced imaging and explain my reasoning to the patient. In the setting of trauma, it is not uncommon for me, especially in the younger patient, to use my clinical examination skills to decide whether the patient has lumbar radiculopathy and would benefit from a lumbar epidural injection, without the need for MRI. Of note, for cervical radiculopathy, obtaining an initial cervical MRI scan should be the standard of care for all patients who may undergo cervical epidural injections.

The provider should explain to the patient that if they fail to improve with initial treatment and tincture of time, the diagnostic workup will be advanced. In the chronic setting and in the absence of radiculopathy, I will sometimes obtain the therapeutic spinal MRI to help reassure the patient that we are leaving no stone unturned. I explain that the scanning may be reassuring or may show age-related wear and tear but that it is not unreasonable to obtain the study given the severity and chronicity of their problem. Patients are often relieved when these studies are reviewed with them. In fairness, I am sometimes surprised by significant findings on an MRI in the absence of radiculopathy, humbling me to remember that no rules in clinical medicine should remain hard and fast.

REFERENCES

1. Gaskin DJ, Richard P. The economic costs of pain in the United States. J Pain 2012;13:715–24.
2. Roland M, Morris R. A study of the natural history of back pain. Part I: development of a reliable and sensitive measure of disability in low-back pain. Spine (Phila Pa 1976) 1983;8:141–4.
3. Wallis BJ, Lord SM, Bogduk N. Resolution of psychological distress of whiplash patients following treatment by radiofrequency neurotomy: a randomised, double-blind, placebo-controlled trial [see comments]. Pain 1997;73:15–22.
4. Lankester BJ, Garneti N, Gargan MF, et al. Factors predicting outcome after whiplash injury in subjects pursuing litigation. Eur Spine J 2006;15:902–7.
5. Radanov BP, Di Stefano G, Schnidrig A, et al. Common whiplash: psychosomatic or somatopsychic? J Neurol Neurosurg Psychiatry 1994;57:486–90.
6. Radanov BP, Sturzenegger M, Di Stefano G. Long-term outcome after whiplash injury. A 2-year follow-up considering features of injury mechanism and somatic, radiologic, and psychosocial findings. Medicine (Baltimore) 1995;74:281–97.
7. Turner MA, Taylor PJ, Neal LA. Physical and psychiatric predictors of late whiplash syndrome. Injury 2003;34:434–7.
8. Schofferman J, Wasserman S. Successful treatment of low back pain and neck pain after a motor vehicle accident despite litigation. Spine 1994;19:1007–10.
9. Swartzman LC, Teasell RW, Shapiro AP, et al. The effect of litigation status on adjustment to whiplash injury. Spine 1996;21:53–8.
10. McDonald GJ, Lord SM, Bogduk N. Long-term follow-up of patients treated with cervical radiofrequency neurotomy for chronic neck pain. Neurosurgery 1999;45: 61–7 [discussion: 67–8].
11. Sapir DA, Gorup JM. Radiofrequency medial branch neurotomy in litigant and nonlitigant patients with cervical whiplash: a prospective study. Spine 2001;26: E268–73.
12. Peterson C, Bolton J, Wood AR, et al. A cross-sectional study correlating degeneration of the cervical spine with disability and pain in United Kingdom patients. Spine 2003;28:129–33.
13. Sterling M, Jull G, Vicenzino B, et al. Development of motor system dysfunction following whiplash injury. Pain 2003;103:65–73.
14. Zuberbier OA, Kozlowski AJ, Hunt DG, et al. Analysis of the convergent and discriminant validity of published lumbar flexion, extension, and lateral flexion scores. Spine 2001;26:E472–8.

15. Curatolo M, Arendt-Nielsen L, Petersen-Felix S. Central hypersensitivity in chronic pain: mechanisms and clinical implications. Phys Med Rehabil Clin N Am 2006; 17:287–302.
16. Staud R, Nagel S, Robinson ME, et al. Enhanced central pain processing of fibromyalgia patients is maintained by muscle afferent input: a randomized, double-blind, placebo-controlled study. Pain 2009;145:96–104.
17. Staud R. Is it all central sensitization? Role of peripheral tissue nociception in chronic musculoskeletal pain. Curr Rheumatol Rep 2010;12:448–54.
18. Smith AD, Jull G, Schneider G, et al. A comparison of physical and psychological features of responders and non-responders to cervical facet blocks in chronic whiplash. BMC Musculoskelet Disord 2013;14:313.
19. Lee KE, Davis MB, Mejilla RM, et al. In vivo cervical facet capsule distraction: mechanical implications for whiplash and neck pain. Stapp Car Crash J 2004;48: 373–95.
20. Lee KE, Thinnes JH, Gokhin DS, et al. A novel rodent neck pain model of facet-mediated behavioral hypersensitivity: implications for persistent pain and whiplash injury. J Neurosci Methods 2004;137:151–9.
21. Stone AM, Vicenzino B, Lim EC, et al. Measures of central hyperexcitability in chronic whiplash associated disorder—a systematic review and meta-analysis. Man Ther 2013;18:111–7.
22. Finsterbush A, Frankel U, Arnon R. Quantitative power measurement of extensor hallucis longus. A simple objective test in evaluation of low-back pain with neurological involvement. Spine 1983;8:206–10.
23. Lord SM, Barnsley L, Wallis BJ, et al. Third occipital nerve headache: a prevalence study. J Neurol Neurosurg Psychiatry 1994;57:1187–90.
24. Lord SM, Barnsley L, Wallis BJ, et al. Chronic cervical zygapophysial joint pain after whiplash. A placebo-controlled prevalence study [see comments]. Spine 1996;21:1737–44 [discussion: 1744–5].
25. Curatolo M, Bogduk N, Ivancic PC, et al. The role of tissue damage in whiplash associated disorders: discussion paper 1. Spine (Phila Pa 1976) 2011;36(25 Suppl):S309–15.
26. Gellhorn AC. Cervical facet-mediated pain. Phys Med Rehabil Clin N Am 2011; 22:447–58, viii.
27. Valenza MC, Valenza G, Gonzalez-Jimenez E, et al. Alteration in sleep quality in patients with mechanical insidious neck pain and whiplash-associated neck pain. Am J Phys Med Rehabil 2012;91:584–91.
28. Verma A, Anand V, Verma NP. Sleep disorders in chronic traumatic brain injury. J Clin Sleep Med 2007;3:357–62.

Opioid Therapy in Chronic Pain

Jane C. Ballantyne, MD, FRCA

KEYWORDS

• Opioid dependence • Addiction • Pain management • Dependence

KEY POINTS

- Not all patients with pain are suitable candidates for chronic opioid therapy (COT).
- Short-term opioid therapy has different goals and purposes and should not progress to COT without reconsideration of goals and purposes.
- Opioid dependence develops in all patients receiving COT, may have a strong psychological component, and is not always easily reversible.
- COT should be goal oriented and discontinued if goals are not met.
- There are significant safety issues that need consideration during COT.

INTRODUCTION

Opioids have a long history of use for the treatment of pain, and despite efforts to find alternatives, they remain the strongest and most effective analgesics available. The downside is that they are addictive and potentially dangerous, especially when used not as prescribed, and there are many complex reasons why opioids used to treat pain in outpatients, who control their own use, may not be taken strictly as prescribed. Throughout history, although recognizing the value of opioids in treating serious pain, especially acute pain and pain at the end of life, there has been caution about using opioids to treat chronic pain. This caution existed because of the perceived increased risk of addiction when opioids are used long term and at home. There has been a surge in prescribing of opioids for chronic pain, especially in the United States, and this surge has been produced by a combination of increased availability, production of new opioids and new formulations that have been aggressively marketed, and changed beliefs about whether the risk of addiction for some should preclude use when it might help the many who do not become addicted.[1] The surge in prescribing for chronic pain has produced a parallel increase in cases of opioid abuse and related deaths,[1–3] and despite what is now more than 2 decades of experience, it is still unclear whether, and under what conditions, opioids can be used to treat chronic

Department of Anesthesiology and Pain Medicine, University of Washington, 1959 NE Pacific St, Seattle, WA 98195, USA
E-mail address: jcb12@uw.edu

Phys Med Rehabil Clin N Am 26 (2015) 201–218
http://dx.doi.org/10.1016/j.pmr.2014.12.001
1047-9651/15/$ – see front matter © 2015 Elsevier Inc. All rights reserved.

pain safely and effectively. Many questions remain, but what this article presents is how opioids should be used to treat chronic pain considering recent concerns about their efficacy and safety.

PATIENT SELECTION

Not all patients are suitable candidates for opioids. In fact, proper selection of candidates for the treatment can do more to improve efficacy and safety than any other aspect of managing the treatment. It is tempting to think that a patient's complaint of severe pain is enough to warrant use of strong pain medications. Recent teaching has been that a report of severe pain warrants treatment with opioids if all efforts to use alternative treatments have failed. But recent evidence shows that for some pain conditions, opioids not only may not work well but also may hinder the progress toward recovery that can be achieved by other means.[4–9] It is becoming clear that this is true for several pain conditions and is particularly true for musculoskeletal pain. Opioids allow people to rest comfortably and are useful for providing comfort.[10] They are also useful during acute onset or acute exacerbations of pain when they can reduce pain enough to start the process of active rehabilitation. With long-term usage, however, they may have a different role. Analgesia is not always maintained long term, and the numbing effect of opioids tends to make people less inclined to move even when exercise, or at least maintained activity, is the intervention most likely to achieve recovery. There are many musculoskeletal conditions and so-called centralized pain states such as nonstructural low back pain or fibromyalgia, where the numbing effects of opioids can actually lessen the likelihood of recovery.[11–15] At the same time, when there is significant damage due to disease, trauma, or surgery, and normal activity is not a realistic goal, the numbing effect of opioids can be helpful and may even improve function in patients with serious functional incapacity. Opioids at low doses can also be helpful in low-risk patients who are intolerant of alternative treatments and cannot realistically be active, for example, the elderly. Choosing candidates for opioid therapy based on their disease state and not on their reported pain severity has several advantages. It allows one to exclude cases that are more likely to recover without opioids. It allows one to target opioids only toward cases that can be improved. It removes the need to make judgments about pain severity and what a report of pain suggests. Past teaching was that because pain is a subjective experience, "pain is what the reporting person says it is." Although this is indisputable, severe pain that would be better managed without opioids should not be treated with opioids simply because of a report of severe pain. Decisions about the suitability of opioid treatment must always be made on an individual patient basis, but **Table 1** attempts to summarize some of the broad categories of suitability for long-term opioid treatment.

BASIC PRINCIPLES OF CHRONIC OPIOID MANAGEMENT

- Decisions about opioid treatment always take place after a full history and physical examination and after reaching and documenting a pain diagnosis.
- Continuous treatment with an opioid for 90 days or longer is COT.[16]
- At 90 days, or preferably sooner, a process of shared decision making needs to occur concerning whether COT is a good choice.[17–21]
- Before offering COT[21]
  - Patient completes a screening instrument for addiction risk.
  - Baseline urine drug toxicology screen is done.
  - If available, active or prior usage is checked in prescription monitoring system.

Table 1 Patient selection principles	
Suitable Candidates	**Rationale**
Arthritis or other pain in the elderly	Low dose can be helpful. Not tolerant of alternative treatment. Frailty may preclude maintenance of activity or rehabilitative exercise
Provision of comfort in cases of serious disease or existential suffering or when persistent attempts to treat without opioids have failed	Reasonable to abandon ideas of functional restoration. Different risk/benefit balance
Acute exacerbations of chronic musculoskeletal pain, including back pain	Short course of opioids may help in initiating rehabilitation
Not Suitable Candidates	**Rationale**
Chronic musculoskeletal pain, including low back pain without a pathoanatomic diagnosis (nonstructural back pain)	Restoration of normal activity, normal social and work functions, and healthy habits (such as diet and exercise) likely to be more effective than opioids. Opioids are deactivating when activity is beneficial
Centralized pain states such as fibromyalgia, irritable bowel disease, and pelvic pain	There are hyperalgesic pain states that can be made worse by opioids. The factors listed under chronic musculoskeletal pain also apply
Headache	Well established that long-term opioid therapy does not help headache and can cause headache in some cases, especially rebound

- Decision to treat is made based on benefit versus risk.
- If COT is chosen, the following safeguards are necessary:
  ○ Patient studies and signs a treatment agreement that includes a statement of agreed goals.
  ○ Patient receives prescriptions in person on a monthly basis or more frequently if high risk.
  ○ Once effective dose is established, dose escalation is avoided.
  ○ Either long-acting opioid or short-acting opioid is used but not both.
  ○ Concomitant sedatives should not be used, especially benzodiazepines or alcohol.
  ○ Goals are reassessed regularly (at least 3 monthly).
  ○ Urine drug test (UDT) is repeated according to clinic standards.
  ○ Opioid is weaned if goals are not met or for noncompliance.
  ○ The lowest effective dose should always be used and should not exceed 100 mg morphine equivalent daily dose (MEDD) (see the "Opioid Medication Choices" section for definition of MEDD).
  ○ Safe-keeping practices and disposal of unused opioid should be encouraged.

Starting Chronic Opioid Therapy

Most COT begins with short-term opioid therapy. For example, the opioid is used to treat an acute exacerbation of chronic back pain or pain after surgery or trauma. Occasionally, administration of opioids is started in the absence of an acute exacerbation. Short-term opioid therapy should not be allowed to become COT without a formal decision that COT is indicated. When using opioids to treat acute pain, the likely duration of pain should be kept in mind and only the amount and duration that is necessary should be prescribed. Most routine surgery and trauma do not require opioids after 3 days. Sometimes longer is needed, but prescribing for acute pain should never be open-ended. Susceptible individuals may rapidly progress to dependence or addiction.[22]

Evidence suggests that patients treated with opioids for 90 days or longer are likely to continue treatment for life.[17–20] Ninety days is also the point at which persistent pain is termed chronic.[16] If opioids have been provided continuously for 90 days, this would be a reasonable stopping place, or a time to define the treatment as COT if the decision is to continue the opioid.

Before starting COT, there must always be a fully documented history and physical examination (repeated if the patient is inherited), culminating in a pain diagnosis. Screening for addiction risk should ideally take place before starting an opioid (ie, before short-term treatment is started), but failing that, screening should take place before starting COT. **Table 2** lists some commonly available screening tools.[23–27] The simplest and most commonly used is the Opioid Risk Tool (**Fig. 1**). A baseline UDT should also be performed before starting COT (see the "Urine Toxicology" section for more details on urine drug toxicology). COT may be contraindicated in patients with high risk of addiction or with illicit drugs in the urine.

Decision to Treat

The decision to use COT should never be considered trivial. COT has huge implications for patients' lives, including the likelihood that they will not return to work,[7,20,28–32] they will be infertile and lose libido,[33–35] they risk becoming dependent,[36,37] they may become cognitively impaired, and pain relief will be partial at best.[38] Ideally, family members should be included in the decision. COT also has huge implications for the prescriber, because neither is COT simple nor are the patients who receive this treatment simple: the treatment can be draining of both resources and time. For the right indications, COT can be tremendously valuable, and worth the effort, but COT should never be undertaken lightly.

Reducing the Risks of Chronic Opioid Therapy

Written agreements
The best way to reduce the risk of COT is to ensure that the patient is well informed about the limitations and risks of COT, as well as the safe keeping of the medications.

Table 2
Commonly used opioid risk screening instruments
Butler et al,[63] 2004	Screener and Opioid Assessment for Patients with Pain (SOAPP) 5-, 14-, or 24-item questionnaire. Completed by patients
Webster & Webster,[25] 2005	Opioid Risk Tool (ORT) 5-item questionnaire. Completed by patients
Passik et al,[26] 2005	Pain Assessment and Documentation Tool (PADT) Assesses 4 domains. Completed by physicians
Belgrade et al,[27] 2006	Scoring system to predict outcome (DIRE) Assesses 4 domains (diagnosis, intractability, risk, efficacy). Completed by physicians
Butler et al,[24] 2007	Current Opioid Misuse Measure (COMM) 17-item questionnaire. Complete by patients

Data from Refs.[24–27,63]

		Female	Male
■ Five-question clinical interview to assess patients			
■ Specifically developed to screen patients with chronic pain who will be using opioids	**Family history of substance abuse**		
	Alcohol	[ ] 1	[ ] 3
	Illegal drugs	[ ] 2	[ ] 3
■ Quantifies the level of risk for patient	Prescription drugs	[ ] 4	[ ] 4
	Personal history of substance abuse		
■ Three risk categories	Alcohol	[ ] 3	[ ] 3
■ Low: 0 - 3 points	Illegal drugs	[ ] 4	[ ] 4
■ Moderate: 4 - 7 points	Prescription drugs	[ ] 5	[ ] 5
■ High: 8 points and above	**Age** (if between 16-45)	[ ] 1	[ ] 1
	History of preadolescent sexual abuse	[ ] 3	[ ] 0
	Psychological disease		
	Attention deficit disorder, obsessive-compulsive disorder, bipolar, schizophrenia	[ ] 2	[ ] 2
	Depression	[ ] 1	[ ] 1
	Scoring Total: _____		

Fig. 1. Stratifying risk: opioid risk tool. (*Adapted from* Webster LR, Webster RM. Predicting aberrant behaviors in opioid treated patients: preliminary validation of the opioid risk tool. Pain Med 2005;6(6):433.)

Written agreements can be useful as educational tools, as well as for documenting patients' acceptance of the terms of treatment and their stated goals. Many other educational tools are available, including more comprehensive written materials, videos, and Web sites, and patients should be encouraged to pursue these. However, a simple and short written agreement in lay language is probably preferable as a starting point. **Box 1** lists the principles that should be present in a written agreement. **Fig. 2** is an example of a written agreement.

> **Box 1**
> **Core features of an opioid care agreement**
>
> 1. Pain medications cannot be refilled early.
> 2. Refills require a clinic visit by appointment.
> 3. No urgent requests for refills. Call to make appointments in advance.
> 4. Lost or stolen pain medications or prescriptions cannot be refilled. They must be safeguarded.
> 5. Never get pain medication for chronic pain from other clinics or emergency rooms.
> 6. If you get any pain medications from another provider for any other reason, you must tell your provider here immediately.
> 7. Do not share, sell, or trade your pain medications with anyone.
> 8. You must allow your urine to be tested for drugs at any time.
> 9. Failure to follow these rules may result in discontinuation of your pain medications.

Urine toxicology

Urine toxicologic tests are imperfect and complex but have become a standard of care during COT. Simple dipsticks that can be used in the clinic are notoriously inaccurate; there is a high rate of both false-positive and false-negative results. Nevertheless, they are much cheaper than the laboratory-based tests, and it is reasonable to use a simple test before progressing to a laboratory test, particularly as a means of familiarizing patients on COT with the process of giving urine and the need to give urine as a routine part of COT. The least likely compounds to give false-positive results are cocaine and amphetamines, so if these are found at initial simple in-house screening, that may be a reason to postpone starting COT until confirmatory tests can be completed and further history sought if necessary. Opioids are the most likely to show false-positive and false-negative results. No action should be taken on dipstick testing, and even after confirmatory laboratory testing, no action should be taken without discussing the result with the laboratory because there are many reasons that an unexpected test result may be due to factors other than taking a nonprescribed substance or not taking the prescribed opioid.

For medical purposes, giving urine is usually done unobserved. Urine specimens can easily be adulterated or swapped. Tampering or swapping can be detected to some extent by shaking the urine to test for frothiness (possible soap contamination), assessing its color, and measuring its temperature and pH immediately after collection.

The appearance of opioid metabolites can be confusing. For example, codeine is metabolized to morphine, hydrocodone may be metabolized to hydromorphone, and oxycodone may be metabolized to oxymorphone. Tests for oxycodone may not have the sensitivity to pick up low levels.

Weaning

It is easy to say if the treatment does not work, stop it. Or if aberrant behaviors arise, stop the treatment. It is not always easy to wean opioids, and in fact, it may not always be appropriate even in the face of poor efficacy or aberrancy. Patients who are given opioids for a long time become dependent on them (see Section "Dependence and Addiction").[37] Not all dependence is addiction, but dependence is often hardwired and difficult to reverse, especially when it accompanies prolonged treatment, which makes it important (1) not to use COT other than for the most refractory of cases in

Patient name: _____   Patient DOB: _____   Patient MRN: _____

Opiate Pain Medicine Agreement
(examples of opiates are: hydrocodone, codeine, oxycodone, hydromorphone, morphine, fentanyl)

- ▪ If I want to get refills of my pain medicine, I have to come to all of my appointments (at least every 6 months).
- ▪ If I miss more than 2 appointments without calling ahead to cancel, my doctor may stop prescribing this medicine for me.
- ▪ I cannot get pain medicine from any other doctor or clinic, unless I am in the hospital or my doctor says it is okay.
- ▪ I should keep my appointments with other doctors, therapists, and other treatments for my pain in order to get refills of my medicine.
- ▪ I will tell my doctor if the medicine is not helping my pain, and will not take more medicine on my own or run out early.
- ▪ To get more medicine, I need a paper prescription. These medicines cannot be called into the pharmacy, or filled on a night, holiday, or weekend.
- ▪ I may get the prescription from my doctor at my regular appointment, or by calling the practice at least 3 business days before I run out. I may not just walk into the office and ask for a refill.
- ▪ I will keep my medicines in a safe place. If my medicine is lost, damaged or stolen, I may not get a new prescription.
- ▪ I agree to have a urine drug test at any time. If I don't take the test, I will stop getting the medicine.
- ▪ If I share, sell or trade my medicine or use illegal drugs or other pain medicines, my doctor may stop giving me this medicine.
- ▪ If I act out at the staff or my doctor, I will not get my medicine, and may be asked to leave the clinic.
- ▪ I understand that this medicine may not work for my pain. If this happens, my doctor may stop giving this type of pain medicine to me.
- ▪ If I do not follow this agreement, my doctor will stop giving me this type of pain medicine.
- ▪ I will get my pain medicine at only one pharmacy.

Pharmacy _____   City _____   Phone _____

I have read this agreement, understand it, and will follow it.

Patient Signature _____ Date_____

Physician Signature_____ Date_____

Fig. 2. Opiate pain medicine agreement. (*Courtesy of* Robin Canada, MD, David Goldman, MD, Craig Wynn, MD. Department of Medicine, University of Pennsylvania School of Medicine, Philadelphia, PA.)

which the treatment can provide comfort and risks are acceptable and (2) to stop COT early or as soon as it becomes evident that it is not meeting goals of treatment.
   Principles of weaning are as follows:

- Patient must agree.
- Structure a weaning protocol (eg, 10% reduction in dose per visit).
- Be prepared to plateau (most patients tolerate a few dose reductions and then stall; it is reasonable to allow a break and then restart the wean later).

- Be prepared to fail (if a wean is not tolerated, be prepared to continue opioid for life).
- If a wean is not tolerated, patient is likely to have complex and persistent dependence[37]; treat this much like addiction, with opioid maintenance and counseling.
- Always consider the possibility of addiction and need for addiction treatment.

DEPENDENCE AND ADDICTION

- There are special considerations when using COT in patients with known risk of substance abuse.
- Dependence or addiction may arise during COT in any patient.[36]

Using Chronic Opioid Therapy in Patients with Risk of or Current Substance Abuse

Neither risk of nor current substance abuse precludes the use of COT. However, in both cases there is a high risk of development or worsening of addiction; this means that COT should not be used without the full understanding of risks by both patients and their families. Full precautions should be taken (eg, only use long-acting opioids, pick up prescriptions weekly or even daily if indicated, use frequent UDTs and random pill counts, involve family in giving medications, involve family in safe keeping of medications, and reevaluate frequently).

Dependence or Addiction Arising During Chronic Opioid Therapy

Dependence on opioids is completely expected during COT, particularly extended COT. Dependence essentially means that there are symptoms of withdrawal if the drug is withdrawn or the dose reduced, when circumstances change and the dose requirement changes, or if tolerance develops and is not satisfied by a dose escalation. For a few patients, withdrawal consists simply of classic withdrawal symptoms such as pupillary dilatation, goose flesh, nausea and vomiting, abdominal pain, tachycardia, worsening pain, and agitation. These physical symptoms of withdrawal usually subside within weeks of discontinuing opioid altogether, although they may recur as circumstances change for a patient receiving COT. But for many patients, there is also a psychological component to withdrawal, which does not reverse easily and may be a strong factor in difficulty weaning patients from opioids, especially when they have been receiving COT for a long time. The combination of physical and psychological dependence can seem much like addiction because the dependence is a strong driver of opioid-seeking behavior, behavior that may even seem compulsive.[39,40] Some patients on COT exhibit clear signs of true addiction, and if they do, they should be referred for specialty treatment. Many fit into a gray zone between clearly not addicted and clearly addicted (**Fig. 3**). These patients are dependent and warrant treatment much like addiction treatment. They may do better if their opioid pain treatment is maintained. As mentioned in "Weaning" section, it is always worth trying to wean if the treatment does not seem to be working well, but if the wean is not tolerated, then it may be better to continue the opioid. The other important aspect of treatment of these patients is counseling. In the United States at least, because of the past 2 decades of gross overprescribing of opioids for chronic pain, there are not enough specialty centers that can handle patients at the intersection of chronic pain and opioid dependence, and there are not enough trained counselors to help busy medical practitioners with counseling. This is another reason to be circumspect about the decision to embark on COT.

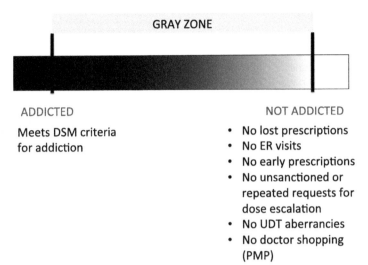

Fig. 3. Spectrum of dependence and addiction. ER, Emergency room; PMP, prescription monitoring program (now available in several states in the United States, in continued development); UDT, urine drug test. Note: Doctor shopping occurs in the United States because many patients have multiple providers, unlike countries with national health systems where patients have a medical "home."

PHARMACOLOGIC AND DOSE CONSIDERATIONS

Opioid choices, restrictions, precautions, and dose equivalences can be found in any drug reference book to which the reader is referred. This article provides only a broad understanding of the available opioids, how they relate to each other, how and why to move from one opioid to another, and how and why to achieve dose limitation.

Opioid Medication Choices

Morphine

- Morphine is the archetypal opioid and the opioid to which all others are compared.
- Morphine is a pure opioid agonist.
- Morphine is a "dirty" drug, meaning it has several active metabolites.
- Dosing of other opioids is often calculated for comparison in terms of MEDD, that being the daily dose of morphine that would be equivalent to the daily dose of the opioid being used.
- Morphine is derived from poppy and accounts for 50% of the active components of opium.
- Morphine utility for chronic pain is related to familiarity with its use and low cost.

Other naturally occurring opioids

- Codeine and thebaine are also naturally occurring constituents of opium.
- Codeine is used as an analgesic but is not useful for chronic pain because it causes constipation and has highly variable metabolism and thus highly variable effects.

Semisynthetic opioids

- Other pure opioid agonists in common usage are oxycodone, hydrocodone, and hydromorphone.
- These compounds are all synthesized from opium constituents.
- Because they have straightforward metabolism and clearance, they are the first choice for COT.

Synthetic opioids

- Fentanyl, meperidine, methadone, and tapentadol are also pure opioid agonists but have limited utility for COT.
- Fentanyl's kinetics mean that it is only available for outpatients as a transdermal patch or various transmucosal forms. There are disadvantages to both, and fentanyl use is not encouraged for COT. Tolerance develops rapidly requiring dose escalation. The ultrarapid onset of transmucosal form is not needed during chronic pain management and is undesirable because of increased risk of addiction.
- Meperidine is not a good choice for COT because it has a toxic metabolite (normeperidine) and tends to be addictive because of its rapid onset.
- Methadone is a complex drug and can be dangerous because of its variable kinetics, which can lead to accumulation, overdose, and subsequent death. Its use for COT is generally discouraged, unless the therapy has been started and stabilized by an expert.
- Tapentadol is a pure opioid agonist with additional noradrenaline reuptake inhibition. It is a good analgesic but has all the same considerations in terms of addiction risk as other pure opioid agonists and is expensive and not covered by all insurance companies.

Mixed agonist/antagonists and partial agonists

- Mixed agonist/antagonists and partial agonists are generally too complicated to use as COT.
- The exception may be buprenorphine, which is a partial agonist/antagonist that is available in patch form for use in chronic pain or sublingual (SL) for addiction treatment.
- It could be argued that buprenorphine, because it has a ceiling dose and rarely causes respiratory depression, should be the first choice for COT.
- Buprenorphine SL is not approved as an analgesic in the United States, restricting use in COT to the patch, which is expensive and not approved by many insurance companies.
- Tramadol is a partial opioid agonist with additional serotonin and noradrenaline reuptake inhibition. It is useful for COT and has a lower risk of addiction than pure agonists, although addiction can still arise.

Dosing Guidance

- The lowest recommended dose should be used when starting opioid treatment in an opioid-naive individual.
- Because there is a great deal of interindividual variation, it may be necessary to increase the dose during the first few visits to reach the effective dose.
- Once the effect dose is established, further dose escalation should always be carefully considered. Periodic pain increases, often related to changes in life events, are to be expected in patients with chronic pain (**Fig. 4**) and often result

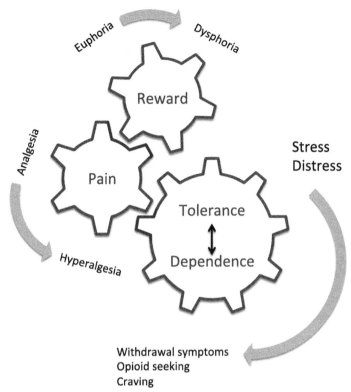

Euphoria   Dysphoria

Reward

Analgesia

Pain

Stress
Distress

Tolerance

Dependence

Hyperalgesia

Withdrawal symptoms
Opioid seeking
Craving

Fig. 4. Interdependence of mood, tolerance/dependence, and pain. Even in normal individuals, pain and mood are interdependent, in part through endogenous opioid mechanisms. Individuals taking exogenous opioids long term and continuously adapt by developing tolerance and dependence. Psychological factors such as stress and distress can alter tolerance and thereby induce withdrawal symptoms. For the dependent individual, the need for more opioid becomes the predominant reaction to stress. Although pain is seen as the primary reason to escalate dose, pain is often secondary to other factors. (*From* Ballantyne JC, Sullivan MD, Kolodny A. Opioid dependence versus addiction: a distinction without a difference. Arch Intern Med 2012;172:1342; with permission.)

in a request for higher dose of opioid in the case of COT. Use of nonopioid interventions rather than dose increase should be encouraged.

- It is widely recognized and supported by evidence that adverse events are more likely to arise when doses are high. In general, doses more than 100 mg MEDD are discouraged.[19,41–46] Even less than this dose, adverse events do occur, so this dose limitation should not be taken to mean that doses less than this level are completely safe. The safest dose is the stable dose that has been established at the start of treatment.

Opioid Switching

- Because of incomplete cross-tolerance at receptor sites, and possibly other factors, switching from one opioid to another can be an effective means of restoring analgesia when effectiveness has diminished because of tolerance.[47]
- When switching to any opioid except methadone or buprenorphine, 50% of the calculated MEDD should be used.

- Switches to methadone or buprenorphine are effective but complicated and should only be undertaken by an expert.
- One should be watchful when switching opioids. Adverse effects are more likely to arise when dose or drug is changed. The conservative dosing recommendation (50% reduction in MEDD) is necessary for safety.
- Switching opioid can be remarkably effective, despite drastic dose reduction.

Long Acting Versus Short Acting

- There is rarely any need to use long-acting together with short-acting opioids during COT.
- In general, for patients at low risk (eg, elderly patients being treated for osteoarthritis pain), occasional and minimal use of short-acting opioid is best and the best way to maintain opioid efficacy.
- For patients at risk of misuse or addiction, or patients with confusion, 2 or 3 times daily-scheduled long-acting opioid may be preferable.
- The concept of breakthrough pain or use of short-acting opioid to supplement long-acting opioid should not apply during COT. It tends to focus attention on pain and obtaining opioid (a particular problem for at-risk patients), leads to unnecessary and unsafe dose escalation, and may lead to unsafe situations whereby overdose can occur.

THE ROLE OF NONMEDICAL AND NONPHARMACOLOGICAL INTERVENTIONS

It is worth mentioning and emphasizing here that there are many approaches to managing chronic pain that are better than COT, and many of these approaches should be used even during COT, to reduce reliance on COT and in hopes to obviate dose escalation. Opioids, as has already been stated, have good analgesic efficacy when first used. All nonopioid interventions, whether pharmacologic, nonpharmacologic, or even nonmedical, take longer to work and require a lot more effort. Opioids are therefore seductive. It may feel as if, in the belief system of patients and their providers, opioids are the only thing that works. But it is now known that analgesia is often not maintained at initial levels over time and that there are many adverse outcomes of COT. Physical pain can be a manifestation of existential suffering, in which case medicine per se may not have any answers. The answer then lies in empowerment by friends, family, priests, and counselors and use of self-management techniques, lifestyle changes, or complementary medical approaches such as acupuncture, yoga, and tai chi. Helpful medical interventions could include injections, dry needling, targeted physical therapy, occupational therapy, nutritional counseling, and nonopioid medications, all of these being particularly helpful given in a multidisciplinary setting. However, there are too few multidisciplinary programs in the United States because of a failure to fund them or to recognize their long-term value. The point to emphasize here is that COT should never be used as sole therapy nor should the decision to initiate COT be taken until all other avenues of treatment have been fully explored. Again, COT is good treatment when it can provide comfort for refractory pain or suffering but not a good choice in the case that functional restoration toward normalcy is the ultimate goal.

CHRONIC OPIOID THERAPY OUTCOMES

Ideally, one wants any medical intervention to be evidence based. However, despite many attempts to mine the literature and develop an evidence base in support of COT, there simply is no such evidence.[48,49] There is a great deal of rhetoric, anecdote, and widely differing opinions but no strong evidence to support either the efficacy or the safety of COT. In fact, the safety of COT has been brought into question because of an accumulation of population studies that have revealed an alarmingly high incidence of life-threatening adverse outcomes.[2,3,50–55] It can be argued that population studies cannot show causation, and that is why responses to such alarming statistics have been slow. Nevertheless, a shift in prescribing toward the more conservative regimens is occurring in response to reports on adverse outcomes for COT in both the medical and nonmedical media.

Efficacy

Short-term efficacy for opioids is supported by both randomized trials and observational studies.[56,57] The establishment of long-term efficacy is much more difficult because there simply are no long-term trials in existence.[48,58] Population studies suggest that COT-treated individuals have more pain, more health care utilization, less return to work, and more adverse effects than nonopioid-treated matched individuals.[57,59,60] This result suggests that at the least, opioids do not achieve the goal of improving pain and function across the entire population. But that does not mean there are not some within the population study cohorts who do well. Difficulty lies in understanding exactly who they are and how to predict good outcomes. There is a strong suggestion from existing but still inadequate evidence that patients with nonstructural back pain, centralized pain states such as fibromyalgia, and headache do better without COT.

Adverse or Side Effects

There are many common adverse effects of opioids, and they are listed in **Box 2**. Most adverse effects diminish over time, but this is not true of the effects on the bowel, including constipation, or on the endocrine system, including testosterone depletion. A bowel regime should always be offered during COT, as should testosterone replacement when necessary for men.

Adverse Outcomes and Events

More concerning perhaps than opioids adverse effects or side effects are adverse outcomes and events that can be catastrophic (**Box 3**). Catastrophic outcomes of COT have become a concern for government agencies such as the Center for Disease

---

Box 2
Adverse or side effects of COT

Respiratory depression

Suppression of bowel mobility, constipation

Nausea

Drowsiness

Pruritus

Dry skin

Infertility

Cognitive impairment

Dependence

> **Box 3**
> **Catastrophic adverse outcomes of COT**
>
> Respiratory arrest and death[a]
>
> Addiction
>
> Ileus
>
> Falls and fractures
>
> Accidents
>
> All these catastrophic outcomes are occurring with increasing frequency in the United States and other countries as reported in the literature (see Refs.[1–3]).
>
> [a] More likely with concomitant administration of benzodiazepines and other sedatives, including alcohol.

Control (**Fig. 5**). Addiction is a catastrophic outcome of COT and underpins many other catastrophic outcomes such as respiratory depression and death, falls and fractures, and cognitive impairment. Losing control of opioid usage is often the reason for accidental overdose. Other factors increase the likelihood of death from opioids, and these are listed in **Box 4**. The likelihood of accidental death can be minimized by reduction of risk factors as suggested in **Box 4**. However, that addiction develops in some treated individuals (best estimate, 12%) is inescapable.[61,62] It may be hard for both patients and their prescribers to recognize and accept that dependence or addiction has arisen. The optimal way to make opioids safer in susceptible individuals is to use safe opioids such as tramadol or buprenorphine patch and to provide strong opioids only in a monitored setting, which would include inpatient settings, methadone or suboxone programs, or responsible family members taking control. Using screening tools and vigilant follow-up are the best methods for identifying individuals at risk, and their use is strongly encouraged.

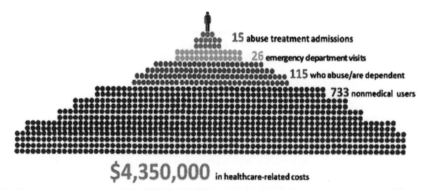

Fig. 5. Adverse outcomes in relation to deaths for prescription opioids. (*From* Frieden T. General session: state policy changes and CDC impacting in prescription drug abuse epidemic. National RX Drug Abuse Summit, Atlanta GA, April 23, 2014. Available at: www.slideshare.net/OPUNITE/wed-gs-frieden. Accessed January 14, 2015.)

Box 4
Risk factors for adverse outcomes of COT

When considering risks, addiction is not the only risk.

Potentially catastrophic outcomes such as respiratory depression (death), constipation (abdominal obstruction), and cognitive impairment (falls and fractures) can be minimized by being aware of their risk factors.

Watch for the following:

- Obesity and sleep apnea
- Use of central nervous system depressants (especially benzodiazepines) and drugs with anticholinergic properties
- Abdominal disease
- Neurologic and cognitive impairment
- History or family history of substance use disorder
- High anxiety (risk of loss of control over use)

SUMMARY

- Carefully select patients for COT. Not all patients are suitable candidates. Patients with nonstructural back pain, centralized pain such as fibromyalgia, and headache are not good candidates.
- Do not let short-term opioid therapy become COT without careful consideration. Most acute pain only warrants a few days opioid therapy; greater than 90 days pain is considered chronic pain, and greater than 90 days opioid therapy is considered COT, but commonly short-term opioid therapy can be stopped much sooner than 90 days.
- Always screen for risk of misuse or addiction before starting COT or ideally before starting short-term opioid therapy.
- Be particularly conservative when risk factors are identified.
- Start at low dose, titrate to effect during initiation, do not dose escalate once stable unless absolutely necessary, and do not exceed 100 mg MEDD.
- Oxycodone, hydrocodone, and hydromorphone are the simplest choice of strong opioid.
- Tramadol or buprenorphine patch may be preferable, especially for patients with known risk, but cost may preclude their use.
- Do not use long-acting and short-acting opioids together during COT. Use long-acting round-the-clock where there are control issues, including confusion, and short-acting as needed in preference when there are no control issues.
- Adhere to the principles of COT outlined in the "Basic Principles of Chronic Opioid Management" section.
- When the treatment is not meeting goals of therapy, or when the dose is too high, discuss tapering with the patient.
- Using these careful precautions, it is hoped that the number of patients taking dangerously high doses of opioids, being dependent on opioids, and having deteriorated quality of life, will go down. In the meantime, there are thousands of patients with the syndrome of chronic pain with opioid dependence, and they need specialty care, which is not always available. In the absence of specialty care, they may need opioid continuation for the treatment of dependence (not pain), together with counseling and maximum use of all suitable nonopioid treatments.

REFERENCES

1. Okie S. A flood of opioids, a rising tide of deaths. N Engl J Med 2010;363:1981–5.
2. Center for Disease Control and Prevention (CDC). CDC grand rounds: prescription drug overdoses - a U.S. epidemic. MMWR Morb Mortal Wkly Rep 2012;61:10–3.
3. Paulozzi LJ, Budnitz DS, Xi Y. Increasing deaths from opioid analgesics in the United States. Pharmacoepidemiol Drug Saf 2006;15:618–27.
4. Deyo RA, Mirza SK, Turner JA, et al. Overtreating chronic back pain: time to back off? J Am Board Fam Med 2009;22:62–8.
5. Deyo RA, Patrick DL. Hope or hype: the obsession with medical advances and the high cost of false promises. New York: AMACOM; 2005.
6. Franklin GM, Rahman EA, Turner JA, et al. Opioid use for chronic low back pain: a prospective, population-based study among injured workers in Washington state, 2002-2005. Clin J Pain 2009;25:743–51.
7. Turner JA, Franklin G, Fulton-Kehoe D, et al. ISSLS prize winner: early predictors of chronic work disability: a prospective, population-based study of workers with back injuries. Spine (Phila Pa 1976) 2008;33:2809–18.
8. Franklin G, Wickizer T, Coe N, et al. Workers' compensation: poor quality health care and the growing disability problem in the United States. Am J Ind Med 2014. [Epub ahead of print].
9. Franklin GM. Opioids for chronic noncancer pain: a position paper of the American Academy of Neurology. Neurology 2014;83:1277–84.
10. Sullivan MD, Ballantyne JC. What are we treating with chronic opioid therapy? Arch Intern Med 2012;172:433–4.
11. Martell BA, O'Connor PG, Kerns RD, et al. Systematic review: opioid treatment for chronic back pain: prevalence, efficacy, and association with addiction. Ann Intern Med 2007;146:116–27.
12. Chaparro LE, Furlan AD, Deshpande A, et al. Opioids compared with placebo or other treatments for chronic low back pain: an update of the Cochrane Review. Spine (Phila Pa 1976) 2014;39:556–63.
13. Levin M. Opioids in headache. Headache 2014;54:12–21.
14. Clauw DJ. Fibromyalgia: a clinical review. JAMA 2014;311:1547–55.
15. Peng X, Robinson RL, Mease P, et al. Long-term evaluation of opioid treatment in fibromyalgia. Clin J Pain 2015;31(1):7–13.
16. Turk DC, Okifuji A. Pain terms and taxonomies. In: Fishman SM, Ballantyne JC, Rathmell JP, editors. Bonica's management of pain. 4th edition. Philadelphia: Lippincott Williams and Wilkins; 2010. p. 14–23.
17. Braden JB, Fan MY, Edlund MJ, et al. Trends in use of opioids by noncancer pain type 2000-2005 among Arkansas Medicaid and HealthCore enrollees: results from the TROUP study. J Pain 2008;9:1026–35.
18. Korff MV, Saunders K, Thomas Ray G, et al. De facto long-term opioid therapy for noncancer pain. Clin J Pain 2008;24:521–7.
19. Martin BC, Fan MY, Edlund MJ, et al. Long-term chronic opioid therapy discontinuation rates from the TROUP study. J Gen Intern Med 2011;26:1450–7.
20. Volinn E, Fargo JD, Fine PG. Opioid therapy for nonspecific low back pain and the outcome of chronic work loss. Pain 2009;142:194–201.
21. Chou R, Fanciullo GJ, Fine PG, et al. Clinical guidelines for the use of chronic opioid therapy in chronic noncancer pain. J Pain 2009;10:113–30.
22. Kreek MJ, Nielsen DA, Butelman ER, et al. Genetic influences on impulsivity, risk taking, stress responsivity and vulnerability to drug abuse and addiction. Nat Neurosci 2005;8:1450–7.

23. Butler SF, Budman SH, Fernandez K, et al. Validation of a screener and opioid assessment measure for patients with chronic pain. Pain 2004;112:65–75.

24. Butler SF, Budman SH, Fernandez KC, et al. Development and validation of the current opioid misuse measure. Pain 2007;130:144–56.

25. Webster L, Webster R. Predicting aberrant behaviors in opioid-treated patients: preliminary validation of the opioid risk tool. Pain Med 2005;6:432–42.

26. Passik SD, Kirsh KL, Whitcomb L, et al. Monitoring outcomes during long-term opioid therapy for noncancer pain: results with the pain assessment and documentation tool. J Opioid Manag 2005;1:257–66.

27. Belgrade MJ, Schamber CD, Lindgren BR. The DIRE score: predicting outcomes of opioid prescribing for chronic pain. J Pain 2006;7:671–81.

28. Webster BS, Verma SK, Gatchel RJ. Relationship between early opioid prescribing for acute occupational low back pain and disability duration, medical costs, subsequent surgery and late opioid use. Spine (Phila Pa 1976) 2007;32:2127–32.

29. Franklin GM, Stover BD, Turner JA, et al. Early opioid prescription and subsequent disability among workers with back injuries: the Disability Risk Identification Study Cohort. Spine (Phila Pa 1976) 2008;33:199–204.

30. Gross DP, Stephens B, Bhambhani Y, et al. Opioid prescriptions in Canadian workers' compensation claimants: prescription trends and associations between early prescription and future recovery. Spine (Phila Pa 1976) 2009;34:525–31.

31. Stover BD, Turner JA, Franklin G, et al. Factors associated with early opioid prescription among workers with low back injuries. J Pain 2006;7:718–25.

32. Franklin GM, Mai J, Wickizer T, et al. Opioid dosing trends and mortality in Washington State workers' compensation, 1996-2002. Am J Ind Med 2005;48:91–9.

33. Daniell HW. Hypogonadism in men consuming sustained-action oral opioids. J Pain 2002;3:377–84.

34. Daniell HW. Opioid endocrinopathy in women consuming prescribed sustained-action opioids for control of nonmalignant pain. J Pain 2008;9:28–36.

35. Finch PM, Roberts LJ, Price L, et al. Hypogonadism in patients treated with intrathecal morphine. Clin J Pain 2000;3:251–4.

36. Ballantyne JC, LaForge SL. Opioid dependence and addiction in opioid treated pain patients. Pain 2007;129:235–55.

37. Ballantyne JC, Sullivan MD, Kolodny A. Opioid dependence vs addiction: a distinction without a difference? Arch Intern Med 2012;172:1342–3.

38. Farrar JT, Portenoy RK, Berlin JA, et al. Defining the clinically important difference in pain outcome measures. Pain 2000;88:287–94.

39. Hyman SE, Malenka RC, Nestler EJ. Neural mechanisms of addiction: the role of reward-related learning and memory. Annu Rev Neurosci 2006;29:565–98.

40. Koob GF, Le Moal M. Drug addiction, dysregulation of reward, and allostasis. Neuropsychopharmacology 2001;24:97–129.

41. Morasco BJ, Duckart JP, Carr TP, et al. Clinical characteristics of veterans prescribed high doses of opioid medications for chronic non-cancer pain. Pain 2010;151:625–32.

42. Edlund MJ, Martin BC, Fan MY, et al. Risks for opioid abuse and dependence among recipients of chronic opioid therapy: results from the TROUP study. Drug Alcohol Depend 2010;112:90–8.

43. Saunders KW, Dunn KM, Merrill JO, et al. Relationship of opioid use and dosage levels to fractures in older chronic pain patients. J Gen Intern Med 2010;25:310–5.

44. Von Korff M, Merrill JO, Rutter CM, et al. Time-scheduled vs. pain-contingent opioid dosing in chronic opioid therapy. Pain 2011;152:1256–62.

45. Weisner CM, Campbell CI, Ray GT, et al. Trends in prescribed opioid therapy for non-cancer pain for individuals with prior substance use disorders. Pain 2009; 145:287–93.
46. Ballantyne JC, Mao J. Opioid therapy for chronic pain. N Engl J Med 2003;349: 1943–53.
47. Pasternak GW. Multiple opiate receptors: deja vu all over again. Neuropharmacology 2004;47(Suppl 1):312–23.
48. Chou R, Ballantyne JC, Fanciullo GJ, et al. Research gaps on use of opioids for chronic noncancer pain: findings from a review of the evidence for an American Pain Society and American Academy of Pain Medicine clinical practice guideline. J Pain 2009;10:147–59.
49. Agency for Healthcare Research and Quality. The effectiveness and risks of long-term opioid treatment of chronic pain. Bethesda, Maryland: US Department of Health and Human Services; 2014. AHCPR Publication No 94-0592 March 1994.
50. Paulozzi LJ, Kilbourne EM, Shah NG, et al. A history of being prescribed controlled substances and risk of drug overdose death. Pain Med 2012;13: 87–95.
51. Gomes T, Mamdani MM, Dhalla IA, et al. Opioid dose and drug-related mortality in patients with nonmalignant pain. Arch Intern Med 2011;171:686–91.
52. Dunn KM, Saunders KW, Rutter CM, et al. Opioid prescriptions for chronic pain and overdose: a cohort study. Ann Intern Med 2010;152:85–92.
53. Bohnert AS, Valenstein M, Bair MJ, et al. Association between opioid prescribing patterns and opioid overdose-related deaths. JAMA 2011;305:1315–21.
54. Fulton-Kehoe D, Garg RK, Turner JA, et al. Opioid poisonings and opioid adverse effects in workers in Washington State. Am J Ind Med 2013;56:1452–62.
55. Hall AJ, Logan JE, Toblin RL, et al. Patterns of abuse among unintentional pharmaceutical overdose fatalities. JAMA 2008;300:2613–20.
56. Ballantyne JC, Shin NS. Efficacy of opioids for chronic pain: a review of the evidence. Clin J Pain 2008;24:469–78.
57. Ballantyne JC. Clinical and administrative data review presented to FDA May 30th and 31st 2012. 2012. Available at: http://www.fda.gov/downloads/Drugs/NewsEvents/UCM307844.pdf.
58. Bruehl S, Apkarian AV, Ballantyne JC, et al. Personalized medicine and opioid analgesic prescribing for chronic pain: opportunities and challenges. J Pain 2013;14:103–13.
59. Eriksen J, Sjogren P, Bruera E, et al. Critical issues on opioids in chronic non-cancer pain. An epidemiological study. Pain 2006;125:172–9.
60. Dillie KS, Fleming MF, Mundt MP, et al. Quality of life associated with daily opioid therapy in a primary care chronic pain sample. J Am Board Fam Med 2008;21: 108–17.
61. Fishbain DA, Cole B, Lewis J, et al. What percentage of chronic nonmalignant pain patients exposed to chronic opioid analgesic therapy develop abuse/addiction and/or aberrant drug-related behaviors? A structured evidence-based review. Pain Med 2008;9:444–59.
62. Fishbain DA, Rosomoff HL, Rosomoff RS. Drug abuse, dependence and addiction in chronic pain patients. Clin J Pain 1992;8:77–85.
63. Butler SF, Budman SH, Fernandez KC, et al. Cross-Validation of a Screener to Predict Opioid Misuse in Chronic Pain Patients (SOAPP-R). J Addict Med 2009; 3:66–73.

Nonopioid Medications for Pain

David Tauben, MD, FACP[a,b,*]

KEYWORDS

- Opioid • NSAID • Acetaminophen • Antidepressant • Anticonvulsant
- Benzodiazepine • Neuropathic pain • Central sensitization

KEY POINTS

- Although there is evidence supporting the analgesic efficacy of opioids, other classes of medications seem to be equally effective, and are often safer to use.
- Nonsteroidal antiinflammatory drugs are most likely to be effective in the setting of nociceptive or inflammatory pain.
- Antidepressants and anticonvulsants are the most effective agents for neuropathic pain or pain from central sensitization.
- Unless there is clear evidence of spasticity, muscle relaxers, including benzodiazepines, and antispasticity agents add limited, if any, benefits in the management of chronic pain.
- Benzodiazepines should not be used in conjunction with opioids.
- An important early target for pharmacologic management should be improvement in the patient's ability to sleep.

INTRODUCTION

Treatment of pain, particularly chronic pain, requires multimodal analgesia that includes pharmacologic and nondrug therapies as well as a large measure of clinician-guided patient self-management. This article emphasizes the point that pain medicine is more than opioid management; that chronic pain treatment should rarely if ever be opioid monotherapy. The conflation of pain care with opioid

Disclosures and Conflicts of Interest: ER/LA Opioid Analgesics REMS Program Companies (CME grant 2015).
[a] Division of Pain Medicine, Department of Anesthesiology and Pain Medicine, UW Center for Pain Relief, University of Washington, 1959 Northeast Pacific Street, Box 356540, Seattle, WA 98195, USA; [b] Division of General Internal Medicine, Department of Medicine, UW Center for Pain Relief, University of Washington, 1959 Northeast Pacific Street, Box 356540, Seattle, WA 98195, USA
* Division of Pain Medicine, Department of Anesthesiology and Pain Medicine, UW Center for Pain Relief, University of Washington, 1959 Northeast Pacific Street, Box 356540, Seattle, WA 98195.
E-mail address: tauben@uw.edu

Phys Med Rehabil Clin N Am 26 (2015) 219–248
http://dx.doi.org/10.1016/j.pmr.2015.01.005
1047-9651/15/$ – see front matter © 2015 Elsevier Inc. All rights reserved.

prescribing has, since the mid 1990s, displaced the initial tenets of multidisciplinary pain care that were fundamentally about functional and behavioral retraining without opioids and other central nervous system depressants. Recent population-based trends document that significant increases in opioid prescribing without increases in other drug categories[1] have directly contributed to the pain-related distress experienced not only by patients with chronic pain but by providers of pain care, and health systems.[2] Understanding the basic pharmacologic principles and comparative effectiveness of so-called adjuvant drugs in the management of chronic pain should increase not only success of pharmacologically based pain treatments but also reduce over-reliance on opioids and the associated challenges of opioid-related side effects such as accidental overdoses, dependency and addiction, and most importantly poor pain care outcomes.

Principles and Definitions

A key principle guides this article: chronic pain is a complex multidimensional disorder that is different from acute pain in both pathoanatomic and psychosocial domains. Although many commonly encountered chronic pain disorders do involve continuing nociceptive triggers (nociceptive pain results when tissue injury or disease leads to stimulation of nociceptors at peripheral sensory nerve endings located in the skin, muscle, joints, and viscera), the persistence of pain beyond 3 to 6 months alters peripheral and central nervous function and, with additional behavioral and functional modifications, adds the insult to the original injury. This pathophysiologic process involves sensitization, whereby the intrinsic neuroplasticity of the nervous system disrupts previously normal (or worsens previously abnormal) neurochemical and structural function of the peripheral and central nervous system, altering neuronal activity, their synapses, and the brain's regional connectivity.[3,4] Current functional imaging data support the emerging understanding that, over time, nearly all chronic nociceptive stimulation, especially persistent and repetitive high input, becomes transformed in a process called chronification.[5] In addition, susceptibility to chronification varies by complex mechanisms determined by an increasingly well-understood overlay of genetic predisposition, epigenetic biological processes, psychological responses, and sociologic exposures.[6] Hence pain, an "unpleasant sensory and emotional experience that is commonly associated with actual or potential tissue damage,"[7] is an emergent experience, shaped by the complex interplay of genetics, past experiences, setting, affect, cognitive context, and cultural and social expectations. Patients with both acute and chronic pain thus present with a wide range of responses to seemingly identical injuries, and effective treatment requires a clinical toolbox capable of multidimensional therapies.

Assessing Effectiveness

Consideration of effectiveness is essential to clinicians' proper selection of pain treatments. An expanded appreciation and more detailed understanding of the complex nature of pain entail multimodal assessment of pain beyond a simple numeric pain intensity score (numerical rating scale [NRS]) of 0 to 10 out of 10. Although pain rating is useful in acute pain, in which reduction in pain intensity can be achieved quickly and effectively with opioids, nerve blocks, and general anesthetics, successful chronic pain care requires demonstration of improved measures of physical, emotional, and social function, and thus overall quality of life. Hence, this article references treatment goals beyond how much it hurts; successful pain management requires careful tracking of outcomes across key domains of physical (including sleep), psychological, and social function.

High-quality multidisciplinary pain care also reduces overall health care costs by adding system value. Literature since the 1970s has supported the positive effects of multidisciplinary pain care on function, mood, and quality of life. Because health care delivery is obliged to move toward value-based care, in which value equals quality of patient satisfaction, family experience, and improved psychosocial outcomes at lower costs, clinically useful knowledge of alternatives to opioids is needed.

ARTICLE OBJECTIVES

1. Understand why chronic pain pharmacologic management should not be opioid monotherapy.
2. Identify the clinical value and potential side effects of nonsteroidal antiinflammatory drugs (NSAIDs), antidepressants, anticonvulsants, and other pain neuromodulators.
3. Optimize use of nonopioid drug options for management of chronic pain.

WHY NONOPIOIDS?

The preceding discussion underpins the consensus recommendation from pain experts: "opioids are (just) part of the plan…"[8] A basic limitation of opioid monotherapy is that, at doses needed to maintain conscious awareness (that is, less than anesthetic levels), the effectiveness of opioids in chronic pain has not been clearly shown.[9] A recent evidence-based literature review of long-term opioid effectiveness by Chou and colleagues[10] concluded that the best available evidence is low quality, and most is insufficient. In the context of the current epidemic of prescription opioid overdoses, deaths (>16,000 in the United States in 2012), and parallel increase in addiction treatment, expertise in nonopioid pain pharmacotherapy is essential.[11] Complications of increased falls,[12] risks with co-occurring medical conditions (especially sleep apnea),[13] and hypogonadism are salient.[14] The recommendation by some pain specialists during the past 20 years that reductions in long-term analgesic effectiveness of opioids (typically because of tolerance) can be overcome by routinely increasing the opioid dose is no longer seen as appropriate, particularly because there is emerging clinical and scientific evidence of opioid-induced hyperalgesia.[15]

Best evidence currently supports multimodal analgesia, which is the use of combinations of analgesic medications with different mechanisms of action.[16] The classes of medications that should be considered are:

- Opioids
- NSAIDs
- Local anesthetics
- Antiepileptics
- Antidepressants
- N-methyl-D-aspartate (NMDA) antagonists
- Cannabinoids

Even when efficacy is limited to just assessment of numeric pain intensity, and acknowledging that the quality of evidence is limited because of problems with study duration, nonrepresentative patient cohorts, and small effect sizes, many nonopioids have effectiveness at least as good or better than opioids in chronic noncancer pain (CNCP) (**Table 1**).

Although the scope of this article does not include extended reviews of multimodal nondrug analgesia, these are included for completeness (**Box 1**). Goals include improved patient self-management by reduced catastrophizing, fear avoidance, and pain anticipation. Nondrug treatments are promoted by deemphasizing medications as a central element for managing pain, empathic listening interwoven with respectful

Table 1
CNCP pain treatment comparative effectiveness

Opioids (%)	30
Antidepressants[a] (%)	30
Anticonvulsants (%)	30
Acupuncture (%)	10+
Cannabis (%)	10–30
CBT/mindfulness (%)	30–50
Physical fitness (%)	7–50
Sleep restoration (%)	40
Hypnosis, manipulations, yoga	Some effect

Based on NRS and qualitative extrapolations from published data.
Abbreviation: CBT, cognitive behavior therapy.
[a] Antidepressants include tricyclics and serotonin-norepinephrine reuptake inhibitors.
Data from Refs.[18–27]

response, sharing development of mutually agreed-on care goals, and self-identification of strategies and support needed to reduce medication-seeking behaviors. Outcomes include an increased ability to tolerate pain to fulfill life roles for family and job to increase overall quality of life. Effective use of these techniques requires a well-integrated team of interprofessionals, including but not limited to physical, occupational, and behavioral therapists and often nurse care educators.

DIAGNOSIS-BASED SELECTION OF PHARMACOTHERAPY

Medical treatment decision making requires a careful, detailed, systematic, structured history and physical examination. Careful empathic listening permits patients to communicate their pain narratives and attributions, and to disclose many domains of relevant history. The history as obtained by interview should be supplemented with evidence-based tools that assess mood and psychiatric diagnoses (ie, personal health questionnaire, 9-item [PHQ-9],[17] generalized anxiety disorder, 7-item [GAD-7],[18] posttraumatic stress disorder [PTSD] screening[19]), sleep (quality and duration), important co-occurring conditions such as sleep apnea (snore, tired, obstructed breathing, high blood pressure, body mass index, age, neck size, gender [STOP-BANG][20]), and risk of drug misuse and addiction (ie, opioid risk tool [ORT], screener and opioid assessment for patients with pain-revised [SOAPP-R], diagnosis, intractability, risk, efficacy [DIRE]).[21] Use of measurement-based tools for assessment of chronic pain is described in detail by this author in the January 2013 *IASP Clinical Update*.[22] Once diagnoses are established across biopsychosocial domains, drug

Box 1
Nondrug multimodal analgesia

- Cognitive: identify distressing negative cognitions and beliefs
- Behavioral approaches: mindfulness, relaxation, biofeedback
- Physical: activity coaching, graded exercise (land and aquatic) with physical training, class, trainer, and/or solo
- Spiritual: identify and seek meaningfulness and purpose of life
- Education (patient and family): promote patient efforts to increase functional capabilities

treatments can be formulated based on type of pain (such as nociceptive and/or neuropathic), behavioral diagnoses, and risk assessments (summarized in **Box 2**).

Improving Sleep Equals Reducing Pain

Sleep management is a key first step to reducing pain intensity and improving quality of life in patients with both acute and chronic pain. Restorative sleep has been reported to predict the resolution of chronic widespread pain.[23] Although sleep treatment is not typically considered analgesic, research has found that sleep loss, and in particular rapid eye movement (REM) sleep loss, are acutely hyperalgesic.[24] For example, compared with insomniacs, individuals with normal sleep patterns rate experimental pain stimuli as 50% less intense, and have pain thresholds that are 50% higher.[25] An important first step to effective pain management is to develop a sleep management program that achieves the patient sleeping at least 6 hours at night. Morin and Benca[26] published an excellent review of insomnia management in *Lancet* 2012.

Nonpharmacologic options typically start with review of so-called sleep hygiene techniques (**Box 3**).[27] Additional supplemental strategies are often needed to support sleep hygiene, such as sleep restriction therapy, which improves sleep efficiency by limiting sleep time to initially conform to the patient's own recorded sleep log; once efficiency is restored, sleep time can then return to 7 to 8 hours nightly. Cognitive behavior therapy for insomnia is a well studied and effective nondrug strategy for insomnia.[28]

Patients with sleep difficulties typically have already tried nonprescription melatonin (1–5 mg), which triggers the sleep circadian cycle, but often take it just before bed, whereas sleep experts recommend that melatonin is more helpful when taken up to 6 hours before bedtime. Patients commonly have tried OTC remedies that include antihistaminic agents; although sedating, antihistamines are not analgesics, even in the setting of interstitial cystitis, for which they are often prescribed.[29] There is limited evidence that diphenhydramine improves insomnia, and routine use is generally not recommended.

Tricyclic antidepressants (TCAs) in general decrease sleep latency, increase total sleep time, but decrease REM sleep duration.[30,31] Gabapentinoids increase REM, total sleep

---

Box 2
Diagnosis-based overview of pharmacologic treatments

- Nociceptive pain
  - Rest, ice, NSAIDs, opioids
- Neuropathic pain
  - Tricyclic antidepressants (TCAs), serotonin-norepinephrine reuptake inhibitor (SNRIs), antiepileptics, opioids
- Co-occurring pain syndromes (functional or central sensitization)
  - TCAs, SNRIs, antiepileptics
- Depression and anxiety
  - Antidepressants, cognitive behavior therapy (CBT)/counseling
- PTSD
  - Prazosin, antidepressants, CBT/dialectical behavioral therapy (DBT)
- Opioid use disorder
  - Substance abuse treatment:
  - Abstinence or medication-assisted treatments (ie, methadone maintenance or Suboxone)

Box 3
Sleep hygiene

- Maintain a regular wake/sleep schedule: fixed bed and wake-up times, regardless of weekday or weekend
- Refrain from taking naps
- No caffeine after noon, if at all
- Exercise, but not within 3 hours of bedtime
- Establish a relaxing routine before bedtime
- No exposure to television or computer screens 2 hours before bedtime
- Use the bedroom for sleep activities
- Set environment (light, noise, temperature) at comfortable levels
- Avoid alcohol close to bedtime

---

time, and slow wave sleep. Although they have not been systematically studied for sleep, clinical experience suggests that they are often useful sleep drugs.[32] Both TCAs and gabapentinoids are sedating and assist sleep initiation and maintenance via different mechanisms: TCAs via antihistaminic side effects, and gabapentinoids by modulating the release of excitatory neurotransmitters. TCAs may be very effective sleep aids, especially those with higher antihistaminic properties, like doxepin (specifically approved for insomnia) and others such as amitriptyline, nortriptyline, and imipramine. Serotonin-norepinephrine reuptake inhibitors (SNRIs) are less antihistaminic, so direct sedative benefits are not expected; they may also disturb sleep by provoking periodic leg movement disorders.[33] Trazodone promotes sleep via 5-hydroxytryptamine (5-HT) 2A antagonism, but analgesic properties have not been shown; prescribing trazodone requires caution when combined with other serotonergic drugs such as selective serotonin reuptake inhibitors (SSRIs), SNRIs, triptans, and tramadol. SSRIs decrease REM sleep, increase REM latency, and fragment sleep.[31] The antidepressant mirtazapine, especially at lower and mostly antihistaminic doses (ie, 7.5–15 mg), is an effective sedative agent, and although not evaluated as an analgesic, would be expected to be so based on its moderate noradrenergic effects. Prazosin is effective at reducing nightmares in patients with PTSD, and can be useful in patients with chronic pain and co-occurring PTSD.[34] Although many prescribers recommend that patients use opioids for sleep, intending to reduce pain-related awakening, opioid medications are associated with dose-related central and obstructive sleep apnea, and are associated with electroencephalogram-demonstrated frequent awakenings, and reduce duration of slow wave sleep, which may be particularly restorative via antiinflammatory mechanisms.[35]

Use of benzodiazepines for sleep is not recommended in chronic pain based on lack of evidence for sustained benefits; rebound insomnia; risk of oversedation, especially when combined with opioids; and the complicating development of tolerance, dependency, and addiction. Benzodiazepines also decrease slow wave sleep as well as REM sleep. The nonbenzodiazepine hypnotic drugs (z-drugs: zolpidem, zaleplon, eszopiclone) risk parasomniac complex behaviors such as sleep walking, sleep eating, and driving unaware; disturb EEG sleep architecture; and their use does not improve patient-reported pain scores, so are of limited value in patients with chronic pain.[36] The Beers criteria for potentially inappropriate medication use in older adults strongly recommend against use of sedative hypnotics in older patients based on moderate quality of evidence, although clinical judgment may find exceptions in the setting of palliative and hospice care.[37] Only a few studies have evaluated long-term effectiveness, although addiction to nonbenzodiazepines is generally considered unlikely.

Acetaminophen

Widely used, inexpensive, and available without prescription (OTC), acetaminophen (paracetamol) is an effective low-potency analgesic and antipyretic agent. Although the mechanism of effect of acetaminophen remains uncertain, its action may be on the transient receptor potential (TRP) A1 ion channel expressed on the central terminals of primary sensory neurons in the dorsal horn of the spinal cord.[38] It has also been cited as either a cyclooxygenase (COX) 2 or 3 inhibitor[39,40] (review of COX actions is presented later), and has been proposed to be more active as a central nervous system analgesic than an antiinflammatory. At doses of less than 4 g daily it is well tolerated and safe for those less than 60 years of age; current recommendations suggest doses at or less than 2 g daily for older patients. Risks of hepatotoxicity increase significantly based on dose, older age, combination with alcohol, and co-occurring liver disease (ie, hepatitis C, alcoholic cirrhosis). Acetaminophen-related hepatic failure is the leading cause of acute liver failure worldwide.[41] Cautious medication review and reconciliation of OTC use of acetaminophen is important for all patients with pain, not only regarding its role as an analgesic but also its presence in combination with a wide range of other minor cold and influenza products. Be alert to acetaminophen in combination with many prescribed opioid analgesics, such as codeine (ie, Tylenol #3), hydrocodone (ie, Vicodin), and oxycodone (ie, Percocet).

Analgesic nephropathy (renal papillary necrosis and interstitial nephritis) is caused by chronic use of phenacetin (a prodrug of acetaminophen) in combination with aspirin, and possibly from chronic high-dose use of acetaminophen and/or NSAIDs, and probably in the setting of underlying chronic kidney disease.

Combination with NSAIDs adds analgesic efficacy, but is also associated with greater risks of gastric and renal injury than with NSAIDs alone.[42,43]

Key points: acetaminophen

- Effective analgesic, without antiinflammatory or coagulation effects
- Mechanism of action still not fully understood
- Caution regarding doses more than 2 g/d
- Be alert to OTC use for colds and fever, and/or presence in combination with other analgesics

---

Nonsteroidal Antiinflammatory Drugs

NSAIDs are the mostly widely used pain relievers, with 60 million US prescriptions yearly, the elderly consuming 3.6 times more than younger adults; they overall account for 25% of adverse drug reactions reported. NSAIDs are available in more than 20 formulations, via oral, intravenous (IV), and transdermal routes of administration. NSAIDs are recommended for nociceptive pain, defined as pain that arises from actual or threatened damage to nonneural tissue and is caused by the activation of nociceptors. They are commonly used for traumatic musculoskeletal pain syndromes, such as muscle, ligament, and or tendon injuries, and joint disorders from traumatic, infectious, or degenerative conditions. Good-quality evidence shows effectiveness for spinal pain from disc, facet, or spinal ligament injuries.[44] Neuritis related to connective tissue disorders also are NSAID responsive.[45] Rheumatic pain syndromes, such as inflammatory myositis, tendonitis, enthesopathy, and autoimmune arthritides, and spondyloarthropathies, as well as crystalline arthritides respond to NSAIDs. NSAIDs are useful in the management of endometriosis pain. NSAIDs may exacerbate preexisting inflammatory bowel disease, complicate diverticulitis, and are associated with collagenous colitis.[46,47]

NSAIDs reduce pain resulting from activation and sensitization of peripheral nociceptors. Phospholipase A_2 releases arachidonic acid from membrane lipids, which then goes on to synthesize the eicosanoid autoacids, hydroperoxidase and endoperoxidase. These cyclized eicosanoids are then converted by COX-1 and COX-2 into key components of the inflammatory cascade: prostaglandins (PGs) and prostacyclins, which go on to sensitize a heterogeneous range of nociceptors,[48] and thromboxanes, which trigger platelet aggregation and leukocyte modulation (**Fig. 1**).

Patients with pseudoallergic NSAID asthma seem to be more susceptible to COX-1 specificity from acquired alterations in arachidonic acid to leukotriene pathways, and do not represent an immunoglobulin E–mediated allergy.[49]

Selective Cyclooxygenase 2 Inhibition

A notable pharmacologic advance in the management of inflammatory pain followed the discovery of the distinct enzymatic categories of COX-1 and COX-2. The subsequent identification of NSAIDs with more or less selective targeting of COX-2 inhibition was heralded as a major therapeutic breakthrough, because COX-1 was thought to be a homeostatic (or constitutive) rather than reactive (or inducible) progenitor of PGs. Subsequent clinical evidence has shown that COX-2 selectivity reduces bleeding risks, because, in contrast with COX-1 agents, it does not reduce thromboxane A_2, a compound required for platelet aggregation. Platelet covalent acetylation with aspirin or other acetylated NSAIDs prevents normal platelet aggregation for the life of the platelet, so restoration of normal coagulation requires about 10 days, which is the

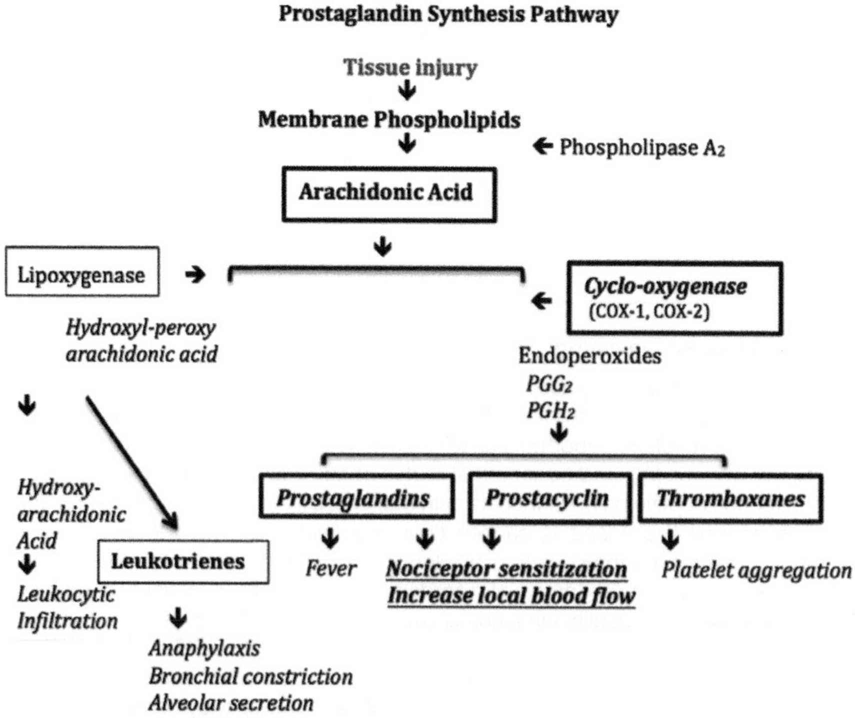

Fig. 1. PG synthesis and effects.

time needed to recover adequate numbers of nonexposed normally functioning platelets. Short-acting nonacetylated NSAIDs require discontinuation for only the half-life of the drug (usually 3–5 days) to prevent thromboxane interference with coagulation, which is an issue when considering at-risk interventional procedures.

Reduced gastric and duodenal mucosal injury side effects of selective COX-2 NSAIDs are important advantages, although incomplete. COX-1 inhibits PG I_1, which does confer cytoprotection of gastric endothelium. However, COX-2 inhibits production of PG E_2 which also plays a significant role in protection of gastric and duodenal mucosa. Although COX-2 selectivity avoids some of the additive COX-2 effects, subclinical endoscopic gastrointestinal (GI) injury of nonselective COX-1 inhibition is only lessened by about half, reduced from between 8% and 18% (nonselective NSAIDs) to between 4% and 12% (selective COX-2).[50] Published evidence supports the addition of any of the widely available proton pump inhibitors or H_2 blockers for patients with a prior history of gastritis or gastroesophageal reflux disease.[51] Misoprostol (Cytotec; a synthetic PG E1 analogue) can be prescribed separately or in combination with diclofenac. Misoprostol is less well tolerated than proton pump inhibitors, because of bloating and other nonspecific abdominal complaints, is contraindicated in pregnancy, and there are concerns in women of child-bearing age because of an abortifacient effect.

Because NSAID use during first and second trimesters have been associated with a variety of fetal risks, as a class they are listed as category C; routine use during early pregnancy is best avoided. NSAIDs are contraindicated in late term pregnancy because of inhibition of closure of the ductus arteriosus, oligohydramnios, and risk of traumatic bleeding at delivery.

Nonsteroidal Antiinflammatory Drugs and Cardiovascular Disease

All NSAIDs, whether COX-2 selective or not, increase risk of cardiovascular (CV) disease, for patients with and without out preexisting risk.[52] This increased risk is likely caused in large part by the well-established increase of 5 mm Hg in normotensive patients and more than 10 mm Hg increase in blood pressure (BP) in hypertensives resulting from PG interference, most likely in the kidney.[53] All NSAIDs interfere, at times significantly, with BP management, countering the effects antihypertensive drugs (especially angiotensin-converting enzymes, angiotensin receptor blockers, and diuretics.) COX-2 selective agents cause prostacyclin activity reduction without COX-1 antiplatelet thromboxane benefits, possibly promoting additional endothelial injury, although celecoxib (a COX-2 selective) at 200 to 400 mg/d seems to present a risk comparable with that of naproxen (a nonselective NSAID). Acetaminophen also increases BP and CV risk. Patients at low CV risk seem to have a very small (<1%/y) dose-related increase in risk of myocardial infarction, congestive heart failure, arrhythmia, and stroke,[54] which is so small an increase that NSAIDs are appropriate when indicated and effective. In patients with known CV disease, risk of new vascular events increases in excess of 0.7%/y from a baseline of 2%.[55] Compared with opioids, NSAIDs seem to increase CV risk by 1.8,[56] although non-CV risks of chronic opioids are higher. Naproxen seems not to present this same increased risk compared with diclofenac, ibuprofen, and celecoxibs, so it can be considered the safest NSAID overall.

Other Major Nonsteroidal Antiinflammatory Drug Risks

Nonsteroidal antiinflammatory drugs and the kidney
Nephrotoxicity from NSAIDs is related to inhibition of glomerular and endothelial renal vasodilation from both COX-1 and COX-2 inhibitors with net lowering of glomerular filtration, more severely so when patients are volume depleted. Risks worsen in older patients, those with preexisting kidney disease, and before procedures involving

radiocontrast agents. NSAIDs also increase potassium levels in patients receiving potassium-sparing antihypertensives.

Reye syndrome

NSAIDs for the treatment of fever in children (aspirin has been shown, but circumstantially all NSAIDs) are associated with Reye syndrome. Acetaminophen management of fever in children is recommended instead.

Nonsteroidal antiinflammatory drugs, bones, and tendons

NSAIDs have a causal relationship with nonunion following bone fracture and spine fusion, although this has not been shown in humans.[57] There is no evidence of poor tendon healing in rodents either.[58]

Nonsteroidal Antiinflammatory Drug-Drug Interactions

NSAIDs displace protein-bound phenytoin and warfarin, increasing their activity. GI bleeding from COX-1 NSAIDs, especially in anticoagulated patients, can be severe and catastrophic. Increased renal toxicity is seen in combination with methotrexate and cyclosporine. Serum levels of lithium are significantly increased when combined with NSAIDs. Although hepatic cytochromes (2C9 and 1A2) metabolize several NSAIDs, this is not a clinically significant concern. Other side effects (especially with aspirin) include dose-related salicylism causing tinnitus and hyperventilation. The sulfonamide structure of celecoxib increases risk of allergic reaction in patients with sulfa allergies.

Transdermal Nonsteroidal Antiinflammatory Drugs

Formulations of diclofenac that are transdermally absorbed show analgesic efficacy that is much less than that of orally administered oral NSAIDs, with demonstrated plasma maximum concentration (C_{max}) bioavailability varying from just 0.2% to 8%. Penetration depth varies with product formulation, but is typically only 3 to 4 mm, although it can be 2-fold deeper with occlusion, so the drugs are unable to reach the synovium and/or periosteum of many joints, which are the inflammatory target sites. Hence, they are recommended for joints proximate to the skin, like phalanges or wrists. Diclofenac with the absorption enhancer dimethyl sulfoxide (Pennsaid) is approved for knee osteoarthritis. Because of low systemic absorption, adverse effects relate mostly to skin site application.

Monitoring Nonsteroidal Antiinflammatory Drugs

Monitoring recommendations with chronic use vary, although it is prudent to obtain a baseline creatinine level for anything more than very short-term use for all prescribed NSAIDs. Cautious prescribing for long-term use merits an annual creatinine level, and with any concerns regarding renal impairment consider either discontinuation or an annual or alternate-year calculation of glomerular filtration or creatinine clearance determination.

Key points: NSAIDs

- Useful for nociceptive pain
- COX-2 selectivity reduces bleeding and GI side effects
- All NSAIDs increase BP and CV risks
- All risks increase with age and dose
- Monitor renal function with prolonged use

Corticosteroids

Brief mention is made of corticosteroids in pain management because they play a limited role as agents effective in acute and subacute pain related to tendon and synovial injuries and inflammatory processes, including those related to cervical or lumbar disc herniation with radiculopathy. Selective injections into joint and tendon sites may also be useful, with or without ultrasonography guidance. A short tapering course of oral prednisone (starting dose of 20–40 mg) or methylprednisolone (starting dose of 24–48 mg) may be considered in an acute radiculopathy without abnormal motor findings before beginning a more detailed imaging evaluation. Long-term use for chronic rheumatologic diseases, such as rheumatoid arthritis, lupus, spondyloarthropathies, and polymyalgia rheumatica, is best reserved for clinicians with special training in management of these chronic conditions. Toxicity includes glucose intolerance, especially in those with established diabetes, even with epidural administration. Sodium retention is a common adverse effect, even with short-term use. Exacerbation of anxiety and depression, sleep disruption, and delirium may occur. Long-term and/or high-dose use raises risks of severe adverse effects on bone mineral metabolism (ie, osteopenia and osteoporosis), and osteonecrosis has been reported with doses greater than or equal to 20 mg/d[59]; cautious use, adequate informed consent, and careful monitoring are strongly advised.

ANTIDEPRESSANTS FOR PAIN

Antidepressants classified as tricyclic (TCAs) and tetracyclic, SNRI, SSRIs, norepinephrine-dopamine reuptake inhibitors, and serotonin modulating drugs are, to varying degrees monoamine (norepinephrine, serotonin, and dopamine) reuptake inhibitors and presynaptic alpha$_2$-adrenergic antagonists that increase availability of norepinephrine and serotonin in the central nervous system. Antidepressant analgesia is multifactorial, because potential sites of action extend across both peripheral and central signaling and transmission systems (**Table 2**).

Antidepressants that increase synaptic norepinephrine are likely to be effective analgesics principally because of their upregulation of the descending noxious inhibitory pain systems, which is a key component in normal human pain modulation. The role of antidepressants in the management of acute and subacute pain is less clear, particularly because antidepressant analgesia may take 2 to 4 weeks to be observed, although more immediate sleep benefits (and arguably muscle relaxant effects) are seen within days. Doses of TCAs for analgesic benefits typically are prescribed at less than antidepressant dosing, avoiding many of the higher dose-related concerns, such as anticholinergic or sedative effects, or effects related to QTc prolongation (discussed later and in **Table 3**).

As a group, antidepressants improve depression and anxiety, and those with sedative side effects also improve sleep, all of which are common disturbances in patients with chronic pain. Antidepressant drug selection for pain, especially neuropathic pain, depends mostly on increasing synaptic levels of norepinephrine, more so than serotonin. Clinical trials show TCA and SNRI, but not SSRI, effectiveness for postherpetic neuralgia (number needed to treat [NNT], 2.7), diabetic peripheral neuropathy (NNT, 1.2–1.5), atypical facial pain (NNT, 2.8–3.4), fibromyalgia (NNT, 1.5–4), and central pain (NNT, 1.7).[60–64] Effectiveness of antidepressants in migraine and tension-type headache is supported by a robust evidence base.[65,66] Low-quality studies also support effectiveness in osteoarthritis[67] and chronic pelvic pain.[68,69]

Gate Control and Descending Pain Modulation

Descending noxious inhibitory pain pathways seem to provide a rationale for the gate-control theory first described by Melzack and Wall[70] more than 50 years ago (**Fig. 2**).

Table 2
Proposed mechanisms of action by category of antidepressants

Mechanism of Action	Site of Action	TCA	SNRI	SRI
Reuptake inhibition of monoamine	Serotonin	+	+	+
	Noradrenaline	+	+	−
Receptor antagonism	Alpha-adrenergic	+	−	−
	NMDA	+	(+) Milnacipran	−
Blocker or activator of ion channels	Sodium channel blocker	+	(+) Venlafaxine-duloxetine	(+) Only fluoxetine
	Calcium channel blocker	+	?	(+) Citalopram fluoxetine
	Potassium channel activator	+	?	−
GABA$_B$ receptor	Increase of receptor function	+ Amitriptyline desipramine	?	+ Fluoxetine
Opioid receptor binding/opioid-mediated effect	μ and δ opioid receptor	(+)	(+) Venlafaxine	(+) Paroxetine
Inflammation	Decrease of PG E$_2$ production	+	?	+ Fluoxetine
	Decrease of TNFα production	+	?	?

+ indicates mechanism of action documented *in vitro* and/or *in vivo*.
(+) indicates mechanism of action documented *in vitro* and/or *in vivo* high concentration.
− indicates no known mechanism of action.
? indicates not investigated/not known.
Abbreviations: GABA, gamma-aminobutyric acid; SRI, selective serotonin reuptake inhibitor; TNFα, tumor necrosis factor alpha.
From Verdu B, Decosterd I, Buclin T, et al. Antidepressants for the treatment of chronic pain. Drugs 2008;68:2614; with permission.

Animal models have identified non–opioid-dependent analgesic effects from lidocaine introduced into the rostral ventral medulla,[71] as well as modulation of dorsal horn inhibitory interneurons by norepinephrine, dopamine, and serotonin.[72] Chronic pain dysregulation in descending pain pathways is shown in studies of spinal cord functional MRI activity in clinical syndromes linked to abnormal descending noxious control.[5,73]

Desirable tricyclic antidepressant drug side effects
Sedative properties of nearly all TCAs can be exploited as an aid for sleep. Because sedation generally wanes as patients become accommodated to the drug, modest dose escalation may be needed, but significant tolerance to sleep benefits is uncommon. Many patients with chronic pain are also anxious and/or depressed so use of an antidepressant agent is also expected to improve this dimension of pain care. In circumstances in which patients are already on a stable SSRI with effective mood control, TCAs can be carefully added because SSRIs are less effective analgesics and are not sedating. Addition of a TCA to SSRI may increase TCA level by 20% to 30% compared with use alone; combination with fluoxetine may double TCA levels because of unique interactions with this SSRI. Maprotiline, a heterocyclic antidepressant that is a selective norepinephrine reuptake inhibitor and so would not be expected to increase serotonin levels, may be the preferred antidepressant in combination with an SSRI or SNRI, especially if the patient is on high-dose SSRI and particularly when the patient is

Table 3
Relative side effects and amine profile of selected antidepressants

Drug	Side Effects			Amine Uptake Profile	
	Sedation	Orthostasis	Anticholinergic	Noradrenaline	Serotonin
Amitriptyline	4+	2+	4+	2+	4+
Doxepin	3+	2+	2+	1+	2+
Imipramine	2+	3+	2+	2+	4+
Nortriptyline	2+	1+	2+	2+	3+
Desipramine	1+	1+	1+	4+	2+
Milnacipran	0	0	0	3+	1+
Duloxetine	0	0	0	2+	3+
Venlafaxine	0	0	0	1+	3+
Trazodone	2+	2+	1+	0	3+
Nefazodone	2+	1+	0/1+	0/1+	5+
Fluoxetine	0/1+	0/1+	0/1+	0/1+	5+
Paroxetine	0/1+	0	0	0/1+	5+
Sertraline	0/1+	0	0	0/1+	5+
Mirtazapine	3+	2+	2+	2+	4+
Bupropion	0	1+	2+	0/1+	0/1+
Maprotiline	2+	3+	2+	4+	0

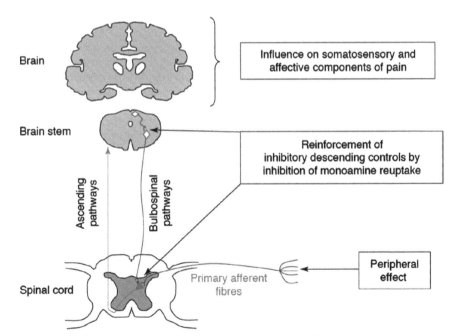

Fig. 2. Descending inhibitory pain system. (*From* Mico JA, Ardid D, Berrocoso E, et al. Antidepressants and pain. Trends Pharmacol Sci 2006;27:352; with permission.)

already on other serotoninergic agents such as trazodone, tramadol, or triptans. Mirtazapine, a presynaptic alpha$_2$-adrenergic antagonist that increases release of norepinephrine and serotonin at higher doses (ie, $\geq$30 mg), is predominantly antihistaminic at low dose, so sedation paradoxically predominates at lower dosages. Like many non-TCAs and SNRIs, mirtazapine's analgesic benefits have not been studied, but by mechanistic extrapolation it could be considered a useful drug in patients with sleep and mood disruption co-occurring with pain.

Undesirable tricyclic antidepressant drug side effects

Principal subjective side effects of TCAs are related to anticholinergic properties of all drugs in this category: dry mouth, constipation, urinary retention (often severe in men with prostatic enlargement), and increased intraocular pressure in patients with glaucoma. Patients with rheumatologic disorders risk exacerbated sicca symptoms. Amitriptyline and imipramine are more anticholinergic than their respective deaminated congeners, nortriptyline and desipramine. Note that cyclobenzaprine (Flexeril) is a tricyclic drug, chemically nearly identical to amitriptyline, although generally classified as an antispasm drug; it shares the side effect profile of the other TCAs and should not be prescribed for patients already on these drugs because of the risk of combined adverse effects.

Cardiovascular risks of TCAs are predominantly related to QTc prolongation caused by delayed cardiac depolarization and increase of the QT interval. SSRIs show less QT period expansion and hence produce lower cardiotoxic side effects.[74] SNRIs have not shown significant QTc prolongation except at high dose,[75] but because neither SNRIs nor SSRIs promote sleep, many experienced clinicians (including this author) choose TCAs at low to moderate dose when sleep initiation and/or maintenance is a clinical issue. There is continuing expert disagreement about whether patients require electrocardiogram monitoring before initiation and/or monitoring during follow-up.[76] If there is a history of clinically significant cardiac arrhythmia, especially in patients prescribed antiarrythmics (most of which prolong QTc), TCAs are best avoided. TCAs in combination with methadone, which at even a moderate dose prolongs QTc, may preclude use, especially in high dose; many other opioids are also associated with QTc prolongation, such as fentanyl, oxycodone, and buprenorphine.

Nausea is a common side effect of SNRIs, occurring in up to 30% of patients, and is an intolerance that often leads to discontinuation. SNRIs and SSRIs may provoke periodic leg movement, and so may disturb sleep.[33] Orthostatic hypotension may also result from adrenoreceptor alpha-1 blockade at moderate and high doses of TCAs. Sexual impairments are notable in the more highly serotoninergic drugs. Reduced seizure threshold is described with use of the TCAs, maprotiline and bupropion (a mixed dopamine-norepinephrine reuptake inhibitor); these are best avoided in patients with history of epilepsy, even when well controlled. Suicide risk is arguably increased in patients, especially adolescents and younger adults, with all categories of antidepressants, so warnings to patients and families about increased suicidal ideation should be routine. Mania may be precipitated in patients with bipolar mood disorders, so collaboration with a psychiatrist is strongly advised when considering antidepressant management for pain control. Older adults are at risk of heightened drug-related side effects of all kinds, including delirium, with any psychoactive drug, so cautious prescribing and regular follow-up are always advised. Mixing antidepressants drugs with alcohol heightens sedation and other adverse effects. Antidepressant discontinuation syndromes occur most commonly when stopping short-acting agents, especially SNRIs, which are very short acting but are usually prescribed as extended-release products. SNRI weaning may require use of a long-acting SSRI, such as fluoxetine, as a bridge to taper. Because TCAs have prolonged half-lives, withdrawal is not a common problem. Monoamine oxide inhibitors are not recommended for management of pain because of the many and severe drug-drug interactions that complicate use of this older drug category (**Box 4**).

Box 4
Analgesic antidepressant dose and schedule

TCAs

Amitriptyline 10–75 mg at bedtime

Nortriptyline 10–50 mg at bedtime

Imipramine 10–50 mg at bedtime

Desipramine 10–50 mg at bedtime

Doxepin 10–75 mg at bedtime

SNRIs

Milnacipran 25–50 mg twice a day

Duloxetine 30 mg up to twice a day

Other

Mirtazapine 7.5–30 mg at bedtime

Maprotiline 25–75 mg at bedtime

Key points: antidepressant analgesia

- Antidepressants that increase synaptic norepinephrine levels (TCAs>SNRIs) are effective analgesics
- Sedating antidepressants are useful agents to improve both sleep initiation and maintenance
- Anticholinergic side effects are most common with TCAs
- Nausea is common with SNRIs
- Dose-related QTc prolongation occurs with TCAs more than SNRIs
- Warn patients and families about risks of suicidality when any antidepressant is prescribed
- Mania may be precipitated by any category of antidepressant

---

NEUROPATHIC PAIN
Some Preliminaries

Drug treatment of neuropathic pain, defined as pain caused by a lesion or disease of the somatosensory nervous system, has robust evidence-based support for TCA, SNRI, and anticonvulsant drugs (ACDs) (see **Table 3**). There are many high-quality studies showing efficacy of ACDs in the management of neuropathic pain. Several of these efficacy trials are included earlier. Note that opioids also seem to be as effective reducing pain intensity in chronic neuropathic pain conditions in only short-term trials,[77] and are not considered first-line therapy because of the many challenges and risks associated with long-term opioid prescribing. Opioids have also been shown to induce allodynia (pain after a stimulation that is not normally painful) in rodent models,[78] the transformation of migraine into chronic daily headache following regular use of opioids,[79] and hyperalgesia (increased level of pain from a stimulus that normally provokes a lower level of pain).[15] Other than misuse of antidepressants with the intention to overdose, and with the exception of addicts drug seeking gabapentin to self-manage opioid and benzodiazepine withdrawal, abuse and addiction to nonopioid analgesics are not clinical problems (**Table 4**).

Central Sensitization

Central sensitization is thought to play an important role in functional pain conditions characterized by widespread pain. Special mention is made of conditions that are difficult to diagnose, especially those that have been exhaustively evaluated often by many different subspecialties without a clearly defined biomedical diagnosis, notably fibromyalgia and other widespread pain syndromes.[3] These diagnoses are syndromic, frequently occur simultaneously, and present with pan-positive review of systems; they include fibromyalgia most notably but also chronic daily headaches, interstitial cystitis, irritable bowel syndrome, and chronic fatigue. Excellent reviews include those by Yunus[80] in 2007 and Clauw[81] in 2014 (**Fig. 3**). High degrees of fibromyalgianess[82] may be a predictor of poor pain outcomes in inflammatory rheumatologic disease and even in routine orthopedic surgery.[83] Of particular relevance is the frequent finding of significant adverse childhood traumas and often overwhelmingly difficult social and psychological problems that may play a secondary or even a primary role in creating altered central nervous system pain processing. Patient assessment of medical and nonmedical circumstances during childhood and adulthood (ie, variety of childhood traumas and abuse,[84] PTSD,[85] elective spine surgery,[86] extended intensive care unit care[87]) is needed for proper diagnosis and management.

Some Caveats Regarding Pharmacotherapy for Neuropathic Pain

Separating the diverse pharmacodynamics of sodium channel ACDs broadly into one category and the calcium channel ACDs into another provides a simplified and practical model for clinicians managing pain involving peripheral, central, and sympathetic nervous systems. This approach takes some liberty with the taxonomy of neuropathic pain because it includes sensitization syndromes associated with abnormal central pain processing as neuropathic pain states. However, this symptom-based approach allows prescribers to select ACDs based on clinical presentations regardless of well-defined pathophysiology. This model was presented by Baron[88] in a 2006 review linking proposed mechanisms of neuropathic pain to targets for pharmacotherapeutic interventions. Until many currently uncertain pain mechanisms and drug pharmacodynamics are better understood, improved clinical decision making requires a pragmatic symptom-based approach to ACD selection.

ANTICONVULSANT DRUGS
Sodium Channel Blockers

Lidocaine, carbamazepine, oxcarbazepine, and lamotrigine have shown efficacy in spontaneous shooting pain of trigeminal neuropathy, diabetic peripheral neuropathy, human immunodeficiency virus–related peripheral neuropathy, and multiple sclerosis.[89–91] A proposed mechanism of pain from these disorders is nociceptor hyperexcitability from ectopic impulse generation in the dorsal root ganglion. These sodium channel blockers selectively enhance slow inactivation and discriminate between resting and depolarized neurons (ie, they are state dependent).[92] Lacosamide may be even more selective, targeting channels that are in a state of depolarization, and although this drug does not have an evidence-based literature to support its use, it may be considered in patients intolerant to other better studied sodium channel blocker ACDs. Mexiletine, an oral lidocaine analogue, has been used by many pain clinicians for decades may also be prescribed, although without quality evidence to support its use; all reports are case series and anecdotal.[93] Other sodium channel blockers include diphenylhydantoin and valproic acid with variably low-quality published evidence, and topiramate with better evidence for migraine and other headache conditions.[94]

Calcium Channel Blockers

The gabapentinoids (gabapentin and pregabalin) have a robust evidence base for efficacy in diabetic peripheral neuropathy and fibromyalgia. Proposed pharmacodynamics of the gabapentinoids (and hypothetically another ACD calcium channel blocker, levetiracetam) seem to target abnormally functioning sensitized presynaptic calcium channels at spinal and supraspinal levels that cause increased synaptic transmission, amplification of C-fiber input, and abnormal gating of A-beta fiber input that generates the clinical presentation of symptomatic spontaneous ongoing pain and dynamic mechanical allodynia. Combining gabapentinoid efficacy data for both the peripheral neuropathy of diabetes and the central sensitization of fibromyalgia, to achieve ~30% reduction in numeric pain rating at 3 months (gabapentin dosed at 1200–2400 mg/d and pregabalin dosed at 300–600 mg/d), the NNT is 4 to 6.[95,96]

Some evidence supports the use of both gabapentinoids and TCAs for chronic pelvic pain when treatment of endometriosis is completed and no active bowel obstructions are present.[97] Sensitization mechanisms would support the use of these neuropathic drug categories for 2 other visceral hyperalgesic functional pain syndromes: interstitial cystitis and irritable bowel disease.[98] There is also emerging evidence for gabapentinoids in thoracoabdominal and post–spinal surgery pain.[99–101]

Side Effects of Anticonvulsant Drugs

ACDs produce a wide range of side effects. Sedation is common, dose related, and can occur at therapeutic doses. Weight gain, edema, global cognitive impairment such as forgetfulness and word-finding difficulty, and sometimes poor balance are common with all ACDs. Gabapentinoid side effects are more straightforward to assess clinically, mostly by patient (and family) history and bedside examination rather than requiring the varying laboratory monitoring protocols recommended for nearly all sodium channel drugs (**Table 5**). Note that no laboratory monitoring is needed for gabapentinoids, with the exception of dose reduction in renal impairment (because there is 100% renal clearance). Note that gabapentin requires an active intestinal transport system, such that it is occasionally poorly absorbed, and pregabalin is more readily (passively) absorbed, so a switch from gabapentin to pregabalin may be useful when therapeutic doses lead to no benefits and no side effects, because this may be caused by poor absorption alone.[102] Otherwise pharmacodynamic targets are near identical, so common side effects to gabapentin generally predict similar side effects to pregabalin. Carbamazepine and oxcarbazepine are strong cytochrome P3A4 inducers, and mexiletine is a strong cytochrome P1A2 (CYP1A2) inducer, so drug-drug interactions are potentially significant; reference or pharmacist review is recommended.

Lidocaine is available in 2 transdermal forms: 5% patches and a eutectic mixture of lidocaine and procaine. Both penetrate skin to a depth of only 4 to 5 mm, so the therapeutic targets are skin nociceptors. Thus, the drugs are recommended for postherpetic neuralgia, predermatologic procedures, and IV needle placement.

Review of Drugs for Neuropathic Pain

Table 4
Summary of efficacy of drugs for neuropathic pain

	Tricyclics	SNRI	Dopamine NRI	Carbamazepine	Diphenylhydantoin	Lamotrigine	Valproic Acid	Gabapentin Pregabalin	Topiramate	Tramadol	Opioids
NNT	1.5–3.7	3.4–14	13–2.1	1.6–2.5	1.5–3.6	3.5–8.1	2.1–4.2	4.0–5.6	4.3–2.8	2.7–6.7	2.0–3.2
NNH	10–25	—	—	13–79	—	—	—	4–30	5–8	2.7–6.7	10–66[a]

[a] Dose related.
Abbreviations: NNH, numbers needed to harm; NRI, norepinephrine reuptake inhibitor.
Data from Sindrup SH, Jensen TS. Efficacy of pharmacological treatments of neuropathic pain: an update and effect related to mechanism of drug action. Pain 1999;83:391.

Mention of tramadol and tapentadol is important in order to recognize that they are SNRIs but also possess weak mu opioid receptor binding and effect. They are included in **Table 6**.

Table 6 Pharmacodynamics of neuropathic pain drugs	
Drug/Drug Class	**Major Effect on Neuropathic Pain**
Tricyclic antidepressants	Inhibition NE>5-HT reuptake, blockade sodium and calcium channels and NMDA receptors
5-HT/NE reuptake inhibitors	Inhibition 5-HT/NE reuptake
Lidocaine	Blockade voltage-dependent sodium channels
Carbamazepine/oxcarbazepine	Blockade voltage-dependent sodium channels
Lamotrigine	Blockade voltage-dependent sodium channels/inhibits glutamate release
Gabapentin/pregabalin	Blockade voltage-gated calcium channel
Tramadol/tapentadol	Opioid agonist, inhibits 5-HT/NE reuptake

Abbreviation: NE, norepinephrine.
Adapted from Finnerup NB, Sindrup SH, Jensen TS. Chronic neuropathic pain: mechanisms, drug targets and measurement. Fundam Clin Pharmacol 2007;21:131.

Key points: ACDs for pain

- ACDs with both sodium and calcium channel blocking effects are effective in a variety of neuropathic pain disorders, fibromyalgia, and headache.
- Sodium channel ACDs have a wide range of potential serious adverse drug effects, including electrolyte disorders, pancytopenias, and skin rashes, and so require routine laboratory monitoring.
- Gabapentinoid side effects are usually clinically evident: cognitive slowing, weight gain, and edema.

BENZODIAZEPINES

Although widely prescribed, benzodiazepines have limited clinical value as skeletal muscle relaxants, especially over long-term use. They are occasionally useful in acute circumstances as short-term sedatives, when required for short-term antianxiety effects, and as sleep aids before transitioning to more effective drugs, as discussed earlier. Stiff person syndrome is an exception, because benzodiazepines are currently recommended treatment of this rare condition; neurologic consultation to confirm diagnosis and support benzodiazepine use is strongly advised before embarking on the exceptionally high doses often needed to achieve an often incomplete response.

Risks are many and nearly always complicate benzodiazepine use in chronic pain management because of rapid development of tolerance, rebound insomnia, respiratory suppression, and accidental prescription overdose death (especially when combined with opioids and other sedating drugs, and alcohol). Benzodiazepine discontinuation also risks potentially life-threatening abstinence syndrome, similar to delirium tremens, so they must always be tapered slowly. Benzodiazepines pose significant risks of misuse, abuse, and addiction that may significantly complicate

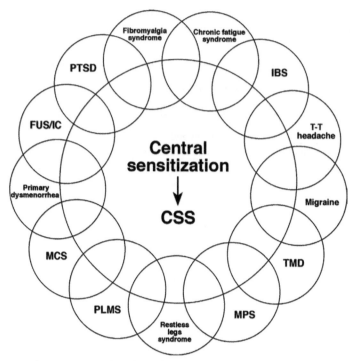

Fig. 3. Proposed co-occurring disorders of central sensitization with common pathophysiology. FUS/IC, functional urologic syndrome/interstitial cystitis; IBS, irritable bowel syndrome; MCS, multiple chemical sensitivity; MPS, myofascial pain disorder; PLMS, periodic leg movement syndrome; T-T headache, tension headache; TMD, temporomandibular disorder. (*From* Yunus MB. Fibromyalgia and overlapping disorders: the unifying concept of central sensitivity syndromes. Semin Arthritis Rheum 2007:36:341; with permission.)

pain management. Current evidence-based pain treatment guidelines strongly recommend against coprescribing benzodiazepines with opioids in CNCP.[103]

Key points: benzodiazepines

- Do not use for chronic pain
- Do not mix with opioids

The Myth of Skeletal Muscle Spasm

Although widely used in chronic musculoskeletal pain, antispasm muscle relaxant drugs show limited analgesic relief and may add to sedating polypharmacy.[104,105] Functioning mostly as sedatives, they do relax the patient, but this is better achieved with drugs that have antianxiety and analgesic effects long term, such as TCAs and SNRIs. As a class, muscle relaxants are safe with the exception of carisoprodol (Soma), which in this author's opinion should never be prescribed. Carisoprodol's active metabolite is meprobamate, a drug that has been withdrawn from the US market (and elsewhere) because of lack of proven efficacy, serious withdrawal symptoms similar to those seen with benzodiazepine discontinuation, and problems with misuse and abuse. Orphenadrine has some demonstrated NMDA antagonist effects, so may

Table 5
Monitoring sodium channel anticonvulsant drug side effects

Drug	Risk	All:
		Increased LFTs
		Low Sodium, Especially With Diuretics
		Neutropenia
		Rash/SJS
		Sedation
		Suicidality
Carbemazepine Oxcarbazepine	Agranulocytosis	
Valproic acid	Hyperammonemia Weight gain	
Lamotrigine	Recommended slow dose up-titration because of higher risk SJS Weight gain	
Topiramate	Weight loss Agitation Metabolic acidosis Glaucoma Kidney stones	
Lacosamide	Prolonged PR, AV block	
Mexiletine	GI upset (up to 40%) QTc prolongation Second-degree or third-degree AV block Proarrhythmia (10%–15% in patients with malignant arrhythmia)	

Abbreviations: AV, atrioventricular; LFT, liver function test; PR, ECG interval from beginning of P-wave to beginning of QRS-wave; SJS, Stevens Johnson syndrome.

be considered differently than other agents such as methocarbamol and metoxazole. As discussed earlier, cyclobenzaprine is a tricyclic drug, although without demonstrated antidepressant effects.

In contrast, antispasticity agents are recommended when true spasticity is present, such as occurs with neurologic disease or injury of upper motor neurons, as seen following spinal cord trauma, multiple sclerosis, and head injuries from trauma or stroke. Intense muscle contractions are painful, and pain relief occurs when this spasm can be pharmacologically controlled. Baclofen, a gamma-aminobutyric acid (GABA) B agonist, is active in the dorsal horn and supraspinally, and when oral dosages of more than 80 to 120 mg/d are either ineffective for control of spasticity (for both functional rehabilitation and pain control) or are poorly tolerated, baclofen can be administered via an implanted intrathecal delivery system after a trial showing efficacy. High-dose baclofen abstinence is a life-threatening condition, because abrupt discontinuation is associated with a rebound hypercontractile state causing hyperpyrexia and rhabdomyolosis[106]; in-patient intensive care management is required when baclofen pumps fail (because of missed reservoir refills, line breakage, or pump failure). The alpha$_2$-adrenergic agonist, tizanidine, has also been shown to be an effective antispasticity drug.[107] Mechanism of effect seems to be at the dorsal root ganglion, which when injured increases coexpression of alpha-2 adrenoreceptors.[108] Tizanidine side effects include a significant dose-related orthostatic hypotensive response (usually with dosages of more than 8 mg/d), dry mouth, and sedation, which leads some clinicians to use it as an off-label sleep aid. Clonidine, another alpha$_2$-adrenergic agonist, increases atrioventricular node block and sinus node dysfunction, especially in combination with β-blockers, and so caution is advised when coprescribing tizanidine with clonidine. When abruptly withdrawn, clonidine has been shown to cause a rebound hypertensive response; by inference, tizanidine may cause these same effects. Tizanidine has been associated with hepatic transaminase level increases in 3% to 5% of patients, so consider monitoring patients with co-occurring underlying liver disease. It is cleared by hepatic CYP1A2 to an inactive metabolite, so drugs that inhibit CYP1A2 may increase tizanidine effects; for this reason coprescribed ciprofloxacin is specifically contraindicated following single-dose studies showing up to 10-fold increases in tizanidine levels with clinically severe hypotensive and sedation response.[109]

Key points: antispasm and antispasticity drugs

- Antispasm drugs have limited evidence for effectiveness, are predominantly sedative, and add polypharmacy to chronic pain management with little benefit.
- Carisoprodol should never be used because of no benefit and high risk.
- When true spasticity is present, as in spinal cord injury and multiple sclerosis, baclofen and tizanidine may be useful.
- Avoid abrupt withdrawal off baclofen because of the potential for severe rhabdomyolysis and fever.

CANNABINOIDS IN PAIN

Despite more than 30 published randomized controlled trials positively supporting moderate efficacy of cannabis in treating pain, albeit most of low quality,[110] and widespread popularity (many American states approve medicinal use and since 2014 3 US states have legalized nonmedicinal use or recreational use), cannabis continues to be designated a schedule 1 drug, which per the US Food and Drug Administration has no medicinal value. This designation has complicated clinical effectiveness research, law enforcement approaches, and patient and prescriber understanding of the potential value and risks of cannabis in the management of pain. The endocannabinoid system includes 2 well-studied receptor types: CB_1 and CB_2.[111,112] Brain and spinal cord G protein–coupled CB_1 receptors exceed opioid receptors 10-fold, and are also present in visceral organs and adipose tissue. CB_2 receptors are found more prominently on hematopoietic and immune cells, although they are present in low concentrations in the periaqueductal gray. At least 60 pharmacologically active cannabinoids have been characterized; the 2 most commonly discussed with attributed analgesic effects are tetrahydrocannabinol (THC), which is most strongly linked to psychoactive effects (including pain), and cannabidiol, which seems mostly to enhance THC effect, possibly via the hepatic cytochrome system. Cannabinoids function as synaptic circuit breakers because CB1 receptor activation inhibits release of acetylcholine, dopamine, and glutamate, and modulates opioid, serotonin, NMDA, and GABA receptors.[113] Most clinical trials use combinations of mixed varieties of cannabinoids and are directed to neuropathic pain.[114] The Guideline Development Subcommittee of the American Academy of Neurology published a recent systematic review.[113] Wade and colleagues[115] reported a 50% pain reduction in patients with multiple sclerosis in a good-quality, open-label, long-term, 1-year follow-up study, following a 10-week randomized controlled trial. Several publications have identified a role of cannabis as an alternative to opioids, with reductions in opioid use[116]; improved opioid pain relief[117]; and, in a recent large state-by-state ecological study, a nearly 25% reduction in mean annual opioid overdose mortality.[118] Significant adverse effects include concern regarding addiction to cannabis and other substances, diminished lifetime activity, increased incidence of motor vehicle accidents, and chronic bronchitis.[119] Wide ranges of provider attitudes and individual clinic-specific policies regarding medical and recreational use of cannabis in the setting of pain abound, in significant part related to legal concerns despite risk/benefit analysis that may favor cannabis use rather than current opioid prescribing practice. A recently published guideline recommends evaluation of cannabis use disorder and, when the diagnosis is present, withholding of opioid prescription for CNCP because of a higher likelihood of opioid misuse from a concurrent addiction diagnosis (Washington State Agency Medical Directors Group [AMDG] opioid guidelines, pending publication, 2015). Note that tobacco use disorder is not considered in a similar rubric despite similar evidence of higher risk and worse outcomes in patients with CNCP on chronic opioids who are addicted to nicotine.[120]

Key points: cannabis use for pain

- Evidence supports use in neuropathic pain conditions
- Demonstrated risks of reduced lifetime achievement, motor vehicle accidents, and addiction
- May reduce opioid requirements and accidental opioid overdose deaths
- Complex regulatory and legal environment

KETAMINE

Ketamine, a potent NMDA receptor antagonist, is a dissociative anesthetic and potent analgesic at subanesthetic doses. Its mechanism of effect is NMDA antagonism, which also interferes with mechanisms of opioid tolerance, voltage-gated calcium channels, and monoamine reuptake.[121] Opioid dose requirements that are significantly lower have been reported in the perioperative setting.[122] Current data cannot be translated into specific treatment regimens. A 2005 Cochrane Review of ketamine found reduced postoperative morphine requirements, reduced postoperative nausea and vomiting, and mild or absent adverse effects.[123] Hallucinations and psychotomimetic adverse effects when they occur can readily be managed emergently in the in-patient setting. Although ketamine is not approved for chronic pain use, based on its demonstrated NMDA antagonism and proposed interference with mechanisms of neuropathic pain, central sensitization, and opioid tolerance, ketamine has been used in a variety of out-patient settings, including oral, buccal, and transdermal compounded formulations.[124] Ketamine infusions have not been found to be effective in fibromyalgia pain.[125] In a 2009 review, Blonk and colleagues[126] concluded that lack of proven effectiveness and high risks "do not support routine use of oral ketamine in chronic pain management. Oral ketamine may have a limited place as add-on therapy in complex chronic pain patients if other therapeutic options have failed." There are reports of a low incidence of ketamine abuse for those seeking "an out-of-body experiences, altered perceptions, prolonged sense of time, and rarely hallucinations."[127]

Key points: ketamine

- NMDA antagonist, approved as a dissociative anesthetic
- Reduces postoperative opioid requirements
- Not approved for chronic pain

OTHER ANALGESIC PRODUCTS

Capsaicin is a transient receptor potential vanilloid (TRPV1) agonist that is useful as a transdermal analgesic and is available in several low-dose products, including OTC (0.025%–0.1%) and prescribed (≥0.25%) creams, gels, and lotions. Its mechanism of effect is defunctionalization of cutaneous nociceptors because of sustained TRPV1 activation.[128] At high dose (8%) it causes temporary neurolysis at the site of application. Because of intense pain with application of this concentrated formulation, the skin area to which it is applied should be pretreated with a topical anesthetic. Capsaicin has been approved for postherpetic neuralgia.

Menthol in combination with methyl salicylate is available as a topical local analgesic, available in several OTC products. Its mechanism of effect is not fully established, with evidence of selective activation of kappa-opioid receptors, reduced nitric oxide release locally, alpha$_{2c}$-adrenergic stimulation following cutaneous transient receptor potential melastatin 8 (TRPM8) activation, and sodium channel blockade.[129–131]

Magnesium is an NMDA antagonist, calcium channel blocker, and inhibits catechol release from peripheral nerve endings. When administered intravenously it has been reported in several small case studies to reduce postoperative pain following nonlaparoscopic abdominal surgery,[132] major lumbar surgeries,[133] and knee arthroscopy.[134] Magnesium taken orally is also a laxative and so can reduce constipation side effects from several routinely used analgesics, including opioids and antidepressants.

REFERENCES

1. Daubresse M, Chang HY, Yu Y, et al. Ambulatory diagnosis and treatment of nonmalignant pain in the United States 2010. Med Care 2013;51:870–8.
2. Von Korff M, Deyo RA. Potent opioids for chronic musculoskeletal pain: flying blind? Pain 2004;109:207–9.
3. Woolf CJ. Central sensitization: implications for the diagnosis and treatment of pain. Pain 2011;152:S2–15.
4. Napadow V, LaCount L, Park K, et al. Intrinsic brain connectivity in fibromyalgia is associated with chronic pain intensity. Arthritis Rheum 2010;62:2545–55.
5. Ossipov MH, Morimura K, Porreca F. Descending pain modulation and chronification of pain. Curr Opin Support Palliat Care 2014;8:143–51.
6. Voscopoulos C, Lema M. When does acute pain become chronic? Br J Anaesth 2010;105(S1):i69–85.
7. Bonica JJ. The need of a taxonomy. Pain 1979;6(3):247–8.
8. Chou R, Fanciullo GJ, Fine PG, et al. Clinical guidelines for the use of chronic opioid therapy in chronic noncancer pain. J Pain 2009;10:113–30.
9. Ballantyne JC, Shin NS. Efficacy of opioids for chronic pain: a review of the evidence. Clin J Pain 2008;24:469–78.
10. Chou R, Deyo R, Devine B, et al. The effectiveness and risks of long-term opioid treatment of chronic pain. Evidence report/technology assessment No. 218. (Prepared by the Pacific Northwest Evidence-Based Practice Center under contract No. 290-2012-00014-I.) AHRQ publication No. 14-E005-EF. Rockville (MD): Agency for Healthcare Research and Quality; 2014. Available at: www.effectivehealthcare.ahrq.gov/reports/final.cfm.
11. Okie S. A flood of opioids, a rising tide of deaths. N Engl J Med 2010;363:1981–5.
12. Saunders KW, Dunn KM, Merrill JO, et al. Relationship of opioid use and dosage levels to fractures in older chronic pain patients. J Gen Intern Med 2010;25:310–5.

13. Walker JM, Famey RJ, Rhondeau SM, et al. Chronic opioid use is a risk factor for the development of central sleep apnea and ataxic breathing. J Clin Sleep Med 2007;15:455–61.
14. Deyo RA, Smith DH, Johnson ES, et al. Prescription opioids for back pain and use of medications for erectile dysfunction. Spine 2013;38(11):909–15.
15. Fishbain DA, Cole B, Lewis JE, et al. Do opioids induce hyperalgesia in humans?: an evidence-based structured review. Pain Med 2009;10:829–39.
16. Argoff CE, Albrecht P, Irving G, et al. Multimodal analgesia for chronic pain: rationale and future directions. Pain Med 2009;10(S2):S53–66.
17. Kroenke K, Spitzer RL, Williams JB. The PHQ-9: validity of a brief depression severity measure. J Gen Intern Med 2001;16:606–13.
18. Spitzer RL, Kroenke K, Williams JB, et al. A brief measure for assessing generalized anxiety disorder: the GAD-7. Arch Intern Med 2006;166:1092–7.
19. Ouimette P, Wade M, Prins A, et al. Identifying PTSD in primary care: comparison of the primary care-PTSD Screen (PC-PTSD) and the general health questionnaire-12 (GHQ). J Anxiety Disord 2008;22:337–43.
20. Chung F, Yegneswaran B, Liao P, et al. STOP questionnaire: a tool to screen patients for obstructive sleep apnea. Anesthesiology 2008;108:812–21.
21. Chou R, Fanciullo GJ, Fine PG, et al. Opioids for chronic noncancer pain: prediction and identification of aberrant drug-related behaviors: a review of the evidence for an American Pain Society and American Academy of Pain Medicine clinical practice guideline. J Pain 2009;10:131–46.
22. Tauben D. Chronic pain management: measurement-based step care solutions. IASP Clin Update 2013;1:1–7.
23. Davies KA, Macfarlane GJ, Nicholl BI, et al. Restorative sleep predicts the resolution of chronic widespread pain. Rheumatology (Oxford) 2008;47:1809–13.
24. Roehrs T, Hyde M, Blaisdell B, et al. Sleep loss and REM sleep loss are hyperalgesic. Sleep 2006;29:145–51.
25. Haack M, Scott-Sutherland J, Santangelo G, et al. Pain sensitivity and modulation in primary insomnia. Eur J Pain 2012;16:522–33.
26. Morin CM, Benca R. Chronic insomnia. Lancet 2012;379:1129–41.
27. Bootzin RR, Epstein DR. Understanding and treating insomnia. Annu Rev Clin Psychol 2011;7:435–58.
28. Smith MT, Perlis ML, Park A, et al. Comparative meta-analysis of pharmacotherapy and behavior therapy for persistent insomnia. Am J Psychiatry 2002; 159:5–11.
29. Sant GR, Propert KJ, Hanno PM, et al, Interstitial Cystitis Clinical Trials Group. A pilot clinical trial of oral pentosan polysulfate and oral hydroxyzine in patients with interstitial cystitis. J Urol 2003;170(3):810.
30. Carette S, Oakson G, Guimont C, et al. Sleep electroencephalography and the clinical response to amitriptyline in patients with fibromyalgia. Arthritis Rheum 1995;38:1211–7.
31. Schweitzer PK. Drugs that disturb sleep and wakefulness. In: Kryger MH, Roth T, Dement WC, editors. Principles and Practice of Sleep Medicine. 4th edition. Philadelphia: Elsevier Saunders; 2005. 542–560; 499–518.
32. Sammaritano M, Sherwin A. Effects of anticonvulsants on sleep. Neurology 2000;54:S16–24.
33. Yang C, White DP, Winkelman JW. Antidepressants and periodic leg movements of sleep. Biol Psychiatry 2005;58:510–4.
34. Dierks MR, Jordan JK, Sheehan AH. Prazosin treatment of nightmares related to posttraumatic stress disorder. Ann Pharmacother 2007;41:1013–7.

35. Denis R, Lavigne G, Smith MT, et al. Pain and Sleep. In: Kryger MH, Roth T, Dement WC, editors. Principles and Practice of Sleep Medicine. 4th edition. Philadelphia: Elsevier Saunders; 2005. p. 1442–51.
36. Sweitzer PK. Drugs that disturb sleep and wakefulness. In: Kryger MH, Roth T, Dement WC, editors. Principles and Practice of Sleep Medicine. 4th edition. Philadelphia: Saunders; 2000. p. 441–61.
37. American Geriatrics Society 2012 Beers Criteria Update Expert Panel. American Geriatrics Society updated Beers criteria for potentially inappropriate medication use in older adults. J Am Geriatr Soc 2012;60(4):616–31.
38. Andersson DA, Gentry C, Alenmyr L, et al. TRPA1 mediates spinal antinociception induced by acetaminophen and the cannabinoid Δ^9-tetrahydrocannabiorcol. Nat Commun 2011;2:551.
39. Ruud LE, Wilhelms DJ, Eskilsson A, et al. Acetaminophen reduces lipopolysaccharide-induced fever by inhibiting cyclooxygenase-2. Neuropharmacology 2013;71:124–9.
40. Chandrasekharan NV, Dai H, Roos LT, et al. COX-3, a cyclooxygenase-1 variant inhibited by acetaminophen and other analgesic/antipyretic drugs: cloning, structure, and expression. Proc Natl Acad Sci U S A 2002;99:13926–31.
41. Bunchorntavakul C, Reddy KR. Acetaminophen-related hepatotoxicity. Clin Liver Dis 2013;17:587–607.
42. Ong C, Seymopur RA, Lirk P, et al. Combining paracetamol (acetaminophen) with nonsteroidal antiinflammatory drugs: a qualitative systematic review of analgesic efficacy for acute postoperative pain. Anesth Analg 2010;110: 1170–9.
43. Kumar G, Hota D, Nahar Saikia U, et al. Evaluation of analgesic efficacy, gastrotoxicity and nephrotoxicity of fixed-dose combinations of nonselective, preferential and selective cyclooxygenase inhibitors with paracetamol in rats. Exp Toxicol Pathol 2010;62:653–62.
44. Roelofs PD, Deyo RA, Koes BW, et al. Non-steroidal anti-inflammatory drugs for low back pain. Cochrane Database Syst Rev 2000;(2):CD000396.
45. Dworkin RH, O'Conner AB, Backonja M, et al. Pharmacologic management of neuropathic pain: evidence-based recommendations. Pain 2007;132:237–51.
46. Gibson GR, Whitacre EB, Ricotti CA. Colitis induced by nonsteroidal anti-inflammatory drugs: report of four cases and review of the literature. Arch Intern Med 1992;152:625.
47. Kefalakes H, Stylianides TJ, Amanakis G, et al. Exacerbation of inflammatory bowel diseases associated with the use of nonsteroidal anti-inflammatory drugs: myth or reality? Eur J Clin Pharmacol 2009;65:963–70.
48. Gold MS, Gebhart GF. Nociceptor sensitization in pain pathogenesis. Nat Med 2010;16:1248–57.
49. Stevenson DD, Sanchez-Borges M, Szczeklik A. Classification of allergic and pseudoallergic reactions to drugs that inhibit cyclooxygenase enzymes. Ann Allergy Asthma Immunol 2001;87:177.
50. Borer JS, Simon LS. Cardiovascular and gastrointestinal effects of Cox-2 inhibitors and NDAIDS: achieving a balance. Arthritis Res Ther 2005;7: S14–22.
51. McCarberg BH, Cryer B. Evolving strategies to improve anti-inflammatory drug safety. Am J Ther 2014;21:441–553.
52. McGettigan P, Henry D. Cardiovascular risk and inhibition of cyclooxygenase: a systematic review of the observational studies of selective and nonselective inhibitors of cyclooxygenase 2. JAMA 2006;296:1633.

53. Grover SA, Coupal L, Zowall H. Treating osteoarthritis with cyclooxygenase-2-specific inhibitors: what are the benefits of avoiding blood pressure destabilization? Hypertension 2005;45(1):92.
54. Trelle S, Reichenbach S, Wandel S, et al. Cardiovascular safety of non-steroidal anti-inflammatory drugs: network meta-analysis. BMJ 2011;342:c7086.
55. Bhala N, Emberson J, Merhi A, et al. Coxib and traditional NSAID Trialists Collaborative. Vascular and upper gastrointestinal effects of non-steroidal anti-inflammatory drugs: meta-analyses of individual participant data from randomised trials. Lancet 2013;382(9894):769.
56. Chan AT, Manson JE, Albert CM, et al. Nonsteroidal antiinflammatory drugs, acetaminophen, and the risk of cardiovascular events. Circulation 2006;113:1578.
57. Dodwell ER, Latorre JG, Parisini E, et al. NSAID exposure and risk of nonunion: a meta-analysis of case-control and cohort studies. Calcif Tissue Int 2010;87(3):193.
58. Dimmen S, Engebretsen L, Nordsletten L, et al. Negative effects of parecoxib and indomethacin on tendon healing: an experimental study in rats. Knee Surg Sports Traumatol Arthrosc 2009;17(7):835.
59. Zizic TM, Marcoux C, Hungerford DS, et al. Corticosteroid therapy associated with ischemic necrosis of bone in systemic lupus erythematosus. Am J Med 1985;79(5):596.
60. Verdu B, Decosterd I, Buclin T, et al. Antidepressants for the treatment of chronic pain. Drugs 2008;68:2611–32.
61. Moore RA, Derry S, Aldington D, et al. Amitriptyline for neuropathic pain and fibromyalgia in adults (review). Cochrane Database Syst Rev 2012;(12):CD008242.
62. McCleane G. Antidepressants as analgesics. CNS Drugs 2008;22:139–56.
63. Saarto T, Wiffen PJ. J Neurol Neurosurg Psychiatry 2010;81:1372–3.
64. O'Malley PG, Balden E, Tomkins G, et al. Treatment of fibromyalgia with antidepressants: a meta-analysis. J Gen Intern Med 2000;15:659–66.
65. Rolan PE. Understanding the pharmacology of headache. Curr Opin Pharmacol 2014;14:30–3.
66. Jackson JL, Shimeall W, Sessums L, et al. Tricyclic antidepressants and headaches: systematic review and meta-analysis. BMJ 2010;341:c5222.
67. Kroenke K, Krebs EE, Bair MJ. Pharmacotherapy of chronic pain: a synthesis of recommendations from systematic reviews. Gen Hosp Psychiatry 2009;31:206–19.
68. Fall M, Baranowski AP, Elnell S, et al. EAU guidelines on chronic pelvic pain. Eur Urol 2010;57:35–48.
69. Ophoven A, Pokupic S, Heinecke A, et al. A prospective, randomized, placebo controlled, double blind study of amitriptyline for the treatment of interstitial cystitis. J Urol 2004;172:533–6.
70. Melzack R, Wall PD. Pain mechanisms: a new theory. Science 1965;150:971–9.
71. De Felice M, Sanoja R, Wang R, et al. Engagement of descending inhibition from the rostral ventromedial medulla protects against chronic neuropathic pain. Pain 2011;152:2701–9.
72. Millan MJ. Descending control of pain. Prog Neurobiol 2002;66:355–474.
73. Rempe T, Wolff S, Riedel C, et al. Spinal fMRI reveals decreased descending inhibition during secondary mechanical hyperalgesia. PLoS One 2014;9(11):e112325.
74. Acikalin A, Sagtat S, Avc A, et al. QTc intervals in drug poisoning patients with tricyclic antidepressants and selective serotonin reuptake inhibitors. Am J Ther 2010;17:30–3.

75. Jasiak NM, Bostwick JR. Risk of QT/QTc prolongation among newer non-SNRI antidepressants. Ann Pharmacother 2014;48:1620–8.
76. Beach SR, Kostis WJ, Celano CM. Meta-analysis of selective serotonin reuptake inhibitor-associated QTc. J Clin Psychiatry 2014;75(5):e441–9.
77. Rowbotham MC, Twilling L, Davies PS, et al. Oral opioid therapy for chronic peripheral and central neuropathic pain. N Engl J Med 2003;348:1223–32.
78. Richebe P, Beaulieu P. Perioperative pain management in the patient treated with opioids: continuing professional development. Can J Anaesth 2009;56: 969–81.
79. Davies P. Medication overuse headache: a silent pandemic. Pain 2012;153:7–8.
80. Yunus MB. Fibromyalgia and overlapping disorders: the unifying concept of central sensitivity syndromes. Semin Arthritis Rheum 2007;36:339–56.
81. Clauw DJ. Fibromyalgia: a clinical review. JAMA 2014;311:1547–55.
82. Schmidt-Wilcke T, Clauw DJ. Fibromyalgia: from pathology to therapy. Nat Rev Rheumatol 2011;7:518–27.
83. Brummett CM, Janda AM, Schueller CM, et al. Survey criteria for fibromyalgia independently predict increased postoperative opioid consumption after lower-extremity joint arthroplasty: a prospective, observational cohort study. Anesthesiology 2013;119:1434–43.
84. McBeth J, Macfarlane GJ, Benjamin S, et al. The association between tender points, psychological distress, and adverse childhood experiences: a community-based study. Arthritis Rheum 1999;42:1397–404.
85. Phifer J, Skelton K, Weiss T, et al. Pain symptomatology and pain medication use in civilian PTSD. Pain 2011;152:2233–40.
86. Deisseroth K, Hart RA. Symptoms of post-traumatic stress following elective lumbar spinal arthrodesis. Spine 2012;37:1628–33.
87. Jones C, Backman C, Capuzzo M, et al. Precipitants of post-traumatic stress disorder following intensive care: a hypothesis generating study of diversity in care. Intensive Care Med 2007;33:978–85.
88. Baron R. Mechanisms of disease: neuropathic pain - a clinical perspective. Nat Clin Pract Neurol 2006;2:95–106.
89. Finnerup NB, Sindrup SH, Jensen TS. Chronic neuropathic pain: mechanisms, drug targets and measurement. Fundam Clin Pharmacol 2007;21:129–36.
90. Vaillancourt PD, Langevin HM. Painful peripheral neuropathies. Med Clin North Am 1999;83:627–42.
91. Attal N, Cruccu G, Baron R, et al. EFNS guidelines on the pharmacological treatment of neuropathic pain: 2010 revision. Eur J Neurol 2010;17:1113–23.
92. Cummins TR, Waxman SG. Sodium channels in pain pharmacology. In: Beaulieu P, Lussier D, Porreca F, et al, editors. Pharmacology of pain. Seattle: IASP Press; 2010. p. 139–62.
93. O'Connor AB, Dworkin RH. Treatment of neuropathic pain: an overview of recent guidelines. Am J Med 2009;122:S22–32.
94. Chong MS, Libretto SE. The rationale and use of topiramate for treating neuropathic pain. Clin J Pain 2003;19(1):59–68.
95. Üçeyler N, Sommer C, Walitt B, et al. Anticonvulsants in fibromyalgia syndrome. Cochrane Database Syst Rev 2013;(16):CD010782.
96. Freeman R, Durso-DeCruz E, Emir B. Efficacy, safety, and tolerability of pregabalin treatment for painful diabetic peripheral neuropathy. Diabetes Care 2008; 7:1448–54.
97. Cheong YC, Smotra G, Williams AC. Non-surgical interventions for the management of chronic pelvic pain. Cochrane Database Syst Rev 2014;(3):CD008797.

98. Piche M, Arsenault M, Poitras P, et al. Widespread hypersensitivity is related to altered pain inhibition processes in irritable bowel syndrome. Pain 2010;148: 49–58.
99. Grosen K, Drewes AM, Hojsgaard A, et al. Perioperative gabapentin for the prevention of persistent pain after thoracotomy: a randomized controlled trial. Eur J Cardiothorac Surg 2014;46:76–85.
100. Poylin V, Quinn J, Messer K, et al. Gabapentin significantly decreases posthemorrhoidectomy pain: a prospective study. Int J Colorectal Dis 2014;29:1565–9.
101. Rivkin A, Rivkin MA. Perioperative nonopioid agents for pain control in spinal surgery. Am J Health Syst Pharm 2014;71:1845–57.
102. Larsen MS, Frolund S, Nohr MK, et al. In vivo and in vitro evaluations of intestinal gabapentin absorption: effect of dose and inhibitors on carrier-mediated transport. Pharm Res 2015;32:898–909.
103. Available at: http://www.cdc.gov/HomeandRecreationalSafety/overdose/guidelines. html. Accessed March 02, 2015.
104. Johnson EW. The myth of skeletal muscle spasm. Am J Phys Med Rehabil 1989; 68:1.
105. Tulder MW, Touray T, Furlan AD, et al. Muscle relaxants for non-specific lowback pain: a systematic review within the framework of the Cochrane collaboration. Spine 2003;28:1978–92.
106. Khorasani A, Peruzzi WT. Dantrolene treatment for abrupt intrathecal baclofen withdrawal. Anesth Analg 1995;80(5):1054–6.
107. Malanga G, Reiter RD, Garay E. Update on tizanidine for muscle spasticity and emerging indications. Expert Opin Pharmacother 2008;9(12):2209–15.
108. Ma W, Zhang Y, Bantel C, et al. Medium and large injured dorsal root ganglion cells increase TRPV-1, accompanied by increased α2C-adrenoceptor coexpression and functional inhibition by clonidine. Pain 2005;113:386–94.
109. Granfors MT, Backman JT, Neuvonen M, et al. Ciprofloxacin greatly increases concentrations and hypotensive effect of tizanidine by inhibiting its cytochrome P450 1A2-mediated presystemic metabolism. Clin Pharmacol Ther 2004;76(6): 598–606.
110. Robinson J. Cannabinoids: efficacy and safety. University of Washington CME. Meeting the challenge of chronic pain management in the primary care setting. Shoreline WA, November 8, 2014.
111. Fontelles M, Garcia CC. Role of cannabinoids in the management of neuropathic pain. CNS Drugs 2008;22:645–53.
112. Starowicz K, DiMarzo V. Non-psychotropic analgesic drugs from the endocannabinoid system: "magic bullet" or "multiple target" strategies? Eur J Pharmacol 2013;716:41–53.
113. Koppel BS, Brust J, Fife T, et al. Systematic review: efficacy and safety of medical marijuana in selected neurologic disorders. Neurology 2014;82: 1556–63.
114. Aggarwal SK. Cannabinergic pain medicine: a concise clinical primer and survey of randomized-controlled trial results. Clin J Pain 2013;29:162–71.
115. Wade DT, Makela PM, House H, et al. Long-term use of a cannabis-based medicine in the treatment of spasticity and other symptoms in multiple sclerosis. Mult Scler 2006;12:639–45.
116. Lucas P. Cannabis as an adjunct to or substitute for opioids in the treatment of chronic pain. J Psychoactive Drugs 2012;44:125–33.
117. Abrams DI, Couey P, Shade SB, et al. Cannabinoid-opioid interaction in chronic pain. Clin Pharmacol Ther 2011;90:844–51.

118. Bachhuber MA, Saloner B, Cunningham CO, et al. Medical cannabis laws and opioid analgesic mortality in the United States, 1999-2010. JAMA Intern Med 2014;174:1668–73.

119. Volkow ND, Compton WM, Weiss SR. Adverse health effects of marijuana use. N Engl J Med 2014;371:879.

120. Hooten WM, Townsend CO, Bruce BK, et al. The effects of smoking status on opioid tapering among patients with chronic pain. Anesth Analg 2009;108(1): 308–15.

121. Ben-Ari A, Lewis MC, Davidson E. Chronic administration of ketamine for analgesia. J Pain Palliat Care Pharmacother 2007;21:7–14.

122. Elia N, Tramer MR. Ketamine and postoperative pain: a quantitative systematic review of randomised trials. Pain 2005;113:61–70.

123. Bell RF, Dahl JB, Moore RA, et al. Peri-operative ketamine for acute postoperative pain: a quantitative and qualitative systematic review (Cochrane Review). Acta Anaesthesiol Scand 2005;49:1405–28.

124. Visser E, Schug SA. The role of ketamine in pain management. Biomed Pharmacother 2006;60:341–8.

125. Noppers I, Niesters M, Swartjes M, et al. Absence of long-term analgesic effect from a short-term S-ketamine infusion on fibromyalgia pain: a randomized, prospective, double blind, active placebo-controlled trial. Eur J Pain 2011;15: 942–9.

126. Blonk MI, Koder B, Van den Bemt P, et al. Use of oral ketamine in chronic pain management: a review. Eur J Pain 2010;14(5):466–72.

127. Bokor G, Anderson PD. Ketamine: an update on its abuse. J Pharm Pract 2014; 27:582–6.

128. Anand P, Bley K. Topical capsaicin for pain management: therapeutic potential and mechanisms of action of the new high-concentration capsaicin 8% patch. Br J Anaesth 2011;107:490–502.

129. Galeotti N, Di Cesare Mannelli L, Mazzanti G, et al. Menthol, a natural analgesic compound. Neurosci Lett 2002;12:145–8.

130. Topp R, Winchester LJ, Schilero J, et al. Effect of topical menthol on ipsilateral and contralateral superficial blood flow following a bout of maximum voluntary muscle contraction. Int J Sports Phys Ther 2011;6:83–91.

131. Haeseler G, Maue D, Grosskreutz, et al. Voltage-dependent block of neuronal and skeletal muscle sodium channels by thymol and menthol. Eur J Anaesthesiol 2002;19:571–9.

132. Moharari RS, Motalbi M, Najafi A, et al. Magnesium can decrease postoperative physiological ileus and postoperative pain in major non laparoscopic gastrointestinal surgeries: a randomized controlled trial. Anesth Pain Med 2013;4: e12750.

133. Levaux C, Bonhomme V, Dewandre PY, et al. Effect of intra-operative magnesium sulphate on pain relief and patient comfort after major lumbar orthopaedic surgery. Anaesthesia 2003;58:131–5.

134. Koinig H, Wallner T, Marhofer P, et al. Magnesium sulfate reduces intra- and postoperative analgesic requirements. Anesth Analg 1998;87:206–10.

Injections for Chronic Pain

Virtaj Singh, MD[a],*, Andrea Trescot, MD[b], Isuta Nishio, MD[c]

KEYWORDS

- Chronic pain • Regenerative injections • Trigger point injections • Botulinum toxins

KEY POINTS

- Even in the setting of chronic pain, various injections can still have a useful role in facilitating a rehabilitation program.
- Spinal injections, such as epidural steroid injections and facet joint injections, are among the most commonly used procedures in most pain practices; but a growing number of practices are considering less common injections, such as trigger point injections, regenerative injections/prolotherapy, and injections using botulinum toxins.

INTRODUCTION

Although interventional procedures should be used cautiously in the setting of chronic pain, there is a role for a variety of injections to facilitate patients' overall rehabilitation program. There are many resources available, including a prior edition of *Physical Medicine and Rehabilitation Clinics of North America*, which discuss the more conventional spinal injections. The focus of this article is on lesser-known injection options for treating chronic pain. The authors separately discuss trigger point injections (TPIs), regenerative injections (prolotherapy), and injections using botulinum toxins (BTx).

TRIGGER POINT INJECTIONS

Myofascial pain syndrome (MPS) is a common musculoskeletal pain syndrome characterized by a myofascial trigger point (MTrP) at muscle, fascia, or tendinous insertions. A MTrP is a hyperirritable tender spot, frequently associated with taut band that, on palpation, is firmer in consistency than adjacent muscle fibers. When compressed, an MTrP may cause patient vocalization or a visible withdrawal (which is known as the jump sign).

[a] Department of Rehabilitation Medicine, Seattle Spine & Sports Medicine, University of Washington, 3213 Eastlake Avenue East, Suite A, Seattle, WA 98102, USA; [b] Pain and Headache Center, 5431 Mayflower Lane, Suite 4, Wasilla, AK 99654, USA; [c] Department of Anesthesiology and Pain Medicine, VA Puget Sound Health Care System, University of Washington, 1660 South Columbian Way, S-112-Anes, Seattle, WA 98108, USA
* Corresponding author.
E-mail address: vsingh@seattlespine.com

Phys Med Rehabil Clin N Am 26 (2015) 249–261
http://dx.doi.org/10.1016/j.pmr.2015.01.004
1047-9651/15/$ – see front matter © 2015 Elsevier Inc. All rights reserved.

Stretching and exercise are the foundation of treatment and management of MPS; however, for refractory cases, needle therapy may be offered. This therapy may include TPIs (using local anesthetics, corticosteroids, and/or BTx), dry needling (DN) (intramuscular stimulation [IMS]), and acupuncture.

Local Anesthetics

Despite the popularity of TPIs, there is no conclusive evidence that demonstrates superior effectiveness of TPIs over DN in the treatment of MPS.[1,2] One systematic review of randomized controlled trials found that direct injection to MTrPs was indeed effective but that the nature of the injected substance did not influence the outcome; hence, the investigators concluded that the beneficial effects of TPIs were likely the result of needle insertion or placebo.[1] However, another review showed short-term benefits of TPIs with lidocaine that were superior to DN or placebo.[3] It is conceivable that local pain and soreness associated with needling can be ameliorated with local anesthetic injection.[2]

Corticosteroids

Although inflammation may play a role in MPS, there is no evidence that the injection of corticosteroid provides any enhanced benefits.[4] In addition, corticosteroids carry the risk of local muscle necrosis and adrenal suppression. Thus, the use of corticosteroids for TPIs is not recommended.

Botulinum Toxin

Botulinum toxin (BTx) is a potent neurotoxin produced by the bacterium *Clostridium botulinum* that blocks acetylcholine release into the neuromuscular junction, leading to prolonged muscle relaxation (typically lasting 3 to 4 months). BTx is used for a variety of pain procedures as discussed separately in this article later. Briefly, the authors discuss the use of BTx in TPIs.

In TPIs, BTx is thought to reduce muscular ischemia and free entrapped nerve endings. Central and peripheral antinociceptive properties of BTx have also been postulated. Despite these mechanisms that could theoretically offer a benefit for patients with MPS, the use of BTx injections for myofascial trigger points is controversial. Meta-analyses of randomized trials in patients with neck pain have found no benefit of BTx intramuscular injections in the short-term (4 weeks) or long-term (6 months) when compared with placebo.[5,6] Although a recent review[7] showed inconclusive evidence regarding the effectiveness of BTx in the treatment of MPS, an older Cochrane review found moderate evidence that BTx injections are *not* effective.[3] In sum, given the high cost of the medication and questionable evidence for its efficacy, cost and clinical value should be carefully assessed before considering BTx injections for MPS.

Dry Needling

Dry needling (DN) (also known as intramuscular stimulation [IMS]) involves the practice of using a small-gauge needle (sometimes acupuncture needles) to irritate the MTrP without injecting any substance (as opposed to those discussed earlier). Systemic reviews and meta-analyses of randomized controlled trials suggest that DN is an effective therapy for MPS.[1,8,9] If DN is used to specifically target MTrPs, it is most effective when a local twitch response (LTR) (brisk contraction of the taut band) is elicited.[10] A fast-in-fast-out technique has been advocated to elicit a maximal number of LTRs. The needle penetrates the taut band of the muscle, is withdrawn to superficial subcutaneous tissue, then redirected to another area in proximity (**Fig. 1**). Deep DN to the

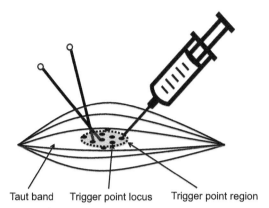

Taut band   Trigger point locus   Trigger point region

Fig. 1. TPIs and DN to myofascial trigger point. (*Courtesy of* Isuta Nishio, MD.)

muscle (eg, 15 mm) has been shown to be more effective than superficial DN (eg, 2 mm).[11]

Acupuncture

Acupuncture is an increasingly popular treatment of a broad spectrum of chronic conditions, including chronic pain. However, the number of needles used, the frequency of sessions, stimulation frequency, and current amplitude to obtain optimal efficacy remains a matter of debate. A Cochrane review found that, in the short-term, acupuncture is more effective for chronic low back pain and neck pain compared to no treatment or sham acupuncture.[12] Other meta-analyses have also demonstrated the effectiveness of acupuncture for chronic pain when compared with no acupuncture or sham (needles placed in non-acupuncture sites).[13,14]

The data suggest that the benefits of acupuncture are clinically relevant and greater than placebo; however, the observed differences in effectiveness between acupuncture and sham acupuncture are smaller than those between acupuncture and no acupuncture. This pattern of findings indicates that the nonspecific physiologic and psychological effects of needling may be more important than the actual acupuncture technique itself.[14,15]

Needing Therapy: Mechanism of Action

The exact mechanism by which DN relieves MTrP and MPS has yet to be fully elucidated. DN has been shown to diminish spontaneous electrical activity when LTR is elicited.[16] Hong and Simons[17] suggested that LTR or referred pain seems to be mediated through a spinal reflex in response to stimulation of a sensitive locus (nociceptor) that is in the vicinity of an active locus (motor end plate). Because DN is most effective when LTR is elicited,[4] it is theorized that DN may relieve MTrP via inhibition of dysfunctional activity in the motor end plate of the skeletal muscle motor neuron.

Acupuncture has been used for various pain conditions in addition to MPS. There is increasing evidence of correlations and similarities between MTrPs and acupuncture points in terms of their distribution and referred pain patterns.[18,19] An electrophysiologic study showed that some acupuncture points are indeed MTrPs.[20] Acupuncture analgesia seems to be a manifestation of integrative processes at different levels of the central nervous system (CNS).[21] The gate control theory (Melzack and Wall[22]) may in part explain these processes; namely, the theory postulates that nonnoxious sensory input (eg, touch, pressure, vibration) into the CNS can modulate pain perception by activating inhibitory interneurons.[22] Furthermore, the possible role of endogenous opioids has been implicated in both TPIs and acupuncture as their analgesic effects can be in part reversed by naloxone.[23,24]

Key Points

- There is no firm evidence that TPIs are superior to DN or acupuncture for MPS; however, TPIs with local anesthetic may offer additional benefits via relieving pain associated with soreness from the needling procedure itself.
- There is no strong evidence to support the use of corticosteroid or BTx in TPIs.
- DN seems to be effective for MPS, especially when LTR is elicited.
- Acupuncture seems to be effective for chronic pain, but nonspecific physiologic and psychological effects may play a significant role in its benefits.
- The mechanism of action in needling therapy seems to be multifactorial, including integrative CNS processes and endogenous opioid peptides.

REGENERATIVE INJECTIONS

Regenerative injection therapy (RIT) encompasses a spectrum of injection treatments designed to stimulate repair of damaged tissue. These injections range from prolotherapy (which provides a mild neurolytic effect followed by a complex restorative process with biochemically induced collagen regeneration), to platelet-rich plasma ([PRP], which uses autologous blood that has been spun down to separate out the platelets), to even stem cells (which can be autologous or banked).

In 1956, George Hackett[25] introduced the term *fibroproliferative therapy* or *prolotherapy*, defined as "the rehabilitation of an incompetent structure by generation of new cellular tissue."[25] He proposed this new name because the term *sclerotherapy* that had been used previously implied scar formation rather than regeneration. In the same text, he published composite pain maps generated from ligaments and tendons, which have unfortunately remained largely unknown to the medical community (**Fig. 2**). Contemporary understanding of the basic science of regenerative medicine is that the regenerative/reparative healing process consists of 3 overlapping phases: *inflammatory*, *proliferative* with granulation, and *remodeling* with contraction (**Fig. 3**). The regenerative and reparative stages extend beyond the proliferative stage. The term RIT was originally coined by Felix Linetskey, MD to replace the name prolotherapy; but authors have used both terms to describe any of the treatments described next.

The first of these techniques, *RIT/prolotherapy* stimulates chemo-modulation of collagen by repetitive induction of inflammatory and proliferative stages, which leads to tissue regeneration and repair. As a result, the tensile strength, elasticity, mass, and load-bearing capacity of collagenous connective tissues increases. The proliferant, which can be any of a number solutions (including dextrose/lidocaine, dextrose/phenol/glycerin, sodium morrhuate, and pumice), creates an inflammatory reaction, thereby generating new tissue at the fibro-osseous junction. Hormones and multiple growth factors mediate this complex process. **Fig. 4** shows rabbit tendon hypertrophy after prolotherapy.[26]

The next technique, *RIT/PRP* relies on the injection of concentrated platelets that release growth factors to stimulate recovery in nonhealing soft tissues. Autologous blood is collected and centrifuged; the portion that contains a high proportion of platelets is syphoned off and injected into the tendon and ligament attachments at the enthesopathy site.

RIT/stem cell injection involves utilization of autologous adult pluripotent mesenchymal stem cells from an individual's bone marrow or adipose tissue as the

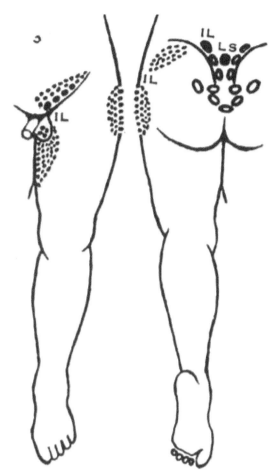

Fig. 2. Example of Hackett pain patterns. (*Courtesy of* Felix Linetsky, MD.)

proliferating solution. Alternatively, banked placental stem cells are beginning to come onto the market, facilitating stem cell procurement.

Indications for RIT are listed in **Box 1**. Appropriate presenting complaints are diverse. These include occipital and suboccipital headaches; pain in the posterior midline and paramedial cervical spine, the cervicothoracic spine, the thoracic spine,

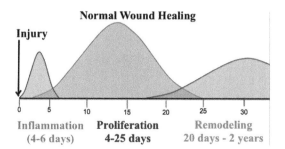

Fig. 3. Stages of wound healing. (*Courtesy of* Andrea Trescot, MD.)

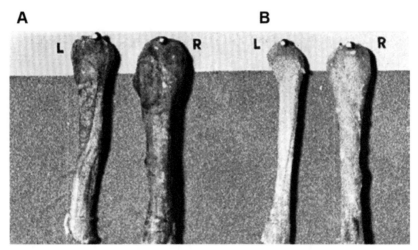

Fig. 4. Rabbit tendons after RIT (the left [L] is the untreated control and the right [R] is the treated side); (*A*) is after 6 weeks and (*B*) is after 3 months. (*Courtesy of* Felix Linetsky, MD.)

the thoracolumbar spine, the lumbar spine, the lumbosacral spine, the scapula, and the shoulder regions; pain between the shoulder blades, in the low back, buttocks, sacroiliac, trochanteric areas, and any combination of the aforementioned complaints.

The onset of pain may be sudden or gradual; the intensity, duration, and quality of pain are variable but usually associated with a traumatic event. Physical examination may reveal postural abnormalities, functional asymmetries, as well as combinations of kyphoscoliosis, flattening of cervical and lumbar lordosis, or arm and/or leg length discrepancies. Variable combinations of flexion/extension, rotation, lateral bending, and/

Box 1
Indications for RIT

1. Painful enthesopathies, tendinosis, or ligamentosis from overuse and occupational and postural conditions known as repetitive motion disorders

2. Painful enthesopathies, tendinosis, or ligamentosis secondary to sprains or strains

3. Painful hypermobility, instability, and subluxation of the axial joints secondary to ligament laxity accompanied by restricted range of motion at reciprocal segments that improve temporarily with manipulation

4. Vertebral compression fractures with a wedge deformity that exert additional stress on the posterior ligamento-tendinous complex

5. Recurrent painful rib subluxations at the costotransverse, costovertebral, and sternochondral articulations

6. Osteoarthritis, spondylosis, and spondylolisthesis

7. Postsurgical cervical, thoracic, and low back pain (with or without instrumentation)

8. Posterior column sources of nociception refractory to steroid injections, nonsteroidal antiinflammatory therapy, and radiofrequency procedures

9. Enhancement of manipulative treatment and physiotherapy

10. Internal disk derangement

or contractions under load can provoke pain. By correcting the ligament laxity that creates the anterior pressure on the disk (causing the disk to bulge posteriorly) and the
facet instability (which causes spondylosis and reflex muscle contracture, leading to
nerve entrapment), the underlying process can be halted and potentially reversed.
These regenerative injections can be, and have been used, to treat painful conditions
from head to toe (**Fig. 5**).

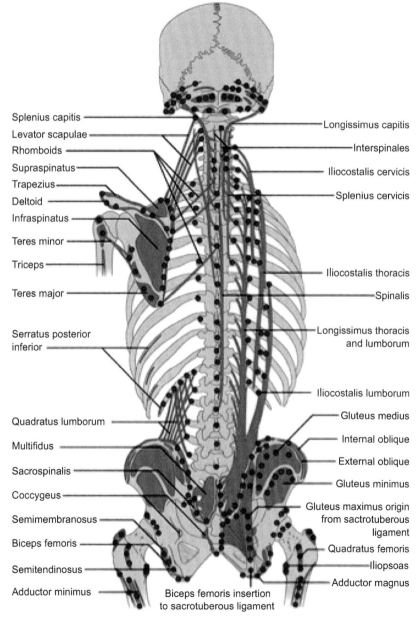

Fig. 5. RIT injection sites. (*Courtesy of* Felix Linetsky, MD.)

The exquisite tenderness at the fibro-osseous junction (enthesis) is the pertinent subjective clinical finding. These areas of tenderness are identified and marked to become the site of infiltration with local anesthetic. The initial needle placement at the fibro-osseous junction usually reproduces the pain, which temporarily worsens during infiltration of the local anesthetic and typically subsides within a few seconds after infiltration. Determination of abolishment or persistence of tenderness, plus the local or referred pain (which objectifies the finding of tenderness), concludes the clinical examination and becomes the basis for clinical diagnosis and further RIT procedures. The proliferant (dextrose/lidocaine for prolotherapy, platelets for PRP, or stem cells) can be injected subsequently or (with the dextrose) at the same time.

RIT has been the subject of multiple published articles, including systematic reviews, randomized trials, and numerous nonrandomized publications, which include prospective and retrospective clinical studies as well as case reports. In a systematic review of prolotherapy injections for chronic low back pain,[27] the investigators included 4 randomized trials[28] that were considered high quality, with a total of 344 patients. Two of the four studies showed significant differences between the treatment and control groups with regard to the proportion of individuals who reported more than 50% reduction in pain or disability; however, the results of these studies could not be pooled. In addition, in one study, co-interventions confounded independent evaluation of results. In the second study of the review, there was no significant difference in mean pain and disability scores between the groups. In the third study, there was little or no difference between the groups with regard to the number of individuals who reported more than 50% improvement in pain and disability. Reporting only mean pain and disability scores, the fourth study showed no difference between groups. The authors of this systematic review concluded that there was conflicting evidence regarding the efficacy of prolotherapy injections in reducing pain and disability in patients with chronic low back pain. They also concluded that, in the presence of co-interventions, prolotherapy injections were more effective than placebo injections, and were yet more effective when both injections and co-interventions were controlled concurrently. In addition, there is substantial evidence for the effectiveness of prolotherapy from nonrandomized prospective and retrospective studies as well as case reports.[29-41] In sum, the extant literature, although it does not offer convincing evidence as to the overall efficacy of prolotherapy, does offer moderate evidence to show its effectiveness in select patients when used with appropriate technique and co-interventions.

Contraindications to RIT include general contraindications that are applicable to all injection techniques; specific contraindications for RIT are listed in **Box 2**. Complications do occur with RIT (as with any injection treatment), but statistically they are rare. There were several serious injuries in the 1950s when untrained providers injected toxic agents into the spinal column.[42-44] The most recent statistical data are from a survey of 450 physicians who perform RIT/prolotherapy.[45] Of the estimated 450,000 patients treated (each with at least 3 visits and at least 10 sites of injection), there were 29 incidences of pneumothorax, 2 of which required chest tube placement (risk of pneumothorax = 1 per 18,333 injections). There were also 24 non–life-threatening allergic reactions; postdural puncture headaches,[46] end plate fractures (after intradiscal dextrose),[47] sterile meningitis,[48] and cervical spine injuries[49] have also been described.

Although risk is inherent in any active intervention, regeneration of worn, frayed, and lax ligaments and tendons holds the promise of treating the cause of the pain rather than just masking it or ablating the nerves that innervate it. Through the use of the body's own healing power, RIT holds the promise of restoration of function and reduction in pain.

Box 2
Contraindications for RIT

General contraindications

Allergy to anesthetic solutions

Bacterial infection, systemic or localized to the region to be injected

Bleeding diathesis secondary to disease or anticoagulants

Fear of the procedure or needle phobia

Neoplastic lesions involving the musculature and osseous structures

Recent onset of a progressive neurologic deficit

Requests for large quantity of sedation and/or opioids before and after treatment

Severe exacerbation of pain or lack of improvement after local anesthetic blocks

Specific contraindications

Acute arthritis (septic, gout, rheumatoid, or posttraumatic with hemarthrosis)

Acute bursitis or tendonitis

Acute nonreduced subluxations, dislocations, or fractures

Allergy to injectable solutions or their ingredients, such as dextrose (corn), sodium morrhuate (fish), or phenol

---

Key Points

- RIT encompasses a spectrum of injection treatments designed to stimulate repair of damaged tissue.
- Contemporary understanding of the basic science of regenerative medicine is that the regenerative/reparative healing process consists of 3 overlapping phases: *inflammatory*, *proliferative* with granulation, and *remodeling* with contraction.
- Appropriate presenting complaints are diverse and include occipital and suboccipital headaches; pain in the posterior midline and paramedial cervical spine, the cervicothoracic spine, the thoracic spine, the thoracolumbar spine, the lumbar spine, the lumbosacral spine, the scapula, and the shoulder regions; pain between the shoulder blades, pain in the low back, buttocks, sacroiliac, trochanteric areas; and any combination of the aforementioned complaints.
- The extant literature, although it does not offer convincing evidence as to the overall efficacy of prolotherapy, does offer moderate evidence to show its effectiveness in select patients when used with appropriate technique and co-interventions.

BOTULINUM TOXIN (BTx) injection

Injectable BTx is frequently used in both physiatric and pain practices. In general physiatry, it is commonly used to treat spasticity, such as that found after a stroke or spinal cord injury. Within pain practices, it is used for a variety of pain syndromes and is often used off-label. The mechanism of action and other theoretic aspects of these toxins are discussed earlier in this article as is their use for TPIs (which is also considered off-label). BTx comes in a variety of formulations, including type A (Botox, Dysport, and Xeomin) and type B (Myobloc). Botox is Food and Drug Administration (FDA) approved for use in migraine headaches (as discussed elsewhere in this edition). For the remainder of the current article, the authors focus on the use of BTx for cervical dystonia, thoracic outlet syndrome, and piriformis syndrome.

In addition to having received FDA approval for migraine headaches, some forms of BTx are FDA approved for use in cervical dystonia. Cervical dystonia, also known as *spasmodic torticollis*, is a cervical spine condition characterized by involuntary contractions of the neck and/or shoulder muscles resulting in abnormal head postures. Neck pain is often an associated symptom in cervical dystonia. BTx injections have been shown in multiple randomized controlled trials to effectively relieve the involuntary contractions, spasms, and pain associated with this condition.[50]

Thoracic outlet syndrome (which may actually be a variant of cervical dystonia) is another condition in which the use of BTx injections may be indicated. Thoracic outlet syndrome is a controversial diagnosis characterized by neurovascular compression within the thoracic outlet. This condition often results from a combination of hypertonic/dystonic muscles, especially the anterior and middle scalenes. Injecting BTx into these muscles has been shown to effectively relieve the symptoms of thoracic outlet syndrome.[51] Although BTx is not FDA approved for the treatment of thoracic outlet syndrome, if the thoracic outlet syndrome is a secondary condition caused by cervical dystonia, then one could make a case for the use of BTx as an FDA approved indication in this scenario.

Piriformis syndrome is another controversial diagnosis. It is characterized by sciatic nerve irritation/compression from presumed hypertonicity of the piriformis muscle. Typical patients describe a deep pain in the buttock and can have symptoms that mimic those associated with a classic L5 and/or S1 radiculopathy. Some clinicians refer to piriformis syndrome as *pseudosciatica*. In addition to piriformis syndrome being a controversial diagnosis, the treatment is similarly controversial, especially with the use of BTx. If priformis syndrome is indeed caused by piriformis hypertonicity, BTx would likely be effective in reducing the hypertonicity and taking pressure off the sciatic nerve. This use is currently off-label, but several studies do demonstrate the effectiveness of BTx for this condition.[52,53]

Key Points

- BTx can be used for various pain diagnoses, including migraines, cervical dystonia, thoracic outlet syndrome, and piriformis syndrome.
- The use of BTx for pain procedures is often off-label, and its use is considered controversial.

SUMMARY

Even in the setting of chronic pain, various injections can still have a useful role in facilitating a rehabilitation program. Spinal injections, such as epidural steroid injections and facet joint injections, are among the most commonly used procedures in pain practices; however a growing number of practices are considering less common injections, such as various TPIs, regenerative injections/prolotherapy, and injections using BTx.

REFERENCES

1. Cumming TM, White AR. Needling therapies in the management of myofascial trigger point pain: a systematic review. Arch Phys Med Rehabil 2001;82:986–92.
2. Scott NA, Guo B, Barton PM, et al. Trigger point injections for chronic nonmalignant musculoskeletal pain: a systematic review. Pain Med 2009;10:54–69.
3. Peloso P, Gross A, Haines T, et al. Cervical overview group. Medicinal and injection therapies for mechanical neck disorders. Cochrane Database Syst Rev 2007;(3):CD000319.

4. Staal JB, de Bie RA, de Vet HC, et al. Injection therapy for subacute and chronic low back pain: an updated Cochrane review. Spine 2009;34:49–59.
5. Langevin P, Lowcock J, Weber J, et al. Cervical overview group. Botulinum toxin intramuscular injections for neck pain: a systematic review and meta-analysis. J Rheumatol 2011;38:203–14.
6. Langevin P, Peloso PM, Lowcock J, et al. Botulinum toxin for subacute/chronic neck pain. Cochrane Database Syst Rev 2011;(7):CD008626.
7. Soares A, Andriolo RB, Atallah AN, et al. Botulinum toxin for myofascial pain syndromes in adults. Cochrane Database Syst Rev 2014;(7):CD007533.
8. Tough EA, White AR, Cummings TM, et al. Acupuncture and dry needling in the management of myofascial trigger point pain: a systematic review and meta-analysis of randomised controlled trials. Eur J Pain 2009;13:3–10.
9. Kietrys DM, Palombaro KM, Azzaretto E, et al. Effectiveness of dry needling for upper-quarter myofascial pain: a systematic review and meta-analysis. J Orthop Sports Phys Ther 2013;43:620–34.
10. Hong CZ. Lidocaine injection versus dry needling to myofascial trigger point. The importance of the local twitch response. Am J Phys Med Rehabil 1994;73:256–63.
11. Ceccherelli F, Rigoni MT, Gagliardi G, et al. Comparison of superficial and deep acupuncture in the treatment of lumbar myofascial pain: a double-blind randomized controlled study. Clin J Pain 2002;18:149–53.
12. Furlan AD, van Tulder M, Cherkin D, et al. Acupuncture and dry-needling for low back pain: an updated systematic review within the framework of the Cochrane collaboration. Spine 2005;30:944–63.
13. Lam M, Galvin R, Curry P. Effectiveness of acupuncture for nonspecific chronic low back pain: a systematic review and meta-analysis. Spine 2013;38:2124–38.
14. Vickers AJ, Cronin AM, Maschino AC, et al. Acupuncture trialists' collaboration. Acupuncture for chronic pain: individual patient data meta-analysis. Arch Intern Med 2012;172:1444–53.
15. Vickers AJ, Linde K. Acupuncture for chronic pain. JAMA 2014;311:955–6.
16. Chen JT, Chung KC, Hou CR, et al. Inhibitory effect of dry needling on the spontaneous electrical activity recorded from myofascial trigger spots of rabbit skeletal muscle. Am J Phys Med Rehabil 2001;80:729–35.
17. Hong CZ, Simons DG. Pathophysiologic and electrophysiologic mechanisms of myofascial trigger points. Arch Phys Med Rehabil 1998;79:863–72.
18. Melzack R, Stillwell DM, Fox J. Trigger points and acupuncture points for chronic pain: correlations and implications. Pain 1977;3:3–23.
19. Dorsher PT. Myofascial referred-pain data provide physiologic evidence of acupuncture meridians. J Pain 2009;10:723–31.
20. Kao MJ, Hsieh YL, Kuo FJ, et al. Electrophysiological assessment of acupuncture points. Am J Phys Med Rehabil 2006;85:443–8.
21. Zhao ZQ. Neural mechanism underlying acupuncture analgesia. Prog Neurobiol 2008;85:355–75.
22. Melzack R, Wall PD. Pain mechanism: a new theory. Science 1965;150:971–9.
23. Fine PG, Milano R, Hare BD. The effects of myofascial trigger point injections are naloxone reversible. Pain 1988;32:15–20.
24. Wang SM, Kain ZN, White P. Acupuncture analgesia: I. The scientific basis. Anesth Analg 2008;106:602–10.
25. Hackett GS. Joint ligament relaxation treated by fibro-osseous proliferation. 1st edition. Springfield (IL): Charles C. Thomas; 1956.
26. Leadbetter WB. Cell-matrix response in tendon injury. Clin Sports Med 1992; 11(3):533–78.

27. Yelland MJ, Del Mar C, Pirozzo S, et al. Prolotherapy injections for chronic low back pain: a systematic review. Spine 2004;29(19):2126–33.
28. Nelemans PJ, deBie RA, deVet HC, et al. Injection therapy for subacute and chronic benign low back pain. Spine (Phila Pa 1976) 2001;26(5):501–15.
29. Topol GA, Reeves KD, Hassanein KM. Efficacy of dextrose prolotherapy in elite male kicking-sport athletes with chronic groin pain. Arch Phys Med Rehabil 2005;86(4):697–702.
30. Scarpone M, Rabago DP, Zgierska A, et al. The efficacy of prolotherapy for lateral epicondylosis: a pilot study. Clin J Sport Med 2008;18(3):248–54.
31. Reeves KD, Hassanein KM. Long-term effects of dextrose prolotherapy for anterior cruciate ligament laxity. Altern Ther Health Med 2003;9(3):58–62.
32. Reeves KD, Hassanein K. Randomized prospective double-blind placebo-controlled study of dextrose prolotherapy for knee osteoarthritis with or without ACL laxity. Altern Ther Health Med 2000;6(2):68–74, 77–80.
33. Rabago D. Prolotherapy for treatment of lateral epicondylosis. Am Fam Physician 2009;80(5):441.
34. Merriman JR. Prolotherapy versus operative fusion in the treatment of joint instability of the spine and pelvis. J Int Coll Surg 1964;42:150–9.
35. Mathews R, Miller M, Bree S. Treatment of mechanical and chemical lumbar discopathy by dextrose 25%. J Minimally Invasive Spinal Technique 2001;1(1):58–61.
36. Linetsky FS, Miguel R, Torres F. Treatment of cervicothoracic pain and cervicogenic headaches with regenerative injection therapy. Curr Pain Headache Rep 2004;8(1):41–8.
37. Klein RG, Eek BC, DeLong WB, et al. A randomized double-blind trial of dextrose-glycerine-phenol injections for chronic, low back pain. J Spinal Disord 1993;6(1):23–33.
38. Klein RG, Dorman TA, Johnson CE. Proliferant injections for low back pain: histologic changes of injected ligaments and objective measurements of lumbar spine mobility before and after treatment. J Neurol Orthop Med Surg 1989;10:123–6.
39. Fullerton BD, Reeves KD. Ultrasonography in regenerative injection (prolotherapy) using dextrose, platelet-rich plasma, and other injectants. Phys Med Rehabil Clin N Am 2010;21(3):585–605.
40. Centeno CJ, Elliott J, Elkins WL, et al. Fluoroscopically guided cervical prolotherapy for instability with blinded pre and post radiographic reading. Pain Physician 2005;8(1):67–72.
41. Carayannopoulos A, Borg-Stein J, Sokolof J, et al. Prolotherapy versus corticosteroid injections for the treatment of lateral epicondylosis: a randomized controlled trial. PMR 2011;3(8):706–15.
42. Schneider RC, Williams JJ, Liss L. Fatality after injection of sclerosing agent to precipitate fibro-osseous proliferation. J Am Med Assoc 1959;170(15):1768–72.
43. Keplinger JE, Bucy PC. Paraplegia from treatment with sclerosing agents. Report of a case. JAMA 1960;173:1333–5.
44. Hunt WE, Baird WC. Complications following injection of sclerosing agent to precipitate fibro-osseous proliferation. J Neurosurg 1961;18:461–5.
45. Dorman TA. Prolotherapy: a survey. J Orthop Med 1993;15:49–50.
46. Yelland MJ, Glasziou PP, Bogduk N, et al. Prolotherapy injections, saline injections, and exercises for chronic low-back pain: a randomized trial. Spine 2004;29(1):9–16 [discussion: 16].
47. Whitworth ML. Endplate fracture associated with intradiscal dextrose injection. Pain Physician 2002;5(4):379–84.

48. Grayson M. Sterile meningitis after lumbosacral ligament sclerosing injections. J Orthop Med 1994;16(3):98–9.
49. Yun HS, Sun HS, Seon HJ, et al. Prolotherapy-induced cervical spinal cord injury -a case report. Ann Rehabil Med 2012;35(4):570–3.
50. Lew MF, Brashear A, Factor S. The safety and efficacy of botulin toxin type B in the treatment of patients with cervical dystonia. A summary of three controlled trials. Neurology 2000;55(12 suppl 5):529–35.
51. Jordan SE, Ahn SS, Freischlag JA, et al. Selective botulinum chemodenervation of the scalene muscles for treatment of neurogenic thoracic outlet syndrome. Ann Vasc Surg 2000;14(4):365–9.
52. Fishman L, Konnoth C, Rozner B. Botulinum neurotoxin type B and physical therapy in the treatment of piriformis syndrome: a dose-finding study. Am J Phys Med Rehabil 2004;83:42–50.
53. Lang AM. Botulin toxin type B in piriformis syndrome. AM J Phys Med Rehabil 2004;83(3):198–202.

Exercise Therapy for Chronic Pain

Heather R. Kroll, MD[a,b]

KEYWORDS

- Exercise • Chronic pain • Physical therapy • Endogenous pain modulation
- Fear-avoidance • Neuroscience education

KEY POINTS

- Exercise has been demonstrated in animal and human studies to diminish pain experience by its effect on the endogenous pain modulatory systems.
- Exercise, in general, is therapeutic for a wide variety of chronic pain diagnoses, but it has been difficult to show that one particular approach is superior to another.
- Patients have multiple barriers to successfully participating in exercise including patient-specific factors, environmental factors, and health care delivery factors.
- Evaluation of a patient before exercise prescription should include a comprehensive bio-psychosocial assessment and determination of the goals of the exercise program.
- Successful exercise prescription requires coordination of care and good communication between physician, therapist, and patient.
- Successful exercise prescription requires patient education regarding the impact of exercise on the nervous system, education targeting fear-avoidance beliefs, and education about the details of how to do the exercise program.

INTRODUCTION

For people with chronic pain, the prospect of doing exercise may seem like an overwhelming and impossible task. And yet, exercise therapy is frequently prescribed for patients with a wide variety of chronic pain problems. Exercise provides multiple benefits for patients including improvements in strength, flexibility, and endurance; decrease in cardiovascular and metabolic syndrome risk; improved bone health; improved cognition and mood; and often most importantly for the patient, improved pain control (**Box 1**). It therefore might seem that patients should be eager to participate in an exercise program. However, patients with chronic pain frequently present with significant levels of fear-avoidance behaviors and are often resistant to

Disclosure: The author has no disclosures to make.
[a] Rehabilitation Institute of Washington, PLLC, 415 1st Ave N, Ste 200, Seattle, WA 98109, USA;
[b] Department of Rehabilitation Medicine, University of Washington School of Medicine, 325 9th Ave, Box 359612, Seattle, WA 98104, USA
E-mail address: hkroll@rehabwashington.com

Phys Med Rehabil Clin N Am 26 (2015) 263–281
http://dx.doi.org/10.1016/j.pmr.2014.12.007

Box 1
Exercise benefits

- Strength
- Flexibility
- Endurance
- Decreased cardiovascular risk
- Better bone health
- Decreased metabolic syndrome
- Improved cognition
- Improved mood
- Improved pain control

---

participating in an exercise program. Prescribing an appropriate exercise program for a person with chronic pain requires an understanding of the person's biopsychosocial circumstances, an armamentarium of different exercise techniques, and good communication with the therapy team.

PATIENT EVALUATION OVERVIEW

Exercise has been found to be beneficial for patients with a wide variety of chronic pain diagnoses including arthritis, fibromyalgia, complex regional pain syndrome (CRPS), chronic neck pain, and chronic low back pain. No matter what the specific diagnosis, the patient evaluation must include an assessment of the biopsychosocial circumstances of the patient. A physical examination does not provide sufficient information. It is necessary to understand the patient's psychological state and beliefs about pain, health, and wellness. It is important to consider the goals of the exercise program (**Box 2**). Goals might be specific correction of impairments (eg, better range of motion), a reduction of disability (eg, walking without a cane), or improvement in participation (eg, return to work). Acute pain and chronic pain present different challenges. In the case of acute injury, assessment includes analysis of functional biomechanical deficits including muscular weakness, inflexibility, scar tissue, muscle strength imbalance, poor coordination, and decreased endurance. Treatment addresses these specific biomechanical deficits through a specifically tailored exercise program. Pain is often a useful guide for determining the intensity and frequency of exercise activities.

A patient with chronic pain may have all of the functional biomechanical deficits and in addition may be dealing with excessive deconditioning, fear-avoidance, depression, centrally mediated pain, loss of role in family and society, and entrenched

---

Box 2
Exercise goals

- Specific correction of impairments (eg, better range of motion)
- Reduction of disability (eg, walking without a cane)
- Improvement in participation (eg, return to work)
- Pain control
- Medical benefits

---

disability. There has typically been a progressive loss of function and diminishing quality of life. Exercise intervention needs to address the biomechanical issues but must do so in the context of these other complicating conditions. Pain is typically a poor guide for determining the frequency and intensity of exercise. Education of the patient plays an important role in facilitating their participation in an exercise program. This education needs to be about the specific biomechanical issues, about the functioning of the nervous system, and about the psychosocial conditions that contribute to the person's pain and disability.

HOW DOES EXERCISE AFFECT PAIN?

It is not always clear what it is about an exercise program that brings benefit to the patient. Exercise impacts the musculoskeletal system, the cardiovascular system, and the brain. The effects on the brain include impact on sensory processing, and improved motor coordination and cognitive and emotional functioning. For the chronic pain patient the impact on the brain may be the most important for improving the patient's function and sense of well-being. A variety of research studies have demonstrated the impact of exercise on the brain. For example, exercise is an effective treatment of depression, which frequently accompanies chronic pain.[1] Research has also shown that specifically targeted exercise programs can improve chronic pain and function, but changes in pain do not correlate well with improvement in physical measures, suggesting that it may be something other than the change in musculoskeletal function that is mediating the pain relief.[2]

Pain perception is brought about by a complex interaction between peripheral nociceptive input and modulatory processes at the spinal and supraspinal level. The nervous system has an endogenous pain modulatory system that has inhibitory and facilitatory functions. Pain modulation occurs in cortical, hypothalamic, midbrain, and brainstem structures, and in the spinal cord. The peripheral nervous system also modulates pain perception. Multiple neurotransmitters are involved in pain perception and pain modulation.[3–5] Studies have been done in animals and humans to try to elucidate the impact of exercise on pain perception and on this endogenous pain modulatory system.

Animal studies have addressed the effects of exercise in models of acute pain and chronic neuropathic pain. Stagg and colleagues[6] evaluated the effect of repeated aerobic exercise on a neuropathic pain model in the rat. They demonstrated that sensory hypersensitivity in a sciatic nerve ligation model of neuropathic pain was reversed by regular moderate aerobic exercise (forced treadmill running). These effects were reversed by naloxone suggesting that endogenous opioids play a role in modulating pain perception in response to exercise. Chen and colleagues[7] studied a rat model of acute postoperative mechanical hypersensitivity caused by skin/muscle incision and retraction. They looked at the effect of 5 day per week treadmill running for 4 weeks on behavioral markers of pain and on levels of substance P and cytokines in the dorsal root ganglion. They demonstrated that mechanical hypersensitivity was alleviated by the treadmill running and was associated with suppression of excess substance P and inflammatory cytokines in the dorsal root ganglion. Mazzardo-Martins and colleagues[8] showed an antinociceptive effect of a swimming exercise in a chemical behavioral model of nociception in mice. This antinociceptive effect was blocked by naloxone and by an inhibitor of serotonin synthesis suggesting that this effect was mediated by the opioid and serotonergic systems. Martins and colleagues[9] studied a mouse model of CRPS-1 and evaluated the effect of high-intensity swimming on mechanical allodynia. There was marked mechanical allodynia in this model of CRPS-1. High-intensity exercise significantly reduced the allodynia shortly after exercise (30 minutes) and at a delayed evaluation (24 hours). They further demonstrated the role of the opioid systems and the adenosine systems in mediating this response.

Multiple studies in humans have looked at the relationship between physical activity and pain sensitivity. Improved pain control is associated with exercise for a variety of painful conditions[10] including chronic low back pain,[11,12] fibromyalgia,[13] osteoarthritis,[14] neuropathic pain,[15] and CRPS.[16] Various studies of healthy individuals have demonstrated a relationship between a person's participation in general physical activity and aerobic exercise and his or her tolerance to pain.[17] Ellingson and colleagues[18] studied a group of healthy women using self-reported and accelerometer measures to determine their degree of sedentary versus active behavior and evaluated the relationship between levels of physical activity and average intensity and unpleasantness of a heat pain stimulus. They found that those participants who met physical activity recommendations (moderate intensity aerobic activity for minimum of 150 minutes per week or vigorous aerobic activity for minimum of 75 minutes per week) had significantly lower pain unpleasantness ratings and pain intensity ratings to noxious thermal stimuli than the participants who did not meet this activity level. Delfa de la Morena and colleagues[19] studied a more localized hypoalgesic response to exercise. They evaluated the effect of repeated eccentric exercise at high intensity on pressure pain thresholds of the wrist extensors in healthy subjects. They demonstrated that an initial bout of high-intensity eccentric exercise resulted in delayed-onset muscle soreness and lowered pressure pain thresholds 24 hours postexercise consistent with hyperalgesia. Subjects underwent a second bout of eccentric exercise after 7 days. The subjects had delayed-onset muscle soreness after this second bout of exercise, but did not show lowered pain pressure thresholds indicating that there had been adaptations that limited the local hyperalgesia. The authors speculated that a combination of neural, mechanical, and cellular adaptations were responsible for this change. Naugle and colleagues[20] sought to determine an intensity threshold for aerobic exercise-induced hypoalgesia. They studied the immediate impact on healthy young men and women of moderate (50% heart rate reserve) and vigorous (70% heart rate reserve) aerobic exercise on pressure and heat pain modulation. Both moderate and vigorous exercise was associated with reduced pain intensity to heat stimulus, and there was a dose response effect with more reduction in pain intensity after vigorous exercise. Vigorous exercise also led to increased pressure pain thresholds.

Researchers have sought to determine how exercise impacts the pain modulatory processes in the central nervous system. Naugle and Riley[21] studied healthy adults and looked at the relationship between self-reported physical activity and pain facilitatory and inhibitory function. They used tests of temporal summation to evaluate pain facilitation and conditioned pain modulation to evaluate endogenous pain inhibition. They found that levels of total and vigorous physical activity predicted pain facilitation and inhibition.[21] Meeus and colleagues[22] also used temporal summation and conditioned pain modulation to evaluate exercise-induced analgesia in female patients with rheumatoid arthritis, chronic fatigue syndrome, and fibromyalgia and sedentary healthy control subjects. Pain assessment was done before and after submaximal exercise on a bicycle ergometer at 75% age-predicted maximal heart rate for up to 15 minutes. The patients with rheumatoid arthritis demonstrated exercise-induced analgesia expressed by reduced temporal summation of experimental pain. Paracetamol reinforced this response to exercise. The patients with chronic fatigue and fibromyalgia had a less clear response with different responses at different experimental pain locations, suggesting that their endogenous pain modulating system is dysfunctional. Ellingson and colleagues[23] tried to determine if conditioned pain modulation was responsible for exercise-induced hypoalgesia. They studied healthy subjects and evaluated heat pain intensity and unpleasantness at rest, after nonpainful aerobic cycling exercise, and after painful aerobic cycling exercise. Both exercise conditions resulted in decreased pain responses, although with a larger magnitude response in the painful, more intense exercise condition. These studies suggest that conditioned pain modulation plays a role in exercise-induced analgesia, but that other mechanisms also contribute.

Studies of motor cortex stimulation allow the evaluation of the hypoalgesic effects of activation of the motor cortex without the concomitant action of the musculoskeletal and cardiovascular systems. All exercise involves motor cortex activation and several studies have tried to evaluate the role that the motor cortex plays in exercise-induced analgesia. Yezierski and coworkers[24] studied the effect of electrical stimulation of the motor cortex in primates showing inhibition of the spinal neuronal responses to noxious pressure and pinch stimuli. A study of transcranial magnetic stimulation of the motor cortex in patients with chronic neuropathic pain using PET imaging for evaluation showed that stimulation induced activity during and after stimulation in multiple brain regions including sensory pathways known to be involved in pain processing. Pain relief correlated with regional blood flow changes.[25] A recent randomized, sham-controlled trial of repetitive transcranial magnetic stimulation of the motor cortex in chronic myofascial pain showed significant reduction in daily pain scores and enhanced corticospinal inhibition.[26] These studies all suggest that activation of the motor cortex contributes to activation of endogenous pain modulatory systems.

There is evidence, however, that endogenous pain modulatory systems may be dysfunctional in at least some chronic pain states. Knauf and Koltyn[27] studied the effect of isometric exercise on pain perception in patients with diabetes with and without diabetic neuropathy. They assessed exercise-induced muscle pain and used an experimental thermal pain protocol to assess temporal summation. Patients with diabetes with and without diabetic peripheral neuropathy performed isometric exercise (grip) at 25% maximum voluntary contraction for 3 minutes. Exercise-induced muscle pain was significantly higher in the patients with peripheral neuropathy and they also rated the exercise as more effortful. Temporal summation was assessed in both groups before exercise and was found to be present in both groups with increasing pain ratings with repeated stimulation. After exercise the patients without peripheral neuropathy showed no temporal summation indicative of the presence of exercise-induced hypoalgesia. The patients with peripheral neuropathy continued to have temporal summation and did not seem to gain any pain-relieving benefit from the exercise.[27] Naugle and colleagues[28] summarized the hypoalgesic effects of exercise in healthy and chronic pain populations in a meta-analytic review. The studies reviewed evaluated the impact of acute exercise on experimentally induced noxious stimulation. Different exercise modalities were studied including aerobic, isometric, and dynamic resistance exercise. Both healthy populations and various chronic pain populations were studied. In the healthy populations the evidence supports that all three types of exercise decrease the perception of experimentally induced pain. In the chronic pain populations the results were more mixed depending on the particular chronic pain condition being studied. For chronic low back pain, findings were similar to healthy participants. For patients with regional chronic pain, exercise of muscles outside the painful region reduced pressure sensitivity of the painful area, but exercise of the painful muscles tended to increase pain sensitivity in those muscles. In fibromyalgia, low-to-moderate intensity activity seems to be effective for eliciting exercise-induced hypoalgesia. However, in some studies of individuals with widespread pain, moderate-to-vigorous activity led to hyperalgesia. Nijs and colleagues[29] also reviewed the literature and came to similar conclusions.

In summary, the literature supports that acute bouts of exercise consistently activate the endogenous pain modulatory systems in healthy adults and have mixed effects on patients with chronic pain depending on the specific diagnosis and type of exercise. The mechanisms involved in exercise-induced hypoalgesia are multifactorial. Likely important contributors to the effect include the release of endogenous opioids and activation of spinal and supraspinal pain inhibitory pathways.

EXERCISE EFFECTS ON SPECIFIC CHRONIC PAIN PROBLEMS

The role of exercise prescribed in a therapeutic manner for the management of a variety of chronic pain conditions has been widely studied. These studies frequently assess function and quality of life, and pain. The effects of exercise for a few of these conditions are summarized next.

Fibromyalgia

Many researchers have evaluated the effects of exercise on patients with fibromyalgia. A 2007 systematic review of 34 studies showed moderate-quality evidence that moderate-intensity aerobic-only exercise training for 12 weeks has positive effects on global well-being, physical function, and possibly on pain and tender points. Results of strength training were less clear, but may improve symptoms of fibromyalgia including improvement in pain and tender points.[30] A 2013 review evaluated the effect of resistance training for managing fibromyalgia. Only five studies met the inclusion criteria. The conclusion was that resistance training was better than a control group for improvement in a multidimensional assessment of function, self-reported physical function, tenderness, and muscle strength. Pain improvement favored aerobic exercise rather than resistance exercise.[31] Hooten and colleagues[32] compared aerobic with strengthening exercise in the context of an interdisciplinary pain management program. Both groups improved in pain severity, strength, pain threshold, and peak oxygen consumption. The only difference between the two groups was a greater increase in oxygen consumption in the aerobic exercise group. McLoughlin and colleagues[33] used functional MRI to evaluate the relationship between physical activity and brain responses to pain in subjects with fibromyalgia. Their results suggested that the fibromyalgia patients who were physically active better preserved their ability to modulate pain compared with their less active peers. In summary, both aerobic and strength training programs are beneficial. However, performing exercise too intensely can precipitate a flare up of symptoms. Therefore, starting at low levels at which the patient can be successful and progressing gradually is more likely to promote benefit from exercise and longer-term adherence to an exercise program.[31]

Osteoarthritis

A wide variety of exercise approaches for osteoarthritis have been studied. A 2012 review of the effectiveness of different exercise approaches for osteoarthritis found strong evidence that aerobic and strengthening exercise programs were beneficial for patients with mild-to-moderate knee and hip osteoarthritis, improving pain and physical function.[14] This comprehensive review did not find differences between types of exercise programs, showing similar improvements in response to aerobic versus strengthening regimens, similar improvements from high- versus low-resistance training, and from dynamic versus isometric training. Bennell and colleagues[34] studied the effect of hip-strengthening exercises on people with medial knee osteoarthritis and varus malalignment, evaluating the impact on pain and function and also the impact on the knee adduction moment. Measures of pain, physical function, and muscle strength improved, but there was no change in knee adduction moment. So, even when exercise does not correct a presumed biomechanical deficit, it can still prove beneficial for improving pain and function. Not surprisingly the benefits of exercise for the patient with osteoarthritis seem to be maintained only as long as the patient continues to participate in an exercise program.[35,36] As with other chronic pain conditions, evaluating the barriers and facilitators of exercise participation is important in guiding exercise prescription to help the patient commit to and participate in ongoing exercise activity.[37]

Complex Regional Pain Syndrome

Exercise intervention for CRPS does not always follow traditional exercise models. The focus of recent studies has been on a process of graded motor imagery (GMI), which is an approach that starts with strategies to activate the motor cortex without actually using muscles. This approach is described by Moseley[38] in a 2004 randomized controlled trial on patients with upper extremity CRPS. The GMI program consisted of three phases. First, participants were shown pictures of hands, and were asked to identify whether each pictured depicted a right hand or a left hand. Then they imagined performing actions shown in pictures of hands. Finally, they engaged in mirror therapy. Participants in the 6-week GMI program demonstrated improved pain ratings and decreased edema compared with the control group.[38] A systematic review in 2009 concluded that GMI should be used to reduce pain in adults with CRPS-1.[39] A more recent systematic review by Cossins and colleagues[40] identified trials showing temporary benefit from repetitive transcranial magnetic stimulation on pain levels and strong evidence for GMI. Sherry and colleagues[16] studied the effect of an intensive exercise program of 14 days mean duration, 5 to 6 hours per day in children with CRPS-1. The treatment philosophy was to re-establish normal use of the affected limb as quickly as possible, primarily through aerobic exercise training. Patients also underwent desensitization. Three-quarters of the families were referred for psychological counseling. A total of 92% of patients had initial complete resolution of pain and return to full function. At long-term follow-up (available for approximately 50% of participants) after a mean of 5 years, 3 months, 88% had no symptoms of CRPS. This type of intense exercise treatment has not been studied in adults with CRPS.

NONSPECIFIC LOW BACK PAIN

The effects of exercise on chronic, nonspecific low back pain have been widely studied. There are many approaches to exercise for back pain including specific exercise protocols targeting specific impairments, general exercise protocols, mind/body techniques of motor control, and multidisciplinary pain management and functional restoration. A 2010 review of 37 randomized controlled trials found that exercise therapy for low back pain, compared with usual care, decreased pain intensity and improved disability and long-term function. There was no evidence that one particular type of exercise was better than another.[41] Mannion and colleagues[42,43] noted a similar difficulty in demonstrating significant differences in outcomes from different exercise approaches to chronic nonspecific low back pain. Smith and Grimmer-Somers[44] summarized evidence of the long-term effectiveness of exercise therapy for chronic low back pain. In reviewing 15 trials using various exercise approaches, they found evidence of ongoing pain reduction and decreased recurrence rates up to 6 months after treatment. Some of the evidence for different exercise approaches for chronic low back pain is summarized next.

Specific Exercise Protocols Targeting Specific Impairments (Spine Stabilization, Direction Specific)

Spine stabilization exercises are commonly prescribed for patients with acute, sub-acute, and chronic low back pain. The goal of this exercise approach is to restore segmental movement and motor control during static and dynamic functional activities. Studies support that these types of exercises have immediate short-term benefit, but limited long-term benefit beyond that of a general exercise program.[45–47] Research has not shown that it is the specific musculoskeletal outcome of the exercise that is causing the benefit to the patient. Mannion and colleagues[2] evaluated the effect of spine stabilization treatment on the voluntary and anticipatory activation of the transverse abdominus before and after 9 weeks of spine stabilization treatment. Outcome measures included pain and disability as measured by the Roland Morris disability score. They found that pain and disability improved. Voluntary, but not anticipatory activation of the transverse abdominus improved. However, there was no correlation between the change in abdominal muscle function and change in disability. Only the reduction in catastrophizing and fingertip-to-floor distance contributed to the variance in the Roland Morris scores. Lomond and colleagues[48] found that general trunk strengthening exercises and specific exercises targeting the trunk stabilizers produced significant improvement in pain and function at 11 weeks and at 6 months after treatment in subjects with chronic low back pain. Muscle activation patterns were similar in the two groups after treatment, but notably were still different from activation patterns in control subjects without low back pain. Wang and colleagues[11] in a meta-analysis of core stability exercise versus general exercise for chronic low back pain found that the stability exercise was more effective at improving pain and disability in the short term, but no significant differences for pain were seen at 6 or 12 months. Steiger and colleagues[49] in a 2012 systematic review asked the question of whether improvements in pain and self-reported disability were contingent on improvement in targeted aspects of performance. Their review included 16 trials, which included a variety of performance measures including mobility, trunk extension strength, trunk flexion strength, and back muscle endurance. They did not find evidence that changes over the course of exercise treatment in these specific parameters were related to changes in pain and self-reported disability.

Another common approach is an exercise protocol based on directional preference, such as the McKenzie approach. These exercises are based on the patient's "directional preference," which is determined by identifying a posture or repeated end range movement in a single direction that immediately decreases midline lumbar pain or reduces referred extremity symptoms. Patients are also instructed in body mechanics and posture. Studies have shown benefit in the very early part of treatment, the first few weeks, but again no consistent benefit in the long term over intensive strengthening, or advice to stay active.[50,51] Hosseinifar and colleagues[52] compared stabilization exercise with McKenzie exercises looking at pain, disability, and stabilizing muscle thickness. Both exercises improved pain equally, although the stabilization exercises improved disability and muscle thickness more. However, the patients doing the McKenzie exercises were randomized to this group and did not perform the exercises based on their particular directional preference. Long and coworkers[53] evaluated the benefit of directional preference–based treatment comparing the effect of treatment matched to patient directional preference with treatment that was not matched. They excluded patients who had been off work for more than a year because of their back pain, but otherwise did not specify whether the patients had acute, sub-acute, or chronic pain. Patients without a directional preference (26% of the initial sample) were excluded from the study. Patients were randomized to matched directionally based care, opposite directionally based care, or evidence-based care consisting of multidirectional, midrange lumbar exercises and stretches for hip and thigh muscles. Over the 2-week trial period, all three treatment groups improved in measures of pain and function. However, the directionally matched group improved significantly more than either of the other groups and also had significantly greater satisfaction with care.[53]

General Exercise Protocols (General Flexibility, Strength and Endurance Training)

General exercise protocols addressing general flexibility, strength, and endurance training have all been used for management of chronic low back pain. A 2005 meta-analysis by Hayden and colleagues[54] found low-to-moderate evidence for the effectiveness of exercise in general for managing chronic low back pain, but the exercise protocols varied over the studies reviewed so it is difficult to point to any one specific treatment as being better than another. Mannion and colleagues[42,43] compared active physical therapy, muscle reconditioning, and low-impact aerobics in patients with chronic low back pain and found that they were equally effective in reducing pain intensity, pain frequency, and disability. These benefits were maintained at long-term follow-up. A systematic review of the effectiveness of walking for low back pain was limited by the number and the quality of the studies. It showed low-to-moderate evidence that walking is an effective intervention strategy for low back pain.[55]

Mind/Body Techniques of Motor Control (Yoga, Alexander Technique, Tai Chi)

In recent years there has been increasing interest in movement approaches other than traditional physical therapy. Although these various approaches may not always fit the common definition of exercise, they all involve whole body movement with an emphasis on mind-body integration and improvement in subtle aspects of motor control. Yoga, Tai Chi, and the Alexander Technique are examples of this nontraditional approach to movement and exercise but do not represent all of the different techniques available.

Several studies of yoga for chronic pain conditions have demonstrated more effectiveness than minimal intervention, such as a self-care book. Cramer and colleagues[56] did a randomized controlled trial of a 9-week yoga course versus a self-care manual of home-based exercises for neck pain for patients with nonspecific neck pain. They found that the yoga group demonstrated greater relief of their neck pain, less disability, improved health-related quality of life, and improved pressure pain thresholds. Tekur and colleagues[57] studied the effects of a 7-day residential program of yoga that included specific poses for back pain and meditation, yogic counseling, and lectures on yoga philosophy. The control group participated in physical therapy exercises for chronic pain and counseling and education sessions. Both groups improved in ratings of pain, depression, and spinal mobility but the improvement was greater in the yoga group. Because of the comprehensiveness of the yoga intervention in this study it is hard to know if it is the specific physical activities that are effective or some combination of the physical, counseling, and educational interventions. Sherman and colleagues[58] randomized adults with chronic low back pain to 12 weekly yoga classes, conventional stretching exercises, or a self-care book. The yoga classes and the stretching provided benefits including better function and decreased symptoms compared with the self-care book. The benefits lasted several months. A 2013 meta-analysis of yoga including eight randomized controlled trials found a medium-to-large effect on pain and functional disability. This improvement was seen despite a wide range of styles and duration of treatment. However, the lack of active control groups made it difficult to assess if yoga had benefit over traditional exercise programs.[59]

The Alexander Technique is a movement education technique that teaches skills for observing the subtleties of overall habits of movement and movement coordination and teaches patients to change their habits of movement and movement patterns to facilitate more efficient movement and better coordination. A large 2008 study compared normal care (control), 6 versus 24 Alexander Technique lessons, six sessions of massage, and an exercise prescription from a doctor with behavioral counseling delivered by a nurse. The main outcome measure was function as measured by the Roland Morris disability score and the number of days in pain. Outcomes were measured at 3 months and 12 months. The researchers found benefit in function and number of days in pain at 3 and 12 months from 6 or 24 Alexander Technique lessons, with the 24 lessons having a larger effect. Six lessons combined with aerobic exercise prescription was nearly as effective as 24 lessons. Although massage provided some benefit at 3 months this was not sustained at long-term follow-up. One of the strengths of this study was the number of participants (579) and the setting including multiple different Alexander Technique teachers.[60]

Tai Chi is a gentle exercise technique that incorporates balance, body awareness, strength, and stretching through repeated patterns of movement that are done slowly and continuously, without strain. Hall and colleagues[61] studied a group of 160 volunteers with persistent nonspecific low back pain. The Tai Chi group participated in 18 Tai Chi sessions over 10-weeks in a group setting. The control group was waitlisted and continued their usual health care. The group that participated in Tai Chi had better improvements than the control group in pain intensity, bothersomeness of symptoms, and self-reported disability. The findings were of a similar magnitude to those found in studies of other exercise interventions for chronic low back pain. They were also statistically significant and clinically meaningful even though only 57% of the participants attended 50% or more of the Tai Chi sessions. A total of 75% of participants said they believed the results were worthwhile.

Multidisciplinary Pain Management Programs/Functional Restoration

Multidisciplinary pain programs, also referred to as functional restoration, are programs of intensive daily treatment that includes quota-based exercise targeting improving strength, stamina, flexibility, and functional abilities. Treatment is typically for 6 to 8 hours per day over the course of 3 to 4 weeks. Treatment includes several hours of active therapy and educational sessions and cognitive behavioral therapy. Medication management is often an important component. This approach to the chronic pain patient with entrenched disability was pioneered by Dr Wilbert Fordyce. In a 1973 article, Dr Fordyce and colleagues[62] described using the approach for selected patients in whom pain was viewed as a learned behavior. The goal of treatment was to diminish pain behaviors and increase well-behaviors and function. Their subjects showed significant improvement in time spent up (not reclining), in distance walked, and exercise tolerance and decreased pain medication use. In the 40 years since this study, there have been multiple studies, meta-analyses, and systematic reviews assessing the benefit of this type of comprehensive treatment with a clear conclusion that this treatment provides benefit for reducing disability, reducing fear-avoidance, decreasing pain, enhancing quality of life, and facilitating return to work.[63–69] Monticone and colleagues[70] found persistence of benefits at 1 year posttreatment.

EXERCISE PRESCRIPTION AND GUIDELINES

From the previous review, it is clear that patient outcomes are better for those patients who exercise than for those who do not. However, based on the data, it can be hard to know exactly which exercise intervention one should choose. The specifics of the exercise regimen likely matter less than the way in which exercise is prescribed and taught and the supportiveness of the environment. If you can get your patients moving, they will typically feel better eventually. The key to effective exercise prescription for chronic pain is identifying and promoting strategies that facilitate actual participation in exercise.

There are multiple barriers to exercise participation for patients with chronic pain (**Box 3**). These can be divided into patient factors, environmental factors, and health care–delivery factors. Patient barriers include pain, fear-avoidance, excessive deconditioning, lack of education and understanding about the benefit of exercise, lack of education and understanding about the neurophysiology of pain and central sensitization, strong beliefs that exercise can be harmful, depression, potential dysfunctional endogenous pain modulation, and lack of self-efficacy. Environmental factors include

---

Box 3
Barriers to exercise participation

Patient factors

- Pain, particularly centrally mediated pain
- Dysfunctional endogenous pain modulation
- Fear-avoidance
- Excessive deconditioning
- Lack of education and understanding about the neurophysiology of pain and central sensitization
- Strong beliefs that exercise can be harmful
- Depression
- Lack of self-efficacy

Environmental factors

- Lack of access to a place to exercise
- Perceived or real lack of time to exercise
- Lack of support for exercise from family and work place
- Variable accessibility of appropriate health care providers

Health care delivery factors

- Overly strong focus on the biomedical model of pain
- Lack of attention to the psychological and central nervous system contributions to pain
- Lack of coordination of care between the physician and therapist
- Poor communication between health care providers and patients regarding the value and importance of exercise
- Poor education of the patient about the meaning of pain
- Lack of sufficient supervision so that the patient feels safe exercising and understands appropriate strategies for progressing exercise

lack of access to a place to exercise, perceived or real lack of time to exercise, lack of support for exercise from family and work place, and variable accessibility of appropriate health care providers. Health care–delivery factors include overly strong focus on the biomedical model of pain with lack of attention to psychological and central nervous system contributions to pain, lack of coordination of care between the physicians prescribing the exercise and the therapist carrying out the prescription, poor communication between health care providers and patients regarding the value and importance of exercise, poor education of the patient about the meaning of pain, and lack of sufficient supervision so that the patient feels safe exercising and understands appropriate strategies for progressing exercise activities. When prescribing exercise, these barriers need to be recognized and addressed.

Exercise prescription for the chronic pain patient needs to attend to the functional biomechanical issues, the cognitive-behavioral issues, and the functioning of the endogenous pain modulatory system to be successful. The patient evaluation should identify if there are specific biomechanical deficits to be addressed, such as lack of flexibility, strength deficits, endurance deficits, or problems with balance and motor control. This evaluation allows the provider to identify the types of specific exercise (eg, aerobic, strength training, stretching, balance, motor control) that will be helpful for correcting these deficits. Patients need specific, detailed advice about the intensity, frequency, and duration of exercise. For example, they need advice about how long to hold a stretch, how many repetitions to do, and how many repetitions to increase. They need to know which qualities of movement to focus on (eg, speed, accuracy, power, or range of motion). They need to understand what system should be used to determine progression of exercise. Should progression be guided by symptoms; by physiologic parameters, such as heart rate; or by quota-based guidelines? Guidelines for progression may be different for different aspects of an exercise program. For example, a patient with upper extremity CRPS may be able to progress aerobic activity on a stationary bike according to physiologic parameters, but need to progress the GMI program for the upper extremity based on symptoms. Giving patients a variety of exercises that address their needs, from which they can choose, adds flexibility to the program and a better sense of control for the patient.

Evaluation should also identify the patient's beliefs and understanding about their pain problem. Most patients with chronic pain still believe that there is a specific problem in their body producing nociceptive input that is driving their pain. They typically believe that if something causes pain, then it is dangerous. Unless these beliefs can be changed, it is unlikely that a patient will persevere enough with an exercise program to succeed. Neuroscience education is a strategy that has shown efficacy for changing patient beliefs and facilitating exercise participation. Louw and colleagues[71] in a 2011 systemic review of eight studies of the effect of neuroscience education for patients with chronic musculoskeletal pain found "there is compelling evidence that an educational strategy addressing neurophysiology and neurobiology of pain can have a positive effect on pain, disability, catastrophization, and physical performance." A practical description of this approach is available from several authors.[72–74]

Education about fear-avoidance has also shown benefit for increasing activity participation. Fear-avoidance promotes persistent pain experience and disability. In the fear-avoidance model, injury leads to a pain experience that in the presence of negative affect and frightening illness information causes pain catastrophizing. This leads to pain-related fear, avoidance (of activity) and hypervigilance (regarding symptoms), disuse, depression, and disability, all of which contribute to an ongoing pain experience.[75] A quota-based approach to exercise with fear-avoidance education studied by Kernan and Rainville[76] led to functional gains and decreased kinesiophobia and improved measures of disability in patients with chronic low back pain. In a primary care setting, education targeting fear-avoidance beliefs and encouraging activation for patients with chronic back pain led to sustained reductions in fear-avoidance beliefs, activity limitations caused by back pain, and days missed from usual activities caused by back pain.[77]

Strategies to facilitate exercise adherence are also important. Cecchi and colleagues[78] found that exercise adherence almost doubled the probability of a favorable response to an exercise program at 1-year follow-up in chronic low back pain patients. Medina-Mirapeix and colleagues[79] assessed factors that predicted adherence to the frequency and duration components of a home exercise program in patients with nonspecific neck and low back pain. They found that self-efficacy (the belief in one's own ability to succeed in a particular situation, in this case exercise) was predictive of adherence to the frequency and duration aspects of a home exercise program. Similarly, Courneya and McAuley[80] found that self-efficacy was an important predictor of physical activity in a sample of young healthy adults. Medina-Mirapeix and colleagues also looked at how the interaction and communication between the physical therapist and the patient impacted home exercise adherence. They found that clarifying doubts and questions from the patient was associated with a higher likelihood of adherence to the recommended frequency of home exercise. Slade and colleagues[81] did a review of patients' beliefs and perceptions about exercise for nonspecific low back pain. They concluded that people prefer and are more likely to participate in exercise activities designed with a consideration of their preferences and consistent with their circumstances, fitness level, and prior exercise experiences. They noted that people did not continue if the exercise program interfered with everyday life, seemed ineffective, or was too difficult to do. Good communication with the therapist was important to patients to allow for questions to be answered and to facilitate making the intervention relevant to the patient. Creating a consultative rather than prescriptive process was important to patients.

One of the barriers to self-efficacy with respect to exercise in the chronic pain patient is prior experience of aggravation of pain symptoms after engaging in exercise or other activity. The quota-based approach to exercise is very valuable for building patients' confidence that they can succeed with exercise (**Box 4**). This approach starts with identifying a baseline level of function that is achievable for the patient. The goal is to start at a level at which the patient can be successful. A rate of progression is determined that is safe and achievable. Each day's activity is based on the specific quota for that day and is not pain-contingent. It is emphasized to the patient that it is important to not do more when feeling good, or less when feeling bad. This approach to

---

Box 4
Quota-based reactivation

- Identify a baseline level of function at which the patient can be successful
- Determine a rate of progression that is safe and achievable
- Do ONLY what is on the schedule for the day, not more if feeling good, or less if feeling bad
- Activity levels are NOT pain-contingent, but based on the predetermined quota for the day
- If patient falls off the progression, go back to an achievable level and resume the process
- Goal is to remove pain as the guiding control of activity and replace control with a rational process that determines a reasonable activity level

exercise has demonstrated effectiveness for patients with chronic low back pain. It allows patients to be successful and therefore build confidence and have reduced fear of reinjury with exercise. This process helps to break patients out of the fear-avoidance cycle.[76] As patients are successful with exercise, their self-efficacy with regard to exercise increases.

Box 5 summarizes decisions to be made when prescribing exercise. An effective exercise prescription starts with education of the patient focusing on neuroscience education so that they better understand the meaning of their pain and also understand the benefits of exercise for improving their pain modulating system. Education must also include specific, detailed exercise recommendations so that the patient understands exactly what they are supposed to do and so that they understand that the exercise activities are safe and are not going to put them at risk of injury or reinjury. Patients typically need frequent reassurance from the physician and the therapist. To prevent confusion, the physician and therapist need to communicate regularly so that the patient is getting the same message from all members of their treatment team. Specific exercise choice needs to make biomechanical sense, but also needs to meet the needs and preferences of the patient. Exercise intensity needs to start at a level and progress at a rate at which the patient can be successful. Through this process the patient learns to differentiate important pain (pain that should be attended to) from unimportant pain (pain that is not providing information about injury or potential for injury). This knowledge allows them to persevere in their exercise activity even when it does not immediately relieve their pain and especially when it flares up their symptoms. Over time, the improvements in strength, flexibility, conditioning, and body mechanics gained through exercise diminish the risk of reinjury and diminish fear-avoidance by helping patients feel in control of their bodies and safe in their daily activities.

SUMMARY

Although there is a lot of research evidence that exercise is helpful for a multitude of chronic pain conditions, it has been difficult to clearly demonstrate the superiority of one approach over another. The benefit of exercise for pain control likely comes

---

Box 5
Decisions to make when prescribing exercise

- Does the program need to address specific biomechanical deficits?
- What types of exercise will be helpful and accepted by the patient?
- What dose of exercise is recommended including intensity, frequency, and duration?
- What quality of movement should be emphasized? Speed, accuracy, power, range of motion?
- What system for progressing exercise? Guide by symptoms? Physiologic changes? Quota-based?
- Are there a range of exercises that can be useful to give the patient as much choice as possible?
- What education does the patient need and who will provide it?
- If multidisciplinary care is needed, but not available, how can the physician and the therapist facilitate a behavioral approach?

from the impact of exercise on the endogenous opioid system and on central pain modulatory systems. Patients with some chronic pain conditions seem to have a dysfunctional endogenous pain modulatory system, which should be considered when prescribing exercise. The prescription of exercise for chronic pain must address the biomechanical issues and the psychosocial factors that contribute to the patient's pain and disability. Patient education, coordination of care within the health care team, and selecting an exercise regimen that is meaningful to and achievable by the patient are all important components to promote a successful rehabilitation program.

REFERENCES

1. Blumenthal JA, Babyak MA, Doraiswamy PM, et al. Exercise and pharmaco-therapy in the treatment of major depressive disorder. Psychosom Med 2007; 69(7):587–96.
2. Mannion AF, Caporaso F, Pulkovski N, et al. Spine stabilisation exercises in the treatment of chronic low back pain: a good clinical outcome is not associated with improved abdominal muscle function. Eur Spine J 2012;21(7):1301–10.
3. Ness T, Randich A. Substrates of spinal cord nociceptive processing. In: Fishman SM, Ballantyne JC, Rathmell JP, editors. Bonica's management of pain. 4th edition. Baltimore (MD): Lippincott, Williams & Wilkins; 2010. p. 35–48.
4. Randich A, Ness T. Modulation of spinal nociceptive processing. In: Fishman SM, Ballantyne JC, Rathmell JP, editors. Bonica's management of pain. 4th edition. Baltimore (MD): Lippincott, Williams & Wilkins; 2010. p. 48–60.
5. Lorenz J, Hauck M. Supraspinal mechanisms of pain and nociception. In: Fishman SM, Ballantyne JC, Rathmell JP, editors. Bonica's management of pain. 4th edition. Baltimore (MD): Lippincott, Williams & Wilkins; 2010. p. 61–73.
6. Stagg NJ, Mata HP, Ibrahim MM, et al. Regular exercise reverses sensory hypersensitivity in a rat neuropathic pain model: role of endogenous opioids. Anesthesiology 2011;114(4):940–8.
7. Chen YW, Tzeng JI, Lin MF, et al. Forced treadmill running suppresses postincisional pain and inhibits upregulation of substance P and cytokines in rat dorsal root ganglion. J Pain 2014;15(8):827–34.
8. Mazzardo-Martins L, Martins DF, Marcon R, et al. High-intensity extended swimming exercise reduces pain-related behavior in mice: involvement of endogenous opioids and the serotonergic system. J Pain 2010;11(12):1384–93.
9. Martins DF, Mazzardo-Martins L, Soldi F, et al. High-intensity swimming exercise reduces neuropathic pain in an animal model of complex regional pain syndrome type I: evidence for a role of the adenosinergic system. Neuroscience 2013;234: 69–76.
10. Sullivan AB, Scheman J, Venesy D, et al. The role of exercise and types of exercise in the rehabilitation of chronic pain: specific or nonspecific benefits. Curr Pain Headache Rep 2012;16(2):153–61.
11. Wang XQ, Zheng JJ, Yu ZW, et al. A meta-analysis of core stability exercise versus general exercise for chronic low back pain. PLoS One 2012;7(12): e52082. http://dx.doi.org/10.1371/journal.pone.0052082.
12. Murtezani A, Hundozi H, Orovcanec N, et al. A comparison of high intensity aerobic exercise and passive modalities for the treatment of workers with chronic low back pain: a randomized, controlled trial. Eur J Phys Rehabil Med 2011;47(3): 359–66.
13. Busch AJ, Webber SC, Brachaniec M, et al. Exercise therapy for fibromyalgia. Curr Pain Headache Rep 2011;15:358–67.

14. Golightly YM, Allen KD, Caine DJ. A comprehensive review of the effectiveness of different exercise programs for patients with osteoarthritis. Phys Sportsmed 2012; 40(4):52–65.
15. Dobson JL, McMillan J, Li L. Benefits of exercise intervention in reducing neuropathic pain. Front Cell Neurosci 2014;8:102.
16. Sherry DD, Wallace CA, Kelley C, et al. Short- and long-term outcomes of children with complex regional pain syndrome type I treated with exercise therapy. Clin J Pain 1999;15(3):218–23.
17. Anshell MH, Russell KG. Effect of aerobic and strength training on pain tolerance, pain appraisal and mood of unfit males as a function of pain location. J Sports Sci 1994;12(6):535–47.
18. Ellingson LD, Colbert LH, Cook DB. Physical activity is related to pain sensitivity in healthy women. Med Sci Sports Exerc 2012;44(7):1401–6.
19. Delfa de la Morena JM, Samani A, Fernandez-Carnero J, et al. Pressure pain mapping of the wrist extensors after repeated eccentric exercise at high intensity. J Strength Cond Res 2013;27(11):3045–52.
20. Naugle KM, Naugle KE, Fillingim RB, et al. Intensity thresholds for aerobic exercise-induced hypoalgesia. Med Sci Sports Exerc 2014;46(4): 817–25.
21. Naugle KM, Riley JL 3rd. Self-reported physical activity predicts pain inhibitory and facilitatory function. Med Sci Sports Exerc 2014;46(3):622–9.
22. Meeus M, Hermans L, Ickmans K, et al. Endogenous pain modulation in response to exercise in patients with rheumatoid arthritis, patients with chronic fatigue syndrome and comorbid fibromyalgia, and healthy controls: a double-blind randomized controlled trial. Pain Pract 2014. http://dx.doi.org/10.1111/papr.12181.
23. Ellingson LD, Koltyn KF, Kim JS, et al. Does exercise induce hypoalgesia through conditioned pain modulation? Psychophysiology 2014;51:267–76.
24. Yezierski RP, Gerhart KD, Schrock BJ, et al. A further examination of effects of cortical stimulation on primate spinothalamic tract cells. J Neurophysiol 1983; 49(2):424–41.
25. Peyron R, Faillenot I, Mertens P, et al. Motor cortex stimulation in neuropathic pain. Correlations between analgesic effects and hemodynamic changes in the brain. A PET study. Neuroimage 2007;34(1):310–21.
26. Dall'Agnol L, Medeiros LF, Torres IL, et al. Repetitive transcranial magnetic stimulation increases the corticospinal inhibition and the brain-derived neurotrophic factor in chronic myofascial pain syndrome: an explanatory double-blinded, randomized, sham-controlled trial. J Pain 2014;15(8):845–55.
27. Knauf MT, Koltyn KF. Exercise-induced modulation of pain in adults wit and without painful diabetic neuropathy. J Pain 2014;15(6):656–63.
28. Naugle KM, Fillingim RB, Riley JL 3rd. A meta-analytic review of the hypoalgesic effects of exercise. J Pain 2012;13(12):1139–50.
29. Nijs J, Kosek E, Van Oosterwijck JV, et al. Dysfunctional endogenous analgesia during exercise in patients with chronic pain: to exercise or not to exercise. Pain Physician 2012;15:ES205–13.
30. Busch AJ, Barber KA, Overend TJ, et al. Exercise for treating fibromyalgia syndrome. Cochrane Database Syst Rev 2007;(4):CD003786. http://dx.doi.org/10.1002/14651858.CD003786.pub2.
31. Busch AJ, Webber SC, Richards RS, et al. Resistance exercise training for fibromyalgia. Cochrane Database Syst Rev 2013;(12):CD010884. http://dx.doi.org/10.1002/14651858.CD010884.

32. Hooten WM, Qu W, Townsend CO, et al. Effects of strength vs aerobic exercise on pain severity in adults with fibromyalgia: a randomized equivalence trial. Pain 2012;153(4):915–23.
33. McLoughlin MJ, Stegner AJ, Cook DB. The relationship between physical activity and brain responses to pain in fibromyalgia. J Pain 2011;12(6):640–51.
34. Bennell KL, Hunt MA, Wrigley TV, et al. Hip strengthening reduces symptoms but not knee load in people with medial knee osteoarthritis and varus malalignment: a randomized controlled trial. Osteoarthritis Cartilage 2010;18(5):621–8.
35. Ettinger WH, Burns R, Messier SP, et al. A randomized trial comparing aerobic exercise and resistance exercise with a health education program in older adults with knee osteoarthritis. The Fitness Arthritis and Seniors Trial (FAST). JAMA 1997;277:25–31.
36. van Barr M, Dekker J, Oostendorp R, et al. Effectiveness of exercise in patients with osteoarthritis of the hip or knee: nine months follow up. Ann Rheum Dis 2001;60:1123–30.
37. Bennell KL, Dobson F, Hinman RS. Exercise in osteoarthritis: moving from prescription to adherence. Best Pract Res Clin Rheumatol 2014;28(1):93–117.
38. Moseley GL. Graded motor imagery is effective for long-standing complex regional pain syndrome: a randomized controlled trial. Pain 2004;108:192–8.
39. Daly AE, Bialocerkowski AE. Does evidence support physiotherapy management of adult complex regional pain syndrome type one? A systematic review. Eur J Pain 2009;13:339–53.
40. Cossins L, Okell RW, Cameron H, et al. Treatment of complex regional pain syndrome in adults: a systematic review of randomized controlled trials published from June 2000 to February 2012. Eur J Pain 2013;17:158–73.
41. van Middelkoop M, Rubinstein SM, Verhagen AP, et al. Exercise therapy for chronic nonspecific low-back pain. Best Pract Res Clin Rheumatol 2010;24: 193–204.
42. Mannion AF, Muntener M, Taimela S, et al. A randomized clinical trial of three active therapies for chronic low back pain. Spine (Phila Pa 1976) 1999;24(23): 2435–48.
43. Mannion AF, Muntener M, Taimela S, et al. Comparison of three active therapies for chronic low back pain: results of a randomized clinical trial with one-year follow-up. Rheumatology 2001;40:772–8.
44. Smith C, Grimmer-Somers K. The treatment effect of exercise programmes for chronic low back pain. J Eval Clin Pract 2010;16:484–91.
45. Liddle SD, Baxter GD, Gracey JH. Exercise and chronic low back pain: what works? Pain 2004;107:176–90.
46. Brennan GP, Fritz JM, Hunter SJ, et al. Identifying subgroups of patients with acute/subacute "nonspecific" low back pain: results of a randomized clinical trial. Spine (Phila Pa 1976) 2006;31:623–31.
47. Koumantakis GA, Watson PJ, Oldham JA. Trunk muscle stabilization training plus general exercise versus general exercise only: randomized controlled trial of patients with recurrent low back pain. Phys Ther 2005;85:209–25.
48. Lomond KV, Henry SM, Hitt JR, et al. Altered postural responses persist following physical therapy of general versus specific trunk exercises in people with low back pain. Man Ther 2014;19(5):425–32.
49. Steiger F, Wirth B, de Bruin ED, et al. Is a positive clinical outcome after exercise therapy for chronic non-specific low back pain contingent upon a corresponding improvement in the targeted aspect(s) of performance? A systematic review. Eur Spine J 2012;21:575–98.

50. Machado LA, de Souza MS, Ferrieira PH, et al. The McKenzie method for low back pain: a systematic review of the literature with a meta-analysis approach. Spine (Phila Pa 1976) 2006;31:E254–62.
51. Peterson T, Kryger P, Ekdahl C, et al. The effect of McKenzie therapy as compared with that of intensive strengthening training for treatment of patients with subacute or chronic low back pain: a randomized controlled trial. Spine (Phila Pa 1976) 2002;27:1702–9.
52. Hosseinifar M, Akbari M, Behtash H, et al. The effects of stabilization and Mckenzie exercises on transverse abdominus and multifidus muscle thickness, pain and disability: a randomized controlled trial in nonspecific chronic low back pain. J Phys Ther Sci 2013;25(12):1541–5.
53. Long A, Donelson R, Fung T. Does it matter which exercise? A randomized control trial of exercise for low back pain. Spine (Phila Pa 1976) 2004;29(23): 2593–602.
54. Hayden JA, van Tulder MW, Malmivaara AV, et al. Meta-analysis: exercise therapy for nonspecific low back pain. Ann Intern Med 2005;142(9):765–75.
55. Hendrick P, Te Wake AM, Tikkisetty AS, et al. The effectiveness of walking as an intervention for low back pain: a systematic review. Eur Spine J 2010;19: 1613–20.
56. Cramer H, Lauche R, Hohmann C, et al. Randomized-controlled trial comparing yoga and home-based exercise for chronic neck pain. Clin J Pain 2013;29: 216–23.
57. Tekur P, Nagaranthna R, Chametcha S, et al. A comprehensive yoga program improves pain, anxiety and depression in chronic low back pain patients more than exercise: an RCT. Complement Ther Med 2012;20(3):107–18.
58. Sherman KJ, Cherkin DC, Wellman RD, et al. A randomized trial comparing yoga, stretching, and a self-care book for chronic low back pain. Arch Intern Med 2011; 171(22):2019–26.
59. Holtzman S, Beggs RT. Yoga for chronic low back pain: a meta-analysis of randomized controlled trials. Pain Res Manag 2013;18(5):267–72.
60. Little P, Lewith G, Webley F, et al. Randomised controlled trial of Alexander technique lessons, exercise, and massage (ATEAM) for chronic and recurrent back pain. Br J Sports Med 2008;42(12):965–8.
61. Hall AM, Maher CG, Lam P, et al. Tai Chi exercise for treatment of pain and disability in people with persistent low back pain: a randomized controlled trial. Arthritis Care Res 2011;63(11):1576–83.
62. Fordyce WE, Fowler RS Jr, Lehmann JF, et al. Operant conditioning in the treatment of chronic pain. Arch Phys Med Rehabil 1973;54:399–408.
63. Flor H, Fydrich T, Turk DC. Efficacy of multidisciplinary pain treatment centers: a meta-analytic review. Pain 1992;49(2):221–30.
64. Guzman J, Esmail R, Karjalainen K, et al. Multidisciplinary rehabilitation for chronic low back pain: systematic review. BMJ 2001;322:1511–6.
65. Proctor TJ, Mayer TG, Theodore B, et al. Failure to complete a functional restoration program for chronic musculoskeletal disorders: a prospective 1-year outcome study. Arch Phys Med Rehabil 2005;86(8):1509–15.
66. Kool JP, Oesch PR, Bachmann S, et al. Increasing days at work using function-centered rehabilitation in nonacute nonspecific low back pain: a randomized controlled trial. Arch Phys Med Rehabil 2005;86(5):857–64.
67. van Geen JW, Edelaar MJ, Janssen M, et al. The long-term effect of multidisciplinary back training: a systematic review. Spine (Phila Pa 1976) 2007;32(2): 249–55.

68. Norlund A, Ropponen A, Alexanderson K. Multidisciplinary interventions: review of studies of return to work after rehabilitation for low back pain. J Rehabil Med 2009;41:115–21.
69. Mayer TG, Gatchel RJ, Brede E, et al. Lumbar surgery in work-related chronic low back pain: can a continuum of care enhance outcomes? Spine J 2014;14:263–73.
70. Monticone M, Ferrante S, Rocca B, et al. Effect of a long-lasting multidisciplinary program on disability and fear-avoidance behaviors in patients with chronic low back pain. Results of a randomized controlled trial. Clin J Pain 2013;29(11): 929–38.
71. Louw A, Diener I, Butler D, et al. The effect of neuroscience education on pain, disability, anxiety, and stress in chronic musculoskeletal pain. Arch Phys Med Rehabil 2011;92:2041–56.
72. Nijs J, van Wilgen CP, Oosterwijck JV, et al. How to explain central sensitization to patients with "unexplained" chronic musculoskeletal pain: practice guidelines. Man Ther 2011;16:413–8.
73. Nijs J, Meeus M, Cagnie B, et al. A modern neuroscience approach to chronic spinal pain: combining neuroscience education with cognition-targeted motor control training. Phys Ther 2014;94:730–8.
74. Butler D, Moseley GL. Explain pain. Adelaide (Australia): NOI Group Publishing; 2003.
75. Vlaeyen JW, Linton SJ. Fear-avoidance model of chronic musculoskeletal pain: 12 years on. Pain 2012;153:1144–7.
76. Kernan T, Rainville J. Observed outcomes associated with a quota-based exercise approach on measures of kinesiophobia in patients with chronic low back pain. J Orthop Sports Phys Ther 2007;37(11):679–87.
77. Von Korff M, Balderson BH, Saudners K, et al. A trial of an activating intervention for chronic back pain in primary care and physical therapy settings. Pain 2005; 113:323–30.
78. Cecchi F, Pasquini G, Paperini A, et al. Predictors of response to exercise therapy for chronic low back pain: result of a prospective study with one year follow-up. Eur J Phys Rehabil Med 2014;50:143–51.
79. Medina-Mirapeix F, Escolar-Reina P, Gascon-Canovas JJ, et al. Predictive factors of adherence to frequency and duration components in home exercise programs for neck and low back pain: and observational study. BMC Musculoskelet Disord 2009;10:155–63.
80. Courneya KS, McAuley E. Are there different determinants of the frequency, intensity, and duration of physical activity? Behav Med 1994;20(2):84–90.
81. Slade SC, Patel S, Underwood M, et al. What are patient beliefs and perceptions about exercise for non-specific chronic low back pain? A systematic review of qualitative studies. Clin J Pain 2014;30(11):995–1005. http://dx.doi.org/10.1097/AJP.0000000000000044.

Psychiatric and Psychological Perspectives on Chronic Pain

Catherine Q. Howe, MD, PhD, James P. Robinson, MD, PhD*,
Mark D. Sullivan, MD, PhD

KEYWORDS

- Major depressive disorder • Dysthymia • Panic disorder
- Posttraumatic stress disorder • Substance use disorders • Illness beliefs
- Coping strategies • Fear avoidance

KEY POINTS

- Several psychiatric disorders are so common among chronic pain patients that physiatrists should be alert to them. They include major depressive disorder, dysthymia, panic disorder, posttraumatic stress disorder, and various substance use disorders.
- A high proportion of chronic pain patients have dysfunctional belief systems about their conditions and/or dysfunctional coping strategies to deal with their conditions. These beliefs and coping strategies can occur in the absence of a diagnosable psychiatric condition and can have significant negative impacts on the patients' response to treatment.
- Physiatrists should consider several factors when they decide whether to refer a pain patient to a psychiatrist or a psychologist. In general, though, an initial referral to a psychiatrist is usually the best strategy.

INTRODUCTION

Physiatrists who treat patients with chronic pain frequently request assistance from mental health practitioners. The 2 types of professionals who typically evaluate these patients are psychiatrists and clinical psychologists. The present article describes the perspectives taken by these 2 professional groups and offers recommendations about when to refer to a psychiatrist versus a psychologist.

THE PSYCHIATRIC PERSPECTIVE

Any discussion of psychiatric disorders in patients with chronic pain is haunted by the concept of psychogenic pain. One is drawn to this concept because it fills the gaps left

Physical Medicine & Rehabilitation, University of Washington, Seattle, WA, USA
* Corresponding author.
E-mail address: jimrob@uw.edu

Phys Med Rehabil Clin N Am 26 (2015) 283–300
http://dx.doi.org/10.1016/j.pmr.2014.12.003   pmr.theclinics.com

when the attempts fail to explain clinical pain exclusively in terms of tissue pathologic abnormality. In fact, psychogenic pain was codified into the pain disorder diagnosis in the fourth edition of the Diagnostic and Statistical Manual of Mental Disorders (DSM-IV). The diagnosis presumes that some pain conditions are solely or predominantly explained by psychological factors rather than medical conditions. Psychogenic pain, however, is an empty concept. Positive criteria for the identification of psychogenic pain, mechanisms for the production of psychogenic pain, and specific therapies for psychogenic pain are lacking. Psychiatric diagnosis of many disorders, such as depression, can be helpful to the clinician and the patient by pointing to specific effective therapies. However, the diagnosis of psychogenic pain too often only serves to stigmatize further the patient who experiences chronic pain.

A notable and welcome change from DSM-IV to DSM-5 is the elimination of the pain disorder diagnosis. The rationale for its removal was given in the introductory section to the chapter, "Somatic Symptoms and Related Disorder," in DSM-5: "The reliability of determining that a somatic symptom is medially unexplained is limited, and grounding a diagnosis on the absence of an explanation is problematic and reinforces mind-body dualism" (American Psychiatric Association, 2013, p. 309).

Epidemiologic evidence supports the use of inclusive rather than exclusive models of psychiatric diagnoses in medical settings that allows for the presence of both medical disease and mental disorders. Medical illness in no way excludes the possibility of a clinically important psychiatric illness. Medically ill patients are, in fact, much more likely to have psychiatric illness than patients without medical illness. Psychiatric illness in no way precludes the possibility of a clinically important medical illness. Psychiatric illness is, in fact, associated with health behaviors and physiologic changes known to promote medical illness.

In the discussion that follows, psychiatric disorders as defined in DSM-5 are used as an organizing strategy. It is important to note, however, that the categorical model of mental disorder favored by psychiatrists and used in DSM-5 can imply more discontinuity between those with and those without a mental disorder than is actually the case. For example, it is common for patients with chronic pain to partially meet criteria for several mental disorders. Therefore, it is sometimes useful to think of these disorders as dimensions rather than categories. The DSM-5 nevertheless provides a well-recognized and systematic template for the discussion of psychiatric disorders in patients with chronic pain.

When asked to evaluate patients at the authors' Center for Pain Relief, they typically consider the following issues: depression, anxiety, trauma and abuse history, posttraumatic stress disorder (PTSD), and substance use disorders. The authors do not usually use a structured interview for psychiatric diagnosis, but some brief, self-administered questionnaires are routinely given to the patients at every visit to screen for major psychiatric symptoms and for outcome tracking in a nonresearch clinical setting. These evaluations include the 9-item Patient Health Questionnaire,[1] the Generalized Anxiety Disorder 7-item scale,[2] and a 4-item Primary Care PTSD Screen.[3]

Depression

One must begin by distinguishing between depressed mood and the clinical syndrome of major depression. It is important to note, especially when working with chronic pain patients, that depressed mood or dysphoria is not necessary for the diagnosis of major depression. Anhedonia, the inability to enjoy activities or experience pleasure, is an adequate substitute. It is common for patients with chronic pain to deny dysphoria but to acknowledge that enjoyment of all activities has ceased, even those without obvious relation to their pain problem (eg, watching television for a patient with low back pain).

The DSM-5 criteria for major depressive episode include both psychological symptoms (worthlessness or guilt, thoughts of death or dying) and somatic symptoms (insomnia or hypersomnia, change in appetite, fatigue, trouble concentrating, psychomotor agitation, or retardation). The presence of 5 or more symptoms is required for diagnosis of a major depressive episode. It is important to note that somatic symptoms count toward a diagnosis of major depression unless they are due to "clearly and fully attributable to a general medical condition" or medication (American Psychiatric Association, 2013, p. 164). The poor sleep, poor concentration, and lack of enjoyment often experienced by patients with chronic pain are frequently attributed to pain rather than to depression. However, because they are not a direct physiologic effect of pain, these symptoms should count toward a diagnosis of depression. In fact, studies of depression in medically ill populations have generally found greater sensitivity and reliability with "inclusive models" of depression diagnosis that accept all symptoms as relevant to the diagnosis than with models that try to identify the cause of each symptom.[4]

Patients with chronic pain often dismiss a depression diagnosis, stating that their depression is a reaction to their pain problem. Psychiatry has long debated the value of distinguishing a "reactive" form of depression caused by adverse life events and an endogenous form of depression caused by biological and genetic factors.[5] Life events are important in many depressive episodes, although they play a less important role in recurrent and very severe or melancholic or psychotic depressions.[6] Previously in DSM-IV, the only life event that excludes someone who otherwise qualifies for a major depression diagnosis is bereavement. This exclusion is eliminated in DSM-5 for several reasons, one of which is that bereavement-related depression responds to the same treatments as non-bereavement-related depression. Determining whether a depression is a "reasonable response" to life's stress may be very important to patients seeking to decrease the stigma of a depression diagnosis, and it has been of interest to pain investigators. It is not, however, important in deciding whether treatment is necessary and appropriate. Indeed, in assessment there is no clarity to be gained from debating whether the depression caused the pain or the pain caused the depression. If patients meet the criteria outlined earlier, they can likely benefit from appropriate treatment.

When considering the diagnosis of depression in patients with chronic pain, important alternatives include bipolar disorder, substance-induced mood disorder, and dysthymic disorder. Patients with bipolar disorder have extended periods of abnormally elevated or irritable, as well as abnormally depressed, mood. These periods of elevated mood need to last several, continuous days (4 days for a hypomanic episode, 1 week for a manic episode) and include features such as inflated self-esteem, decreased need for sleep, increased goal-directed activity, and racing thoughts. A history of manic or hypomanic episodes predicts an atypical response to antidepressant medication and increases the risk of antidepressant-induced mania. Bipolar disorder is less common (12-month prevalence in the general population 2.6 vs 6.7%)[7] than unipolar depression, but it is important to recognize because it requires a different treatment approach.

Substance-induced mood disorders can also occur in those with pain. Patients with chronic pain may be taking medications such as steroids, dopamine-blocking agents (including antiemetics), or sedatives (including "muscle relaxants") that produce a depressive syndrome. Patients' current medication lists should be scrutinized for potential depressogenic medications. For patients with a pure substance-induced mood disorder, symptoms can persist for up to a month after discontinuation of the substance but will eventually resolve. It should be noted that some patients with an underlying mood disorder "self-medicate" with other substances (drugs, alcohol); hence, establishing the temporal relationship (as much as possible) between the onset of mood symptoms and substance abuse is important for diagnosis and treatment planning.

Dysthymic disorder is a chronic form of depression lasting 2 years or longer. Individuals with dysthymia are at high risk to develop major depression as well. This combined syndrome has often been called "double depression."[8] It is important to note that dysthymia is frequently invisible in medical settings, often dismissed as "just the way that patient is." Dysthymia has been shown to respond to many antidepressants, including the selective serotonin reuptake inhibitors. Treatment of double depression can be particularly challenging because of treatment resistance and concurrent personality disorders.[9] Psychiatric consultation may be useful when any of these disorders is suspected.

Twelve-month prevalence rates for major depression and dysthymia in the general population are 6.7% and 1.5%, respectively.[10] Among individuals endorsing one or more chronic pain conditions in the general population (back/neck, arthritis, migraine/chronic headaches), 12-month rates are generally higher, 10% to 30%.[11–14] Prevalence rates of depression among patients in pain clinics have varied widely depending on the method of assessment and the population assessed. Rates as low as 10% and as high as 100% have been reported.[15] The reason for the wide variability may be attributable to several factors, including the methods used to diagnose depression (eg, interview, self-report instruments), the criteria used (eg, cutoff scores on self-report instruments), the set of disorders included in the diagnosis of depression (eg, presence of depressive symptoms, major depression), and referral bias (eg, higher reported prevalence of depression in studies in psychiatry clinics compared with rehabilitation clinics). Overall, chronic pain increases depression risk by 2-fold to 5-fold.[16–20]

Studies of primary care populations have revealed several factors that seem to increase the likelihood of depression in patients with chronic pain. Patients with 2 or more pain complaints were much more likely to be depressed than those with a single pain complaint.[21] Number of pain conditions reported was a better predictor of major depression than pain severity or pain persistence. Von Korff and colleagues[22] developed a 4-level scale for grading chronic pain severity based on pain disability and pain intensity: (1) low disability and low intensity, (2) low disability and high intensity, (3) high disability-moderately limiting, and (4) high disability-severely limiting. Depression, use of opioid analgesics, and doctor visits all increased as chronic pain grade increased.

Patients with chronic pain often feel they are battling to have their suffering recognized as real. They resist a depression diagnosis if they see it as a way to dismiss their suffering. Even if clinicians are sensitive to these issues, they must recognize that legal proceedings, insurance companies, and workers' compensation boards can look on a depression diagnosis with prejudice. Traditional and industrial societies seem to hold individuals less responsible for somatic symptoms than for psychological symptoms. This difference may be especially prominent in modern Western biomedicine, whereby symptom complexes are validated or invalidated through their correspondence with objective disease criteria.[23] Pain is a more acceptable reason for disability than depression in many cultures. Therefore, cultural incentives exist for translation of depression into pain. Because depressed patients have many physical symptoms, these can become the focus of clinical communication and concern. Giving patients with chronic pain permission to talk of distress in the clinical setting using nonsomatic terms can facilitate treatment as long as they do not feel that somatic elements of their problem are being neglected or discounted. The authors try to validate depression as an understandable response to a chronic pain problem.

Anxiety Disorders

It is not unusual for patients with symptoms of pain to be anxious and worried; however, this is not synonymous with a psychiatric diagnosis of an anxiety disorder. When patients with chronic pain do suffer from an anxiety disorder, it is rare that this is their sole psychiatric diagnosis. Most patients with pain and chronic anxiety also meet criteria for either major depression or dysthymia. In these cases, treatment should be directed toward the mood disorder. With successful treatment of the mood disorder, the anxiety should be relieved as well. Benzodiazepines are best avoided because of their association with tolerance, dependence, and withdrawal. Prolonged use may promote inactivity and cognitive impairment.

Panic disorder

Panic disorder is a common, disabling psychiatric illness associated with high medical service utilization and multiple medically unexplained symptoms. In the pain clinic setting, panic disorder should be considered especially in patients with chest pain, abdominal pain, or headaches. The diagnosis of panic disorder requires that recurrent, unexpected panic attacks be followed by at least a month of worry about having another panic attack, about the implications or consequences of the panic attacks, or behavioral changes related to the attacks. A panic attack is defined as a discrete period of intense fear or discomfort in which 4 or more symptoms are present. As with major depression, DSM-5 criteria include symptoms that are somatic (increased heart rate, palpitations, sweating, shortness of breath, chest pain, trembling, dizziness, chills or hot flushes, nausea, feeling of choking, paresthesias) and psychological (fear of dying, fear of losing control, or going crazy). These attacks should not be the direct physiologic consequence of a substance or other medical condition. The panic attacks should not be better accounted for by another mental disorder, such as PTSD (described later) or obsessive-compulsive disorder. At least 2 unexpected attacks are required for the diagnosis, although most patients have more.

One of the most common problems with panic disorder is the fear of undiagnosed, life-threatening illness. Patients with panic disorder can receive extensive medical testing and treatment of their somatic symptoms before the diagnosis of panic disorder is made and appropriate treatment is initiated. Lifetime prevalence of panic disorder throughout the world is estimated to be 1.5% to 4.7%.[7] One-year prevalence rates are from 1% to 2.7%.[10] Panic disorder is 2 to 3 times more common in women than in men. Age of onset is variable, but most cases typically occur between late adolescence and the mid-30s. Of all common mental disorders in the primary care setting, panic disorder is most likely to produce moderate to severe occupational dysfunction and physical disability.[24] It is also associated with the greatest number of disability days in the past month.

Panic disorder is commonly associated with *agoraphobia,* or fear of public places. Patients with panic disorder learn to fear places where escape might be difficult or help may not be available in case they have an attack. Major depression is another common comorbidity in patients suffering from panic disorder. The differential diagnosis of patients presenting with panic symptoms in the medical setting includes thyroid, parathyroid, adrenal, and vestibular dysfunction, seizure disorders, cardiac arrhythmias, and drug intoxication or withdrawal. Patients with panic disorder typically present in the medical setting with cardiologic, gastrointestinal, or neurologic complaints.[25]

Chest pain is one of the most common complaints presented to primary care physicians, but a specific medical cause is identified in only 10% to 20% of cases. From

43% to 61% of patients with normal coronary arteries at angiography and 16% to 25% of patients presenting to emergency rooms with chest pain have panic disorder. Several of these patients eventually receive the diagnoses of vasospastic angina, costochondritis, esophageal dysmotility, or mitral valve prolapse. High rates of psychiatric disorders have been found in some of these groups as well.[26] Many of these patients remain symptomatic and disabled 1 year later despite reassurance concerning coronary artery disease.[27]

Approximately 11% of primary care patients present with the complaint of abdominal pain to their physician each year. Less than a one-fourth of these symptoms are associated with a definite physical diagnosis in the following year. Among the most common reasons for abdominal pain is irritable bowel syndrome. It is estimated that irritable bowel syndrome accounts for 20% to 52% of all referrals to gastroenterologists. Various studies have found that 54% to 74% of these patients with irritable bowel syndrome have associated psychiatric disorders. Patients with irritable bowel syndrome have much higher current (28 vs 3%) and lifetime (41 vs 25%) rates of panic disorder than a comparison group with inflammatory bowel disease,[28] suggesting that the psychiatric disorder was not simply a reaction to the abdominal distress. Other studies have suggested that migraine headache is most strongly associated with panic attacks.[29] Often anxiety symptoms precede the onset of the headaches, whereas depressive symptoms often have their onset after the headaches. Some authors have suggested that people with panic attacks have a common predisposition to headaches (especially migraines and chronic daily headache), anxiety disorders, and major depression.

Posttraumatic Stress Disorder

Previously classified as an anxiety disorder in DSM-IV, PTSD is now in the new category of trauma-related and stress-related disorders in DSM-5. Following direct or indirect exposure to an extreme traumatic event, some individuals develop a syndrome that includes re-experiencing the event, avoidance of stimuli associated with the event, persistent heightened arousal, and negative cognitions or emotion. PTSD was originally described following exposure to military combat, but it is now recognized that it occurs following sexual or physical assault, natural disasters, accidents, life-threatening illnesses, and other events that induce feelings of intense fear, hopelessness, or horror. Persons may develop the disorder after experiencing or just witnessing these events. DSM-5 diagnostic criteria require that the person either experienced or witnessed an event that involved actual or threatened death, serious injury, or threat to the physical integrity of the self or others. Posttraumatic symptoms must last more than 1 month. The event can be re-experienced in the form of recurrent nightmares, flashbacks, or intense psychological distress or physical reactivity in response to internal or external cues resembling the event. Persistent avoidance can present as avoiding thoughts or memories about the event, or avoiding people, places, or situations that arouse memories of the event. Two or more symptoms of negative alterations in cognitions and affect (inability to recall important aspects of the trauma, exaggerated negative beliefs about oneself or others, distorted cognitions about the cause or consequences of the trauma, persistent negative emotional state, diminished interest in activities, a feeling of detachment from others, and inability to experience positive emotions) and 2 or more symptoms of increased arousal (eg, disturbed sleep, irritability, self-destructive behavior, hypervigilance, increased startle response, difficulty concentrating) should also be present.

Up to 80% of Vietnam veterans with PTSD report chronic pain in limbs, back, torso, or head.[30] Increased physical symptoms, including muscle aches and back pain, are also more common in Gulf War veterans with PTSD than in those without PTSD.[31] The

12-month prevalence of PTSD in the general population is 3.5%.[10] The prevalence of PTSD in medical populations has been shown to be quite high. Averaging the prevalence rates of PTSD across several studies reveals that following motor vehicle accidents sufficiently severe to require medical attention, 29.5% of patients met the criteria for PTSD.[32] For more than one-half of these patients, the symptoms resolved within 6 months. In one study, 15% of patients seeking treatment of idiopathic facial pain were found to have PTSD.[33] In another study, 21% of patients with fibromyalgia were found to have PTSD.[34] Case reports have associated reflex sympathetic dystrophy (complex regional pain syndrome) with PTSD. Other studies suggest that 50% to 100% of patients presenting at pain treatment centers meet the diagnostic criteria for PTSD.[35] Pain patients with PTSD have been shown to have more pain and affective distress than those without PTSD,[36] so it is not surprising that PTSD rates among patients with pain increase in more specialized treatment settings.

The relationship between pain and PTSD is multifaceted. Pain and PTSD may both result from a traumatic event. Sometimes acute pain can constitute the traumatic event, such as in a case of traumatic eye enucleation,[37] and in cases of implantable cardioverter defibrillator discharges.[38] PTSD also appears to permit induction of an opioid-mediated, stress-induced analgesia. PTSD-related stimuli can result in a naloxone-reversible decreased sensitivity to noxious stimuli in affected individuals.[39]

The relation between childhood abuse and chronic pain has received plenty of attention in recent years. Multiple studies have demonstrated higher rates of childhood maltreatment in patients with chronic pain than in comparison groups. They have also shown poorer coping among abused patients with pain.[40] However, the relationship between childhood psychological trauma and adult somatic symptoms is complex.[41] PTSD, dissociation, somatization, and affect dysregulation represent a spectrum of adaptations to trauma. They may occur together or separately.[42] The best way to incorporate information about childhood maltreatment into the treatment of the adult patient with chronic pain is as yet unclear. It may signal to caregivers the potential challenges in establishing a therapeutic alliance. It may also mean that additional psychotherapeutic interventions are necessary beyond the coaching of pain management skills. However, chronic pain treatment trials have not yet grouped patients by trauma history or attempted treatment matching.

Substance Use Disorders

DSM-5 no longer distinguishes between substance dependence and substance abuse, as did DSM-IV. The essential feature of any substance use disorder is continued use of a substance despite a cluster of cognitive, behavioral, and physiologic problems. It is characterized by impaired control, social impairment, risky use, and the development of tolerance and withdrawal.

Diagnosis of substance use disorders in patients with chronic pain is controversial, because it is difficult to achieve consensus on what constitutes a *maladaptive* pattern of substance use, especially with regard to prescription opioids. Traditionally, opioids have been considered appropriate for terminal cancer pain, with tolerance, dependence, and dose escalation limited in their importance by the impending death of the patient. However, they have been considered problematic for the chronic noncancer patient with pain whose long-term function is an essential issue. A large percentage of patients referred to multidisciplinary pain centers report taking opioids at the time of assessment. Following treatment, most of these patients report significantly reduced pain concurrent with elimination of opioid medication.[43–45] Portenoy[46] and others have argued forcefully that chronic opioid therapy can be appropriate and beneficial in *some* patients with chronic noncancer pain. One of the current, unanswered questions is what factors characterize those patients who are likely to benefit from long-term opioids without problems of addiction, tolerance, or increased disability. To date, there have been no long-term, double-blind studies that help to select the group for whom long-term opioids are beneficial. Nevertheless, in recent years, there has been a marked increase in the use of opioids for chronic noncancer pain. Several recent studies have found that individuals with underlying depressive, anxiety, or substance use disorders are more likely than those without these disorders to receive opioids for noncancer pain.[47] Hence, screening for and treating these disorders in individuals on, or being considered for, opioid therapy are important.

The lifetime and 12-month prevalences of substance use disorders in the general population are 14.6%[7] and 3.8%,[10] respectively. Prevalence rates for substance abuse in patients with chronic pain are variable because of differences in definitions used and populations assessed. Overall, persistent pain seems to increase the risk of problem substance use by 2-fold to 5-fold.[48,49] Studies completed to date suggest that substance use disorders occur in a minority of chronic pain patients on opioids. They do not answer the more difficult question of whether opioids are, on balance, beneficial treatment for these patients in terms of reduction and improvement of function.

Because small amounts of alcohol use can retard response to antidepressant medication, it is important to inquire about alcohol use that may not otherwise meet criteria for abuse in patients who are candidates for antidepressant medication. The authors encourage patients they place on antidepressant medication to limit alcohol use to 1 or 2 drinks per week. Significant others and other third parties can provide useful information about substance use. The authors also encourage the use of urine toxicology screens in any patients with histories of substance use. Often this is the only way to be sure about the cause of a patient's altered mental status, such as affective lability, cognitive impairment, and treatment nonresponse.

THE PSYCHOLOGICAL PERSPECTIVE

Clinical psychologists and psychiatrists both treat chronic pain patients with behavioral problems, but they approach this task from different perspectives. As a branch of medicine, psychiatry focuses on mental disorders, some of which are common among pain patients. In contrast, psychologists, including clinical psychologists, attempt to understand general principles that govern the behavior of all people and then apply these principles to gain insights into behavioral abnormalities that some pain patients demonstrate.

One way to frame this difference in perspective is to note the obvious point that chronic pain creates stress and challenges the coping resources of patients. Some patients meet these challenges admirably, so that their psychological coping allows them to function much better than one would expect on the basis of the biology of their medical condition. At the opposite extreme, some pain patients adapt to their condition very poorly, and their psychological dysfunction plays a major role in amplifying their disability and/or delaying their recovery. Psychologists are interested in both the successful and the unsuccessful ways in which patients manage their pain.[50,51] Pain patients with the kinds of psychiatric disorders described above are likely to cope poorly with their pain. However, although many of the poor copers meet DSM-5 criteria for a mental disorder, some do not. Psychologists are interested in helping the poor copers manage their pain problems better, regardless of whether or not they meet criteria for a mental illness.

Multiple psychological processes influence the ways in which people cope with chronic pain. Psychologists have not agreed on a comprehensive list of psychological processes or psychological problems relevant to chronic pain. Also, there is no consensus about a model of behavior that shows how various psychological processes are related to each other. Different psychologists have emphasized classical (Pavlovian) conditioning, operant conditioning, psychodynamic theories, and various cognitive theories to explain the behavior of pain patients. The psychological model that informs the present discussion is the stress and coping model originally articulated by Lazarus[52] and amended by multiple authors since then.[53]

As articulated by Lazarus, coping starts with appraisals of a stressful situation. For a patient with chronic pain, these appraisals must occur in several domains, for the simple reason that chronic pain creates challenges in several domains. The process of appraisal is an iterative one, because challenges associated with chronic pain unfold over time. Broadly speaking, appraisals are classified into 2 main classes: characterizing the threats that the pain poses, and identifying coping strategies that address the threats.

The appraisals that patients make regarding threats posed by their pain and the options available to meet these threats reflect their beliefs about their condition. Pain patients often have beliefs regarding their conditions that impede their recoveries. For example, they might be convinced that prolonged inactivity will facilitate recovery, or that they cannot return to normal activities until structural abnormalities identified on imaging studies have been corrected, or that discomfort during activities implies that they have seriously aggravated their problem.

A substantial body of psychological research has addressed various beliefs that are associated with effective and ineffective coping. For example, Jensen and colleagues[54] reviewed 7 studies that examined associations between beliefs and indices of physical and psychological functioning among spinal cord injury (SCI) patients with chronic pain. The authors summarized their findings as follows: "7 beliefs were associated with more positive scores on criterion measures: (1) belief in control over pain, (2) belief in a medical cure for pain, (3) belief in global self-efficacy (ability to engage in a range a daily tasks despite SCI), (4) belief in pain-related self-efficacy, (5) belief in general control over life (6) disease benefit (item example, 'Dealing with my illness has made me a stronger person'), and (7) internal pain control." Six beliefs were associated with poorer outcomes: (1) belief in oneself as necessarily disabled by pain, (2) belief that pain is an indication of physical damage and that activity should be avoided, (3) belief that emotions influence pain, (4) belief that others should be solicitous in response to pain, (5) global helplessness, and (6) external pain control.

Beliefs of patients about whether they can control their pain have been shown to be especially important in determining their adaptation to their conditions.[55] Patients who perceive themselves as having control are described as experiencing self-efficacy in relation to their pain.[53] Various scales have been developed to assess self-efficacy among pain patients.[56] Research using these scales has generally found that patients with high self-efficacy show better adaptation to their pain problems than ones with low self-efficacy.[57,58] Also, considerable experimental research has been done on the effects of providing versus not providing subjects with the perception that they can control an aversive stimulus; this has shown that subjects given control find the stimuli to be less aversive than ones without such control.[59,60]

Patients' beliefs about whether they will recover from injuries have also been found to be clinically important. For example, Carroll[61] reviewed literature showing that among patients with whiplash disorders, ones who expected a good recovery did in fact recover better than ones with the opposite expectation. A related body of research has consistently demonstrated that among injured workers, those who report that their injuries make it impossible to return to work do in fact have lower return to work rates than ones with the opposite perception.[62–64]

Appraisal is a cognitive process. In theory, pain patients could appraise their conditions and develop coping strategies without experiencing much emotion. In fact, though, pain patients typically have intense emotional reactions to their conditions, and these reactions can greatly influence how they cope with their pain.[65,66] The relationship between cognitive processes (eg, beliefs about the significance of pain and the most appropriate strategies for dealing with it) and emotional reactions has occupied psychologists and physiologists for more than a century. For our purposes, it is enough to say that cognitive appraisals (eg, that a situation is highly threatening) can provoke intense emotion, and, conversely, that emotion can strongly influence cognition.[67]

Some pain patients experience undifferentiated emotional distress. However, most of them have emotional reactions that can be described as fear/anxiety, depression, or anger. In recent years, psychologists have done considerable research on fear. The fear-avoidance model articulated by Vlaeyen and colleagues[68] postulates that some patients develop significant fear after they have injured themselves, either of pain itself or of the reinjury that they think episodes of pain signify. Such individuals avoid activity. This avoidance, in turn, creates a dysfunctional pattern of deconditioning and disability. Several studies have shown that low-back-pain patients with high levels of fear are more likely than ones with low fear levels to be disabled by their conditions.[69,70]

A related body of research has examined catastrophizing among chronic pain patients. Catastrophizers have been described as people who have a tendency to magnify or exaggerate the threat value or seriousness of pain sensations.[71] Catastrophizing can be seen by examination of items on the Pain Catastrophizing Scale, the instrument that is used to identify catastrophizing.[72] One item is: "When I am in pain, I feel I can't stand it any more." Another item is: "When I am in pain, it's terrible, and I think it's never going to get any better." Various theories have been proposed to explain why people catastrophize and what role catastrophizing plays in their adaptation to pain. These theories include that catastrophizing represents a form of cognitive distortion, that it causes heightened attention to pain cues, that it reflects sensitization based on earlier life traumas, and that it functions as a means of social communication designed to elicit support.[72] For the purposes of this discussion, it is important to note that although catastrophizing might be construed as a cognitive process, it is closely linked to fear, and, as a practical matter, patients who score high on the PCS also get high scores on questionnaires designed to assess pain-related fear.[73] There is consistent evidence that chronic pain patients who catastrophize demonstrate greater disability and poorer response to treatment than ones who do not catastrophize.[54,74–76]

Depression is also common among chronic pain patients. It was discussed in detail above.

Anger has received less research attention than depression or fear, but there is evidence that it can affect the adaptation that patients make to their pain. Correlational studies have shown that anger and a sense of injustice are associated with high levels of pain and pain-related disability.[77,78] There is also evidence that individuals who suppress anger are more likely to experience pain than ones who express it.[79]

The appraisals that pain patients make form the basis of the coping strategies they adopt to deal with their plights. Broadly speaking, patients must cope in the sense of altering their environments, and also in the sense of mitigating the intensity of their pain and their emotional reactions to the pain. In this article, the first kind of coping is referred to as external coping, and the second kind of coping is referred to as internal coping. Examples of external coping would be making a choice about the physician from whom to seek care, or deciding whether to go off work because of pain. This type of coping has not received much attention in psychological research, largely because it is very difficult to identify and classify the many practical decisions that pain patients must make as they try to improve their situations. In contrast, a substantial body of research exists on internal coping mechanisms, and various scales have been developed to assess them.[80] The most widely used scale is the Coping Strategies Questionnaire (CSQ),[81] a 48-item instrument that was designed to assess the extent to which patients used 8 different strategies: diverting attention, reinterpreting pain sensations, ignoring pain sensations, coping self-statements, praying and hoping, catastrophizing, increasing activity level, and increasing pain behaviors. A more recent instrument for assessing coping strategies is the Chronic Pain Coping Inventory (CPCI).[82] It also identified 8 different kinds of coping strategies, but, as indicated in **Table 1**, most of them were different from those identified by the developers of the CSQ. The limited overlap between coping strategies designated by these 2 instruments could reflect subtle differences in the labels used to describe coping strategies, but it more likely signals the fact that there is an enormous range of strategies that patients can use to cope with their pain; there is nothing like a list that psychologists accept as a definitive one.

Research has generally supported the conclusion that coping strategies affect the functional status of chronic pain patients, as indicated by associations between various strategies and outcome variables such as self-reported disability and work status.[62] For example, Jensen and colleagues[82] found that guarding, resting, and asking for assistance were associated with high scores on the Pain Discomfort Scale and a depression scale, whereas task persistence was associated with low scores on these instruments.

Several researchers have grouped coping strategies into active ones, such as exercising or making coping self-statements, and passive ones, such as guarding or asking for assistance. Their research has generally supported the conclusion that passive coping is associated with poor outcomes.[83–86]

It is plausible to anticipate that a patient's beliefs are related to his coping strategies. Thus, for example, one would expect a patient with catastrophic beliefs about the significance of his condition to avoid physical activity, whereas one who perceives himself

Table 1
Coping strategies identified in the coping strategies questionnaire and the chronic pain coping inventory

CSQ	CPCI
Diverting attention	
Reinterpreting pain sensations	
Ignoring pain sensations	
Coping self-statements	Coping self-statements
Praying and hoping	
Catastrophizing	
Increasing activity level	Exercise/stretch
Increasing pain behaviors	
	Guarding
	Asking for assistance
	Relaxation
	Task persistence
	Seeking social support
	Resting

Strategies that are common to the 2 instruments are shown in the same rows.

as able to control his pain would be more likely to engage in physical activity. Although the issue of associations between beliefs and coping strategies has not been studied extensively, there is some evidence that people who anticipate severe or prolonged pain following an accident are relatively likely to adopt passive coping strategies.[87]

It should be noted that there is enormous subtlety and variation in the beliefs that pain patients develop about their conditions, and the internal coping strategies they use to comfort themselves and limit the toll that pain takes on them. Because of this, there is a risk that when researchers study beliefs and coping strategies in large groups of patients, they miss nuances that are crucial to the ways in which individual patients conceptualize their problem and attempt to cope with it. Qualitative studies on coping among pain patients underscore the complexity of the strategies that the patients use.[57,88,89] One practical consequence of the idiosyncratic nature of coping is that psychologists who treat pain patients need to be sensitive to the ways in which individual patients construe their conditions and mobilize their coping resources to deal with them. The focus of psychologists on the idiosyncrasies of beliefs and coping behaviors of patients stands in contrast to the focus of psychiatrists on placing patients into broad categories based on their DSM-5 diagnoses.

Psychological Treatments

Psychologists have a limited set of procedures that they can use to help chronic pain patients. Their scope of practice does not include pharmacologic management, injections, or any other procedures (such as massage) that involve physical contact with the patient. However, within these limitations, there are several different methods that psychologists use when they treat patients with chronic pain. In a recent review article, Jensen[90] identified the following different methods: (1) hypnosis, (2) relaxation interventions, (3) mindfulness meditation training, (4) operant treatment, (5) graded exposure in vivo, (6) motivational interviewing, (7) cognitive therapy and cognitive-behavioral therapy (CBT) interventions, and (8) acceptance-based CBT interventions. As Jensen points out, these therapies are rationalized on the basis of a variety of different models of how psychological dysfunction can impact negatively on the functional status of pain patients. Thus, it is not possible to rationalize all of them on the basis of concepts of stress and coping. It should be noted, though, that some of the above therapies are congruent with a model of psychological dysfunction that emphasizes stress and coping. In particular, therapists practicing motivational interviewing, cognitive therapy and CBT interventions, and acceptance-based CBT interventions all focus on assessing the belief systems and coping strategies of patients, and helping the patients develop ones that are more conducive to recovery. Also, relaxation treatments can be construed as interventions designed to assist patients in internal coping (ie, to help them find ways to mitigate the distress that pain tends to cause).

Given the multiple kinds of psychological therapies and the multiple types of chronic pain that are treated with such therapies,[91] it is difficult to draw overall conclusions about the effectiveness of the therapies. As a broad summary, there is at least some evidence to support all the therapies described by Jensen,[90] and there is robust evidence that CBT, the most widely used psychological therapy, has positive effects on patients with a variety of chronic pain problems.[92,93]

RECOMMENDATIONS FOR MAKING REFERRALS

Physiatrists should strongly consider referring chronic pain patients to a psychiatrist or a psychologist when they think that the patients have psychiatric disorders that impede recovery or think that the patients have dysfunctional beliefs or coping strategies. The question of the appropriateness of referral to a psychologist versus referral to a psychiatrist is a complex one that raises several issues.

1. Several practical considerations related to the organization of health services and the policies of insurance companies come into play. For example, if a physiatrist refers a patient to a mental health clinic in which psychiatrists and psychologists work together, he or she can be reasonably sure that staff at the clinic will steer the patient to the appropriate clinician and thus he or she does not have to ponder about which type of clinician would be appropriate. Another issue is that insurance coverage may greatly favor one type of referral over the other. The authors' experience has been that psychiatric treatment is more likely than psychological treatment to be authorized by insurance companies.
2. Psychiatrists are more focused than psychologists on establishing DSM-5 diagnoses for patients. In contrast, psychologists are more likely than psychiatrists to evaluate in detail the behaviors, beliefs, and coping strategies of pain patients.
3. If a patient has a major psychiatric disorder, such as schizophrenia, bipolar disorder, or profound depression, referral to a psychiatrist is preferable. There are 2 reasons for this. First, psychiatrists are more likely than psychologists to have experience dealing with these kinds of patients. Second, patients with severe mental illness often need medical therapies such as pharmacologic treatment or electroshock treatment.
4. Psychiatrists rely largely on pharmacologic treatment for patients with chronic pain. Their pharmacologic interventions are by no means uniformly successful. However, when patients are responsive to psychopharmacologic treatment, they usually respond fairly quickly—in a matter of a few days to a few weeks. Thus, a trial of pharmacologic management is often appropriate before a patient embarks on the more arduous and protracted task of psychological treatment.
5. Some patients have gone through multiple unsuccessful trials on psychotropic agents and express antipathy for additional trials. These patients might be more amenable to psychological treatment.
6. Patients vary enormously in their verbal fluency and their willingness to talk in depth about feelings, beliefs, and coping strategies relevant to their pain. Psychologists do their best work with patients who are verbal and introspective. They are less likely to help patients who, for whatever reason, do not readily discuss their beliefs and feelings toward their pain.
7. Some pain patients do not have evidence of a psychiatric disorder, are introspective, and express an interest in getting counseling as a way of coping better with their pain. These patients are most appropriately referred to a psychologist and may be coping quite well with their pain problem.

A simple strategy that usually works is to make an initial referral to a psychiatrist who collaborates with psychologists. The psychiatrist would be able to decide whether the patient warranted a DSM-5 diagnosis and would consider pharmacologic therapy. Depending on the outcome of the psychiatric evaluation, a secondary referral to a psychologist could then be considered.

REFERENCES

1. Spitzer RL, Kroenke K, Williams JB. Validation and utility of a self-report version of PRIME-MD: the PHQ primary care study. Primary care evaluation of mental disorders. Patient health questionnaire. JAMA 1999;282(18):1737–44.

2. Spitzer RL, Kroenke K, Williams JB, et al. A brief measure for assessing generalized anxiety disorder: the GAD-7. Arch Intern Med 2006;166(10):1092–7.

3. Ouimette P, Wade M, Prins A, et al. Identifying PTSD in primary care: comparison of the primary care-PTSD screen (PC-PTSD) and the general health questionnaire-12 (GHQ). J Anxiety Disord 2008;22(2):337–43.

4. Koenig HG, George LK, Peterson BL, et al. Depression in medically ill hospitalized older adults: prevalence, characteristics, and course of symptoms according to six diagnostic schemes. Am J Psychiatry 1997;154(10):1376–83.

5. Frank E, Anderson B, Reynolds CF 3rd, et al. Life events and the research diagnostic criteria endogenous subtype. A confirmation of the distinction using the Bedford College methods. Arch Gen Psychiatry 1994;51(7):519–24.

6. Brown GW, Harris TO, Hepworth C. Life events and endogenous depression. A puzzle reexamined. Arch Gen Psychiatry 1994;51(7):525–34.

7. Kessler RC, Berglund P, Demler O, et al. Lifetime prevalence and age-of-onset distributions of DSM-IV disorders in the National Comorbidity Survey Replication. Arch Gen Psychiatry 2005;62(6):593–602.

8. Keller MB, Hirschfeld RM, Hanks D. Double depression: a distinctive subtype of unipolar depression. J Affect Disord 1997;45(1–2):65–73.

9. Rush AJ, Thase ME. Strategies and tactics in the treatment of chronic depression. J Clin Psychiatry 1997;58(Suppl 13):14–22.

10. Kessler RC, Chiu WT, Demler O, et al. Prevalence, severity, and comorbidity of 12-month DSM-IV disorders in the National Comorbidity Survey Replication. Arch Gen Psychiatry 2005;62(6):617–27.

11. Braden JB, Zhang L, Fan MY, et al. Mental health service use by older adults: the role of chronic pain. Am J Geriatr Psychiatry 2008;16(2):156–67.

12. McWilliams LA, Cox BJ, Enns MW. Mood and anxiety disorders associated with chronic pain: an examination in a nationally representative sample. Pain 2003; 106(1–2):127–33.

13. Stang PE, Brandenburg NA, Lane MC, et al. Mental and physical comorbid conditions and days in role among persons with arthritis. Psychosom Med 2006; 68(1):152–8.

14. Von Korff M, Crane P, Lane M, et al. Chronic spinal pain and physical-mental comorbidity in the United States: results from the national comorbidity survey replication. Pain 2005;113(3):331–9.

15. Romano JM, Turner JA. Chronic pain and depression: does the evidence support a relationship? Psychol Bull 1985;97(1):18–34.

16. Carroll LJ, Cassidy JD, Cote P. The Saskatchewan Health and Back Pain Survey: the prevalence and factors associated with depressive symptomatology in Saskatchewan adults. Can J Public Health 2000;91(6):459–64.

17. Gureje O, Simon GE. The natural history of somatization in primary care. Psychol Med 1999;29(3):669–76.

18. Kroenke K, Price RK. Symptoms in the community. Prevalence, classification, and psychiatric comorbidity. Arch Intern Med 1993;153(21):2474–80.

19. Patten SB. Long-term medical conditions and major depression in a Canadian population study at waves 1 and 2. J Affect Disord 2001;63(1–3):35–41.

20. Von Korff M, Dworkin SF, Le Resche L, et al. An epidemiologic comparison of pain complaints. Pain 1988;32(2):173–83.

21. Dworkin SF, Von Korff M, LeResche L. Multiple pains and psychiatric disturbance. An epidemiologic investigation. Arch Gen Psychiatry 1990;47(3):239–44.

22. Von Korff M, Ormel J, Keefe FJ, et al. Grading the severity of chronic pain. Pain 1992;50(2):133–49.

23. Fabrega H Jr. The concept of somatization as a cultural and historical product of Western medicine. Psychosom Med 1990;52(6):653–72.

24. Ormel J, VonKorff M, Ustun TB, et al. Common mental disorders and disability across cultures. Results from the WHO Collaborative Study on Psychological Problems in General Health Care. JAMA 1994;272(22):1741–8.

25. Zaubler TS, Katon W. Panic disorder and medical comorbidity: a review of the medical and psychiatric literature. Bull Menninger Clin 1996;60(2 Suppl A):A12–38.

26. Carney RM, Freedland KE, Ludbrook PA, et al. Major depression, panic disorder, and mitral valve prolapse in patients who complain of chest pain. Am J Med 1990; 89(6):757–60.

27. Beitman BD, Kushner MG, Basha I, et al. Follow-up status of patients with angiographically normal coronary arteries and panic disorder. JAMA 1991;265(12):1545–9.

28. Walker EA, Gelfand AN, Gelfand MD, et al. Psychiatric diagnoses, sexual and physical victimization, and disability in patients with irritable bowel syndrome or inflammatory bowel disease. Psychol Med 1995;25(6):1259–67.

29. Stewart W, Breslau N, Keck PE Jr. Comorbidity of migraine and panic disorder. Neurology 1994;44(10 Suppl 7):S23–7.

30. Beckham JC, Crawford AL, Feldman ME, et al. Chronic posttraumatic stress disorder and chronic pain in Vietnam combat veterans. J Psychosom Res 1997; 43(4):379–89.

31. Baker DG, Mendenhall CL, Simbartl LA, et al. Relationship between posttraumatic stress disorder and self-reported physical symptoms in Persian Gulf War veterans. Arch Intern Med 1997;157(18):2076–8.

32. Blanchard EB, Hickling EJ. After the crash: psychological assessment and treatment of survivors of motor vehicle accidents. 2nd edition. Washington, DC: American Psychological Association; 2003.

33. Aghabeigi B, Feinmann C, Harris M. Prevalence of post-traumatic stress disorder in patients with chronic idiopathic facial pain. Br J Oral Maxillofac Surg 1992; 30(6):360–4.

34. Amir M, Kaplan Z, Neumann L, et al. Posttraumatic stress disorder, tenderness and fibromyalgia. J Psychosom Res 1997;42(6):607–13.

35. Sharp TJ, Harvey AG. Chronic pain and posttraumatic stress disorder: mutual maintenance? Clin Psychol Rev 2001;21(6):857–77.

36. Geisser ME, Roth RS, Bachman JE, et al. The relationship between symptoms of post-traumatic stress disorder and pain, affective disturbance and disability among patients with accident and non-accident related pain. Pain 1996; 66(2–3):207–14.

37. Schreiber S, Galai-Gat T. Uncontrolled pain following physical injury as the core-trauma in post-traumatic stress disorder. Pain 1993;54(1):107–10.

38. Bhuvaneswar CG, Ruskin JN, Katzman AR, et al. Pilot study of the effect of lipophilic vs. hydrophilic beta-adrenergic blockers being taken at time of intracardiac defibrillator discharge on subsequent PTSD symptoms. Neurobiol Learn Mem 2014;112:248–52.

39. Pitman RK, van der Kolk BA, Orr SP, et al. Naloxone-reversible analgesic response to combat-related stimuli in posttraumatic stress disorder. A pilot study. Arch Gen Psychiatry 1990;47(6):541–4.

40. Spertus IL, Burns J, Glenn B, et al. Gender differences in associations between trauma history and adjustment among chronic pain patients. Pain 1999;82(1):97–102.

41. Walker EA, Unutzer J, Katon WJ. Understanding and caring for the distressed patient with multiple medically unexplained symptoms. J Am Board Fam Pract 1998; 11(5):347–56.

42. van der Kolk BA, Pelcovitz D, Roth S, et al. Dissociation, somatization, and affect dysregulation: the complexity of adaptation of trauma. Am J Psychiatry 1996; 153(7 Suppl):83–93.

43. Flor H, Fydrich T, Turk DC. Efficacy of multidisciplinary pain treatment centers: a meta-analytic review. Pain 1992;49(2):221–30.

44. Hooten WM, Townsend CO, Sletten CD, et al. Treatment outcomes after multidisciplinary pain rehabilitation with analgesic medication withdrawal for patients with fibromyalgia. Pain Med 2007;8(1):8–16.

45. Rome JD, Townsend CO, Bruce BK, et al. Chronic noncancer pain rehabilitation with opioid withdrawal: comparison of treatment outcomes based on opioid use status at admission. Mayo Clin Proc 2004;79(6):759–68.

46. Portenoy RK. Chronic opioid therapy in nonmalignant pain. J Pain Symptom Manage 1990;5(1 Suppl):S46–62.

47. Sullivan MD, Edlund MJ, Zhang L, et al. Association between mental health disorders, problem drug use, and regular prescription opioid use. Arch Intern Med 2006;166(19):2087–93.

48. Larson MJ, Paasche-Orlow M, Cheng DM, et al. Persistent pain is associated with substance use after detoxification: a prospective cohort analysis. Addiction 2007; 102(5):752–60.

49. Martell BA, O'Connor PG, Kerns RD, et al. Systematic review: opioid treatment for chronic back pain: prevalence, efficacy, and association with addiction. Ann Intern Med 2007;146(2):116–27.

50. Pulvers K, Hood A. The role of positive traits and catastrophizing in pain perception. Curr Pain Headache Rep 2013;17(5):1–14.

51. Stewart DE, Yuen T. A systematic review of resilience in the physically ill. Psychosomatics 2011;52:199–209.

52. Lazarus RS. Psychological stress and the coping process. New York: McGraw-Hill; 1966.

53. Bandura A. Self-efficacy: the exercise of control. New York: W.H. Freeman and Company; 1997.

54. Jensen MP, Moore MR, Bockow TB, et al. Psychosocial factors and adjustment to chronic pain in persons with physical disabilities: a systematic review. Arch Phys Med Rehabil 2011;92(1):146–60.

55. Main CJ, Foster N, Buchbinder R. How important are back pain beliefs and expectations for satisfactory recovery from back pain? Best Pract Res Clin Rheumatol 2010;24(2):205–17.

56. van Hartingsveld F, Ostelo RW, Cuijpers P, et al. Treatment-related and patient-related expectations of patients with musculoskeletal disorders: a systematic review of published measurement tools. Clin J Pain 2010;26(6):470–88.

57. Snelgrove S, Liossi C. Living with chronic low back pain: a metasynthesis of qualitative research. Chronic Illn 2013;9(4):283–301.

58. Woby SR, Roach NK, Urmston M, et al. The relation between cognitive factors and levels of pain and disability in chronic low back pain patients presenting for physiotherapy. Eur J Pain 2007;11(8):869–77.

59. Vancleef LM, Peters ML. The influence of perceived control and self-efficacy on the sensory evaluation of experimentally induced pain. J Behav Ther Exp Psychiatry 2011;42(4):511–7.

60. Rokke PD, Fleming-Ficek S, Siemens NM, et al. Self-efficacy and choice of coping strategies for tolerating acute pain. J Behav Med 2004;27(4):343–60.

61. Carroll LJ. Beliefs and expectations for recovery, coping and depression in whiplash-associated disorders. Spine 2011;36(25S):S250–6.

62. Laisné F, Lecomte C, Corbière M. Biopsychosocial predictors of prognosis in musculoskeletal disorders: a systematic review of the literature (corrected and re-published)*. Disabil Rehabil 2012;34(22):1912–41.
63. Mondloch MV, Cole DC, Frank JW. Does how you do depend on how you think you'll do? A systematic review of the evidence for a relation between patients' recovery expectations and health outcomes. CMAJ 2001;165(2):174–9.
64. Iles RA, Davidson M, Taylor NF. Psychosocial predictors of failure to return to work in non-chronic non-specific low back pain: a systematic review. Occup Environ Med 2008;65(8):507–17.
65. Rainville P, Bao QV, Chrétien P. Pain-related emotions modulate experimental pain perception and autonomic responses. Pain 2005;118(3):306–18.
66. Lumley MA, Cohen JL, Borszcz GS, et al. Pain and emotion: a biopsychosocial review of recent research. J Clin Psychol 2011;67(9):942–68.
67. Schachter S, Singer JE. Cognitive, social, and physiological determinants of emotional state. Psychol Rev 1962;69:379–99.
68. Vlaeyen JW, Kole-Snijders AM, Boeren RG, et al. Fear of movement/(re)injury in chronic low back pain and its relation to behavioral performance. Pain 1995; 62(3):363–72.
69. Vlaeyen JW, Linton SJ. Fear-avoidance and its consequences in chronic musculoskeletal pain: a state of the art [review]. Pain 2000;85(3):317–32.
70. Crombez G, Eccleston C, Van Damme S, et al. Fear-avoidance model of chronic pain: the next generation [review]. Clin J Pain 2012;28(6):475–83.
71. Chaves JF, Brown JM. Spontaneous cognitive strategies for the control of clinical pain and stress. J Behav Med 1987;10:263–76.
72. Sullivan M. The pain catastrophizing scale. Available at: http://sullivan-painresearch.mcgill.ca/pdf/pcs/PCSManual_English.pdf. Accessed August 31, 2014.
73. Campbell P, Bishop A, Dunn KM, et al. Conceptual overlap of psychological constructs in low back pain. Pain 2013;154(9):1783–91.
74. Edwards RR, Cahalan C, Mensing G, et al. Pain, catastrophizing, and depression in the rheumatic diseases. Nat Rev Rheumatol 2011;7(4):216–24.
75. Walton DM, Macdermid JC, Giorgianni AA, et al. Risk factors for persistent problems following acute whiplash injury: update of a systematic review and meta-analysis. J Orthop Sports Phys Ther 2013;43(2):31–43.
76. Miles CL, Pincus T, Carnes D, et al. Can we identify how programmes aimed at promoting self-management in musculoskeletal pain work and who benefits? A systematic review of sub-group analysis within RCTs. Eur J Pain 2011;15(8): 775.e1–11.
77. Scott W, Trost Z, Bernier E, et al. Anger differentially mediates the relationship between perceived injustice and chronic pain outcomes. Pain 2013;154:1691–8.
78. Sullivan MJ, Scott W, Trost Z. Perceived injustice: a risk factor for problematic pain outcomes. Clin J Pain 2012;28(6):484–8.
79. Burns JW, Gerhart JI, Bruehl S, et al. Anger arousal and behavioral anger regulation in everyday life among patients with chronic low back pain: relationships to patient pain and function. Health Psychol 2014, August 11. Advance online publication. http://dx.doi.org/10.1037/hea0000091.
80. Kato T. Frequently used coping scales: a meta-analysis. Stress Health 2013. http://dx.doi.org/10.1002/smi.2557.
81. Rosenstiel AK, Keefe FJ. The use of coping strategies in chronic low back pain patients: relationship to patient characteristics and current adjustment. Pain 1983;17:33–44.

82. Jensen MP, Turner JA, Romano JM, et al. The chronic pain coping inventory: development and preliminary validation. Pain 1995;60(2):203–16.

83. Jones GT, Johnson RE, Wiles NJ, et al. Predicting persistent disabling low back pain in general practice: a prospective cohort study. Br J Gen Pract 2006; 56(526):334–41.

84. Jensen MP, Turner JA, Romano JM. Changes after multidisciplinary pain treatment in patient pain beliefs and coping are associated with concurrent changes in patient functioning. Pain 2007;131(1–2):38–47.

85. Ramond A, Bouton C, Richard I, et al. Psychosocial risk factors for chronic low back pain in primary care–a systematic review. Fam Pract 2011;28(1):12–21.

86. Tan G, Teo I, Anderson KO, et al. Adaptive versus maladaptive coping and beliefs and their relation to chronic pain adjustment. Clin J Pain 2011;27(9):769–74.

87. Ferrari R, Russell AS. Correlations between coping styles and symptom expectation for whiplash injury. Clin Rheumatol 2010;29(11):1245–9.

88. Carroll LJ, Rothe JP, Ozegovic D. What does coping mean to the worker with pain-related disability? A qualitative study. Disabil Rehabil 2013;35(14):1182–90.

89. Krohne K, Ihlebaek C. Maintaining a balance: a focus group study on living and coping with chronic whiplash-associated disorder. BMC Musculoskelet Disord 2010;11:158.

90. Jensen MP. Psychosocial approaches to pain management: an organizational framework. Pain 2011;152(4):717–25.

91. Sturgeon JA. Psychological therapies for the management of chronic pain. Psychol Res Behav Manag 2014;7:115–24.

92. Ehde DM, Dillworth TM, Turner JA. Cognitive-behavioral therapy for individuals with chronic pain: efficacy, innovations, and directions for research. Am Psychol 2014;69(2):153–66.

93. Hofmann SG, Asnaani A, Vonk IJ, et al. The efficacy of cognitive behavioral therapy: a review of meta-analyses. Cognit Ther Res 2012;36(5):427–40.

Sleep

Important Considerations in
Management of Pain

Lina Fine, MD, MPhil

KEYWORDS

• Sleep • Pain • Fragmentation • Nociception • Mood • Circadian rhythm • Insomnia

KEY POINTS

- Sleep patterns share common pathways with nociceptive stimuli.
- Causes for sleep fragmentation include (1) sleep disordered breathing; (2) abnormal leg movements, including restless legs syndrome, occurring while the patient is awake, and periodic limb movements that occur while the patient is asleep; (3) underlying mood disorder, which may be exacerbated by physical symptoms; (4) hormonal changes.

SUMMARY AND OBJECTIVES

1. Sleep patterns share common pathways with nociceptive stimuli. Several important factors are reviewed in considering connections between sleep and pain.
2. Causes for sleep fragmentation include:
   a. Sleep disordered breathing, which may present with snoring, witnessed apneas, daytime sleepiness, and also with more subtle symptoms like morning headache and anxiety. Home sleep testing or more extensive in-laboratory polysomnography may be used for diagnosis of this condition. Treatment options include use of continuous positive airway pressure (CPAP); oral advancement devices (OAD); weight loss; surgical interventions; and, most recently, US Food and Drug Administration (FDA)–approved upper airway stimulation devices.
   b. Abnormal leg movements, including restless legs syndrome (RLS), occurring while the patient is awake and periodic limb movements that occur while the patient is asleep.
   c. Underlying mood disorder, which may be exacerbated by physical symptoms.
3. Identification and management of insomnia includes the definition of the condition, pharmacologic interventions, the role of circadian rhythms and clock adjustments, and the use of cognitive behavior therapy (CBT) for insomnia.

Swedish Sleep Medicine, Swedish Neuroscience Institute, Swedish Medical Center, 500, 17 Ave, Seattle, WA 98122, USA
E-mail address: lina.fine@swedish.org

Phys Med Rehabil Clin N Am 26 (2015) 301–308
http://dx.doi.org/10.1016/j.pmr.2015.01.002
1047-9651/15/$ – see front matter © 2015 Elsevier Inc. All rights reserved.

Pain and sleep disorders share a reciprocal relationship: pain interferes with sleep quality and, in turn, poor and truncated sleep perpetuates pain symptoms. Furthermore, nociceptive pathways and sleep-wake pathways may share common central serotonergic transmission. A survey of 18,980 individuals from 5 European countries showed that significantly more participants with chronic painful conditions (eg, limb or joint pain, backache, gastrointestinal pain, and headache) than those without pain experienced insomnia. Compared with individuals without chronic pain conditions, those with pain were 3 times more likely to report difficulties with initiating sleep, maintaining sleep, early morning awakenings, and nonrestorative sleep.[1] There may be confounding factors, such as underlying mental illness and the onset of menopause. These confounding factors are often important and need to be considered when addressing sleep difficulties in patients with pain. Menopause is an important physiologic change in women that has both physiologic and psychological implications. As **Fig. 1** shows, sleep difficulties arise during this period that may layer on the nocturnal symptoms associated with pain.

Average adults require 7 to 8 hours sleep, with less than 6 and more than 9 hours correlating with adverse health outcomes. Insomnia encompasses the inability to initiate sleep, maintain sleep, or reach a state of restfulness and refreshment on awakening. It may be associated with daytime symptoms of fatigue, memory deficits, social/vocational/academic performance deficits, mood changes, daytime sleepiness, lack of motivation, vulnerability to accidents, somatic symptoms, and a preoccupation with sleep that perpetuates the cycle of insomnia. Thirty percent of the working population in the United States sleeps for less than 6 hours a day. Sleep deprivation may lead to a one-third reduction in glucose metabolism[2] and increase in C-reactive protein and interleukin-6 levels.[3] Sleep for longer than 9 hours seems to have similar effects. Onen and colleagues[4] found that men showed hyperalgesia to mechanical stimuli following 40 hours of total sleep deprivation and a robust analgesic effect after selective slow wave sleep recovery.

Sleep deprivation may be dictated by the individual's lifestyle and habits, but several identifiable sleep conditions may magnify pain symptoms and trigger awakenings. When assessing an individual who has sleep difficulties it is helpful to have a checklist of potential conditions that need to be ruled out or addressed. The first important step in such assessment is to evaluate the patient for sleep disordered breathing. Snoring, awakenings with gasping, palpitations, panic, and dry mouth/sore throat are common symptoms of sleep apnea syndrome. In addition, there are often more subtle symptoms, such as morning headache, anxiety, and poor daytime concentration, that point to potential sleep disordered breathing (**Table 1**).

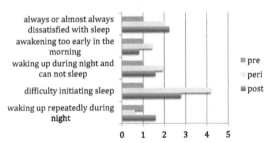

Fig. 1. Odds ratios for self-reported sleep problems among premenopausal, perimenopausal, and postmenopausal women (n = 589). (*Data from* Young T, Rabago D, Zgierska A, et al. Objective and subjective sleep quality in premenopausal, perimenopausal, and postmenopausal women in the Wisconsin Sleep Cohort Study. Sleep 2003;26(6):670. Available at: http://www.ncbi.nlm.nih.gov/pubmed/14572118.)

Table 1 Sleep deprivation symptoms	Men	Women
Snoring/apneas	***	*
Sleepiness	***	**
AM Headaches	*	***
Depressive features	*	**
Apnea frequency	**	*
Hypopnea frequency	*	**

* Qualitative index comparing findings in males and females.
Adapted from Kapsimalis F, Kryger MH. Gender and obstructive sleep apnea syndrome, part 1: Clinical features. Sleep 2002;25(4):411. Available at: http://www.ncbi.nlm.nih.gov/pubmed/12071542.

Using a quick screening tool such as the STOP BANG questionnaire is a helpful way to screen many patients.

Snoring (yes/no)
Tired (yes/no)
Observed apneas (yes/no)
Pressure, treatment of blood pressure (yes/no)
Body mass index greater than 35 (yes/no)
Age more than 50 years (yes/no)
Neck circumference greater than 40 cm (yes/no)
Gender male (yes/no).

Answering "Yes" to more than 3 of these questions suggests a high risk of sleep apnea.[5] Patients at risk can then be assessed with a polysomnogram in a sleep laboratory setting or with a home sleep test device, which is especially helpful in severe cases of sleep apnea. If sleep apnea is diagnosed, treatment options include CPAP, oral appliance, weight loss, and surgical intervention. Resultant improvement in sleep continuity and daytime energy level facilitates improved coping with a range of pain symptoms.

The next important step is to assess for abnormal leg movements during sleep and for RLS (**Fig. 2**).

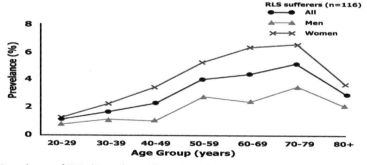

Fig. 2. Prevalence of RLS. (*Data from* Allen RP, Walters AS, Montplaisir J, et al. Restless legs syndrome prevalence and impact: REST general population study. Arch Intern Med 2005;165(11):1289.)

Patients may describe grabbing sensations, sensations that feel creepy-crawly or shocklike, sensations that feel like worms moving, or bubbling in the veins. RLS results in disturbed sleep and sleep onset insomnia and is also associated with a higher risk of depression, anxiety, and somatic pain.[6]

Diagnostic criteria for RLS include:

1. Urge to move: irresistible, involving both legs and may involve arms and trunk
2. Worsening symptoms at rest (body position should not matter)
3. Relief with movement (no symptoms during movement)
4. Worsening in the evening or at night (circadian fluctuation)

RLS may mimic positional discomfort, cramps, positional ischemia, neuropathy, radiculopathy, or hypnic jerks, and should be carefully distinguished from these conditions.[7] RLS is 4 times more likely in first-degree relatives. A polysomnogram is typically unnecessary unless the patient is unable to articulate symptoms.

Although RLS is a condition that the patient is able to report to the provider, periodic limb movements of sleep is a condition diagnosed in the sleep laboratory with recorded periodic episodes of repetitive and highly stereotyped limb movements that occur during sleep and lead to impairment in sleep quality or daytime functioning. Periodic limb movement disorder is defined by the presence of periodic limb movements, electrographic arousals on a sleep study that result in broken sleep, and daytime symptoms of fatigue. Pharmacologic treatments of RLS and periodic limb movement disorder are similar.

Some patients with RLS develop symptoms when ferritin levels decrease to less than 50 ng/mL, and supplementation with iron may improve the symptoms. Other conditions associated with RLS are pregnancy (more commonly the second half), renal insufficiency/failure, neuropathy (Charcot-Marie-Tooth type II only), lumbosacral radiculopathy, anxiety, Parkinson disease, and multiple sclerosis. Dopamine agonists, such as ropinirole and pramipexole, and gamma-aminobutyric acid (GABBA)–ergic (GABA normalizing and increasing) medications are the first approach to the management of restless legs as well periodic limb movements. Long-term use of carbidopa/levodopa may have limited efficacy because of augmentation, which is the process of diminishing efficacy despite dose escalation as frequency of movements, number of duration, body parts affected, and intensity of restlessness worsen with increasing doses. These patients should be cautious in their use of selective serotonin reuptake inhibitors, serotonin-norepinephrine reuptake inhibitors, antihistamines, alcohol, and caffeine because these agents may exacerbate restless legs.

The next step is to assess underlying psychological factors, including pain and mood, which can affect sleep. Patients with pain and/or mood disorders may have excess central autonomic activity triggered by pain as well as peripheral autonomic hyperactivity, including tachycardia, hypertension, mydriasis, vasoconstriction in extremities, and hyperreflexia. Such states of hyperarousal can interfere with the normal process of relaxation that precedes sleep.[8,9] Because of the difficulty of assessing the direction of cause and effect between insomnia and mood, it is often most effective to manage these conditions by using both pharmacologic and nonpharmacologic approaches.

Pharmacologic approaches to the treatment of insomnia can be split into hypnotic and psychotropic medications that can be used to induce or maintain sleep.

Hypnotics and benzodiazepines carry the risk of dependence and respiratory suppression at high doses, especially if combined with opioid agents. For this reason, careful medication selection is especially critical in patients with pain (because of frequent coadministration of opioids, antiepileptic agents, neuropathic agents, and muscle relaxants). In patients at low risk for addiction, these medications may be a helpful for managing acute insomnia (symptoms lasting less than 30 days). Over-the-counter antihistamines may also be of modest efficacy.

Benzodiazepine receptor agonists are among the most common prescription sleeping aids and include eszopiclone and zaleplon. These agents are highly selective for the alpha-1 subunits of the GABA-a receptors, which facilitates a specific sedative effect. However, adequate time (6–8 hours, depending on the agent) must be allowed to pass between dose administration and the next morning awakening. When blood levels of eszopiclone were checked 8.5 hours after administration, driving impairment equivalent to that of an individual with blood alcohol concentration of 0.5% was observed.[10] Other concerning side effects include daytime sedation, risk of falls (especially in the elderly), confusion, exacerbation of underlying breathing difficulties (most concerning in patients who are also on opioid medications), and short-term memory issues. Sleep walking and sleep eating have been reported with zolpidem specifically but are possible with other hypnotics in the same class.

Benzodiazepines specifically targeting sleep include temazepam, triazolam, and estazolam. Concern remains regarding the effect of benzodiazepines and hypnotics on cognition. A recent case-control study by Billioti de Gage and colleagues[11] found that benzodiazepine use may be associated with higher risk of developing Alzheimer disease (the study tracked individuals more than 66 years of age over 5 years after starting benzodiazepines).

Other medications to consider in the treatment of sleep problems:

- Antidepressant medications with sedative properties include tricyclic antidepressants (doxepin, nortriptyline, amitriptyline), the tetracyclic antidepressant mirtazapine, and the selective serotonin reuptake inhibitor trazodone.
- In 2014 the FDA approved a novel sleeping aid called suvorexant. It blocks orexin receptors in lateral hypothalamus. Orexin is required for alertness and blocking this pathway may help with sleep induction (the sleep initiation effect is dose related).
- Another agent with a unique mechanism of action is ramelteon, which is a melatonin receptor (MT-1 and MT-2) agonist that can be used for sleep initiation difficulties. MT-1 binding inhibits circadian-mediated wake-promoting activity, thereby allowing the brain to turn off. MT-2 receptors are involved in the timing of sleep.
- Melatonin (discussed further later) has an important role in sleep initiation because it advances individual circadian clocks by inducing drowsiness earlier in the night, thus allowing earlier sleep onset when used to advance a person's biological clock.

Sleep-wake cycles are intricately linked to multiple environmental and internal stimuli. These circadian rhythms dictate when an individual may become drowsy or wake up. Melatonin is a biogenic amine that is found in humans, animals, and plants. In mammals, melatonin is produced by the pineal gland. Secretion of melatonin increases in darkness and decreases with exposure to light (**Fig. 3**).

Melatonin production begins gradually after sunset, peaks in the earlier part of the night, and drastically diminishes by early morning. Hence, if a melatonin supplement is used to address insomnia, it is advisable to take a low dose several hours before bedtime. Because its concentration increases with dimming of light, it is advisable to keep lights dim following a dose of melatonin. This supplement should be used cautiously in patients who have nightmares because it may cause vivid, although not necessarily disturbing, dreams. Some individuals, often known as night owls,

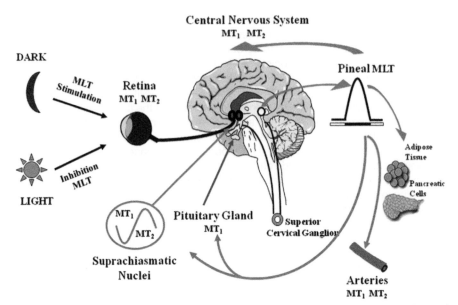

Fig. 3. Regulation of melatonin production and receptor function. Melatonin is synthesized in the pineal gland and in the retina. In the pineal gland, melatonin (MLT) synthesis follows a rhythm driven by the suprachiasmatic nucleus, the master biological clock. Neural signals from the SCN follow a multisynaptic pathway to the superior cervical ganglia. Norepinephrine released from postganglionic fibers activates $\alpha1$- and $\beta1$-adrenoceptors in the pinealocyte, leading to increases in second messengers (i.e., cAMP and inositol trisphosphate) and the activity of AA-NAT, the rate-limiting step in melatonin synthesis. The system is dramatically inhibited by light, the external cue that allows entrainment to the environmental light/dark cycle. The photic signal received by the retina is transmitted to the SCN via the retinohypothalamic tract, which originates in a subset of retinal ganglion cells. Pineal melatonin thus serves as the internal signal that relays day length, allowing regulation of neuronal activity (MT_1) and circadian rhythms (MT_1, MT_2) in the SCN (Dubocovich, 2007), of neurochemical function in brain through the MT_1 and MT_2 receptors (Dubocovich, 2006), of vascular tone through activation of MT_1 (constriction) and MT_2 receptors (dilation) in arterial beds (Masana et al., 2002), and seasonal changes in reproductive physiology and behavior through activation of MT_1 receptors in the pars tuberalis (Duncan, 2007). The pars tuberalis of the pituitary gland interprets this rhythmic melatonin signal and generates a precise cycle of expression of circadian genes through activation of MT_1 receptors. Melatonin synthesis in the photoreceptors of the retina follows a similar circadian rhythm generated by local oscillators (Tosini et al., 2007). Activation of MT_1 and MT_2 melatonin receptors regulate retina function and hence transmission of photic information to the brain (Dubocovich et al., 1997). (*Adapted from* Dubocovich ML, Masana M. Melatonin receptor signaling. In: Henry H, Norman A, editors. Encyclopedia of hormones and related cell regulators. San Diego: Academic Press; 2003; with permission.)

experience a delay in their melatonin production (and other physiologic processes, including nocturnal temperature regulation). Specific genetic mutations have been isolated in so-called clock genes (including Per2, Per 3, and aralkylamine N-acetyltransferase [AANAT]) that may explain the predilection for different sleep-wake schedules.[12] When faced with distracting external stimuli, as well as the burden of physical ailments, such patients are prone to develop sleep initiation insomnia (ie, their sleep-wake phases become delayed, resulting in later bedtimes and further difficulty awakening in the morning). In addition to using melatonin in these patients, keeping lights dim in the evening can help to advance the sleep schedule, thereby allowing sensations of drowsiness to occur earlier in the evening. With evening sleep phase delay (later bedtime) may also come later awakening times. These individuals must maintain regular wake up times with morning light exposure to help regulate this cycle and enhance morning alertness. Sunlight or light boxes (10,000 lx) are the most effective methods.

Circadian shifting ideally should be combined with CBT to address disrupted sleep. When applied independently and in coadministration with hypnotic zolpidem to address insomnia, CBT alone was the most effective long-term treatment at 6-month follow up. Note that a hypnotic was helpful when used briefly during the first stages of insomnia.[13] The cognitive component of CBT includes addressing dysfunctional beliefs about sleep and catastrophizing thoughts about next-day performance. Behavioral components focus on healthy sleep habits, including avoidance of caffeine in the later part of the day, avoidance of television in bed, and avoidance of excessive time in bed without sleep. There is evidence to suggest that both components are important for the management of insomnia.[14]

Just as it is important to use a broad range of tools to address individual pain symptoms, it is essential to adopt a nuanced approach to diagnosis and management of insomnia. Such an approach, which reflects the common physiologic pathways and unique psychological forces that dictate patterns of sleep, is best suited to interrupting dysfunctional pain/sleep cycles.

REFERENCES

1. Ohayon MM. Relationship between chronic painful physical condition and insomnia. J Psychiatr Res 2005;39(2):151–9.
2. Spiegel K, Leproult R, Van Cauter E. Impact of sleep debt on metabolic and endocrine function. Lancet 1999;354(9188):1435–9.
3. Patel SR, Zhu X, Storfer-Isser A, et al. Sleep duration and biomarkers of inflammation. Sleep 2009;32(2):200–4. Available at: http://www.pubmedcentral.nih.gov/articlerender.fcgi?artid=2635584&tool=pmcentrez&rendertype=abstract.
4. Onen SH, Alloui A, Gross A, et al. The effects of total sleep deprivation, selective sleep interruption and sleep recovery on pain tolerance thresholds in healthy subjects. J Sleep Res 2001;10(1):35–42. Available at: http://www.ncbi.nlm.nih.gov/pubmed/11285053.
5. Chung F, Yegneswaran B, Liao P, et al. STOP questionnaire: a tool to screen patients for obstructive sleep apnea. Anesthesiology 2008;108(5):812–21.
6. Allen RP, Picchietti D, Hening WA, et al. Restless legs syndrome: diagnostic criteria, special considerations, and epidemiology. A report from the restless legs syndrome diagnosis and epidemiology workshop at the National Institutes of Health. Sleep Med 2003;4(2):101–19. Available at: http://www.ncbi.nlm.nih.gov/pubmed/14592341.
7. Hening WA, Allen RP, Washburn M, et al. The four diagnostic criteria for restless legs syndrome are unable to exclude confounding conditions ("mimics"). Sleep Med 2009;10(9):976–81.
8. Latremoliere A, Woolf CJ. Central sensitization: a generator of pain hypersensitivity by central neural plasticity. J Pain 2009;10(9):895–926.
9. May A. Chronic pain may change the structure of the brain. Pain 2008;137(1):7–15.

10. Gustavsen I, Hjelmeland K, Bernard JP, et al. Individual psychomotor impairment in relation to zopiclone and ethanol concentrations in blood–a randomized controlled double-blinded trial. Addiction 2012;107(5):925–32.

11. Billioti de Gage S, Moride Y, Ducruet T, et al. Benzodiazepine use and risk of Alzheimer's disease: case-control study. BMJ 2014;349:g5205. Available at: http://www.pubmedcentral.nih.gov/articlerender.fcgi?artid=4159609&tool= pmcentrez&rendertype=abstract.

12. Lamont EW, James FO, Boivin DB, et al. From circadian clock gene expression to pathologies. Sleep Med 2007;8(6):547–56.

13. Morin CM, Vallières A, Guay B, et al. Cognitive behavioral therapy, singly and combined with medication, for persistent insomnia: a randomized controlled trial. JAMA 2009;301(19):2005–15.

14. Harvey AG, Bélanger L, Talbot L, et al. Comparative efficacy of behavior therapy, cognitive therapy, and cognitive behavior therapy for chronic insomnia: a randomized controlled trial. J Consult Clin Psychol 2014;82(4):670–83.

Nutrition and Pain

Heather Tick, MD[a,b],*

KEYWORDS

- Nutrition • Inflammation • Micronutrients • Diet • Antioxidants • Microbiome
- Healing • Integrative pain medicine

KEY POINTS

- Macronutrients such as proteins, carbohydrates, and fats provide the calories in food. Micronutrients such as vitamins, minerals, flavonoids, and other antioxidants are also essential for health.
- Heavily processed foods are high in calories and poor in micronutrients, leading to calorie excess and micronutrient deficiency in many Americans.
- An antiinflammatory diet can reduce the prevalence of many of the chronic diseases that are associated with pain: diabetes, cardiovascular disease, and obesity.
- Research into nutrients does not mirror drug research randomized controlled trials (RCTs) because nutrients, which bodies are programmed to use, work more slowly and physiologically than do drugs, which are "new-to-nature" molecules that often have dramatic effects and side effects.

INTRODUCTION

There is growing literature documenting the effects that lifestyle choices have on overall health outcomes by changing host susceptibility and the propensity to heal.[1] The European Prospective Investigation Into Cancer and Nutrition (EPIC), Potsdam study, evaluated the effects of 4 lifestyle factors on health (never smoking; body mass index [BMI], calculated as the weight in kilograms divided by height in meters squared, less than 30; physical activity for at least 3.5 hours a week, and eating a healthy diet with vegetables, fruits, whole-grain bread, and low quantities of meat). The study revealed benefits for these 4 lifestyle factors that no drugs or procedures can remotely approximate. A total of 23,000 participants were followed up for 7.8 years. Participants with all 4 factors at baseline, when compared with those without a healthy factor, had a 78% lower risk of developing a chronic disease: specifically 93% reduced risk of diabetes, 81% reduction in myocardial infarction, 50% less chance of strokes, and 36%

[a] Department of Family Medicine, University of Washington, C408 Health Sciences, 1959 NE Pacific St, Seattle, WA 98195-6390, USA; [b] Department of Anesthesiology and Pain Medicine, University of Washington, Box 356540, 1959 NE Pacific Street, BB-1469, Seattle, WA 98195-6540, USA
* Department of Anesthesiology and Pain Medicine, University of Washington, Box 356540, 1959 NE Pacific Street, BB-1469, Seattle, WA 98195-6540, USA
E-mail address: htick@uw.edu

Phys Med Rehabil Clin N Am 26 (2015) 309–320
http://dx.doi.org/10.1016/j.pmr.2014.12.006
1047-9651/15/$ – see front matter Published by Elsevier Inc.

reduction in cancer.[2] The common denominator of all these chronic conditions is inflammation: all the 4 factors studied reduce body-wide inflammation, which in turn can influence the course of chronic diseases. Each of these chronic diseases can affect pain, but the reduction of inflammation itself can affect the experience of pain.

A diet of processed foods tends to be high in calories with an abundance of unhealthy fat, refined carbohydrates, salt, and chemicals such as pesticides, stabilizers, antibiotics, and preservatives. Almost 80% of processed foods contain added sugar.[3] Such a diet is poor in fiber, micronutrients, and antioxidants and is proinflammatory. Pain-specific studies are lacking in this area, but a month of following this practice (either for the practitioner or their patients) will convince most practitioners that "you are what you eat." There are studies looking at the influence of diet on inflammatory markers showing that diets high in fiber, healthy oils, fruits, and vegetables and low in sugars, starchy carbohydrates, and unhealthy oils can reduce inflammation and disease.[4–8]

The United States is faced with an obesity epidemic, and it is estimated that 1 in 3 Americans will become diabetic in their lifetime and that the figure increases to 1 in 2 for those of Latin American descent, African Americans, and American Indians. At present, in the preteen population, there is an increasing prevalence of obesity, diabetes and coronary artery disease and the attendant complications of other chronic diseases and pain syndromes.

PATIENT EVALUATION

We persist, as a nation, to subsidize grains instead of fruits and vegetables and have made fast foods and processed foods cheap, whereas fresh foods are unaffordable for much of the nation. There are food deserts in the United States where people cannot find fresh produce in their local stores. There are movements to reverse these trends, such as The Family Dinner Project,[9] Slow Food,[10] and Food Inc.[11] Against the vigorous lobbying of food industries, a host of governmental and nongovernmental organizations are trying to improve school lunches and reduce the high-sugar, high-fat, empty calorie junk foods available in schools.

Taking a detailed dietary history must be done carefully to maximize patients' openness about eating habits that may be causing embarrassment or guilt, especially if patients are poor, have been overweight, or had eating disorders. People can be simultaneously obese and malnourished. Many people do not know what real food is: things that come from a farm are food; things that come from a factory are usually not food anymore. This conversation can lead to a worthwhile discussion about how to seek out health-promoting foods.

It can be easiest to go through an example of the patient's meal cycle: breakfast, lunch, dinner, and snacks. (For example, for breakfast, I ask specific details such as specifically what types of starches, cereal, and bread they eat; how much and what type of sweetener they use in their beverage; and whether they use cream or chemical-laden creamer.) Other important parameters are numbers of vegetables (in handfuls) and fruits, amounts of sugar or artificially sweetened beverages, amount of other sugars in the diet such as candy or pastries, and an idea of the relative amounts of processed foods versus homemade "from-scratch" foods.

> People's tastes become desensitized to sweet if they over ingest sweets. Very often, removing sweets from their diet for a week allows their palates to reregulate and they will use less added sweeteners of all kinds. The same holds true for salt.

MACRONUTRIENTS AND MICRONUTRIENTS

Macronutrients include proteins, simple and complex carbohydrates, and fats. These macronutrients provide the calories in food. Micronutrients are vitamins, minerals, enzymes, and antioxidants that are abundant in unprocessed fruits, vegetables, beans, legumes, nuts, seeds, and whole grains. Americans overconsume animal sources of protein and neglect the vegetable sources.[12] The result is an overconsumption of unhealthy fats and reduction of the nutrient-replete plant sources of food. Americans are also heavy consumers of grains and their processed derivative foods.

It has been estimated that junk food makes up one-third of the average American diet.[13]

Americans each eat an average of 68 kg of sugar[14] and 68 kg of refined flour each year. These are high-glycemic foods that spike blood sugar quickly, usually resulting in a reactive drop in blood sugar that then precipitates food cravings, irritability, and increased inflammation.[15] Chronic inflammation is associated with medical and psychiatric disorders, including cardiovascular diseases, metabolic syndrome, cancer, autoimmune diseases, schizophrenia, and depression, all of which adversely affect health and life expectancy and can exacerbate pain.[16] A processed foods diet also promotes low pH, which in turn reduces the activity of essential physiologic enzyme reactions in the body (the optimal enzyme function pH is 6.5–7.5).[17] Refined foods, sugar, meat, and dairy lower pH. Green vegetables, lentils, and most fruits raise the pH.

Eat, Drink, and be Healthy[18] by Willett, MD, of Harvard is an excellent resource for practitioners and patients, outlining the evidence base of the health-promoting effects of a proper diet. Willett provides an alternative food pyramid to that of the United States Department of Agriculture. At its base are whole grains and plant oils, followed at the next tier by unlimited vegetables and 2 to 3 fruits per day. Nuts and legumes are the next most abundant food group followed by fish, poultry, and eggs, with dairy or calcium supplementation above that. At the very top, with the advice to use sparingly, are red meat, butter, and white food—white bread, pasta, potatoes, and rice along with soda and sweets.

Moderate use of coffee, tea, wine, and dark chocolate is sanctioned under the antioxidant banner. Awareness of the sources and quality of the products is essential, because all the above-mentioned foods tend to be produced with heavy pesticide use and can be chemically altered under certain circumstances. The Environmental Working Group is a watchdog group that compiles lists of contaminants and sources of least and most contaminated foods and makes these available to the public.[19]

Merely understanding and explaining glycemic index (GI) and glycemic load to patients goes a long way to convincing them that they should pay attention to recommendations. GI refers to the rate of rise of the blood sugar after eating a certain food measured against the standard of a glucose load, which scores 100. A high-glycemic food is one with GI greater than 55. Low-GI foods produce only small fluctuations in blood glucose (BS) and insulin levels. Large fluctuations in BS begin the path to insulin resistance and the increase in inflammation that is now recognized as a factor in the development of most known chronic degenerative diseases.[20] The glycemic load is (GI × the amount of carbohydrate) divided by 100 and takes into account the amount of carbohydrate intake as well as GI.

SUPPLEMENTATION
Drugs and Nutrients: Relative Safety

The safety profiles of nutritional supplements continue to be monitored and evaluated. There is the potential for adverse effects, interactions with drugs, and interactions between supplements. However, the statistics speak for themselves when comparing adverse effects from supplements with the adverse effects from commonly used medications and frequently performed procedures. A review of the Institute of Medicine reports *To Err is Human*[21] and *Shorter Lives Poorer Health*[22] and the works of Starfield,[23] James,[24] and Volkow and colleagues[25] point out the significant morbidity and mortality from conventional medicines. In contrast, the National Poison Data System, which tracks deaths from drugs and supplements, reported no deaths due to multiple vitamins, A, B, C, D, and E, or any other vitamin, and no deaths attributable to amino acid or other dietary supplements in their 2010 report.[26]

In family medicine, orthopedic, pain, rheumatology, sports, and physical medicine practices, there are many commonly used, nonlifesaving drugs that are associated with significant morbidity and mortality. Nonsteroidal antiinflammatories have been estimated to kill more than 16,500 patients per year within the diagnostic categories of osteoarthritis (OA) and rheumatoid arthritis alone.[27] In addition, they may contribute to nutritional deficiencies from intestinal malabsorption and disruption of the microbiome: the masses of microorganisms that inhabit the body and outnumber the individual's human cells in numbers of cells by 10:1.[28] The balance of microorganisms can determine health or disease by affecting the absorption of nutrients, causing or preventing excessive gut permeability, affecting the function of the immune system, and stimulating unhealthy fermentation within the gut and may be responsible for some forms of abdominal pain. (The National Institutes of Health [NIH] have a consortium devoted to the study of the microbiome called the Human Microbiome Project. A PubMed search on "human microbiome" displayed 13,662 articles dating back to the 1950s with 12,565 published in the past 10 years.) The microbiome is also adversely affected by processed foods and many other drugs commonly used in physical medicine and rheumatology practices such as proton pump inhibitors (PPIs), antibiotics, steroids, and hormones. PPIs now carry a warning from the US Food and Drug Administration saying they are risks in the development of osteoporosis, *Clostridium difficile* infection, food poisoning, nutritional deficiencies of vitamin B_{12} and protein, as well as potential life-threatening deficiency of magnesium. It has been known since the 1990s that gut bacterial imbalances can cause abnormal colonic fermentation and present as irritable bowel syndrome.[29]

SPECIFIC SUPPLEMENTS

It is impossible to review research on the merits of all the vitamins, minerals, antioxidants, and botanicals in this article. This article focuses on supplements that are readily available, affordable, and have been proved in practice to be highly efficacious[30,31] in improving inflammation, pain, and healing.

Vitamin D

Studies repeatedly show that the population in the northern hemisphere is vitamin D deficient.[32,33] More significant deficiencies are recorded in the chronic pain populations,[34–36] and there can be improvement of pain with the mere supplementation of vitamin D.[37] Grimaldi and colleagues[38] have also shown that vitamin D improves muscle strength in men and women. The extensive study of vitamin D is impressing upon us that it is more of a hormone than a vitamin and is necessary for every system and cell type that has so far been studied. Deficiencies are associated with inflammation and susceptibility to illness, and sufficient levels are necessary for a healthy immune system.

In some patients, it is difficult to achieve optimal levels despite usual levels of supplementation, and therefore being guided by serum levels of 25-hydroxyvitamin D is helpful. It is known that deficiencies are more common in the elderly, the obese, and in those with more skin pigment. It is generally regarded as safe for people to take 2000 IU/d orally and the no adverse effect level, an international standard, has been set at 4000 IU daily.

Omega-3 Oils

Omega-3 and omega-6 polyunsaturated fatty acids (PUFAs) are essential nutrients that must be obtained from the diet. The North American diet is generally too high in omega-6 PUFAs and deficient in omega-3 PUFAs. Linoleic acid is the predominant omega-6 PUFA that promotes inflammation.[39] The omega-3 PUFAs are alpha-linolenic acid, which comes from plants such as flax, and docosahexaenoic acid (DHA) and eicosapentaenoic acid (EPA), which come from fish, organic free-range eggs, and grass-fed beef. Omega-3 PUFAs promote antiinflammatory pathways and are being investigated for their effects on headache.[39] An RCT was conducted in which 56 of 67 patients completed a dietary intervention increasing n-3 and reducing n-6 fatty acids resulting in "reduced headache pain, altered antinociceptive lipid mediators, and improved quality of life in this population."[40] Lee and colleagues[41] found nonsteroidal antiinflammatory drug (NSAID)-sparing effects with omega-3 oils in the treatment of rheumatoid arthritis, and Goldberg and Katz[42] found an analgesic effect with supplementation for inflammatory joint pain. Maroon and Bost[43] showed a 60% reduction in pain with the addition of 1200 mg of purified omega-3 fish oil in discogeneic pain. The doses used in many studies are 3000 to 4000 mg of combined EPA and DHA, which can usually be found in 6000 to 8000 mg of fish oil. (In most good-quality, microdistilled fish oil preparations there will be at least half the amount made up by the sum of the amount of DHA and EPA. For example, a 1000-mg capsule may have 230 mg of EPA and 270 mg of EPA for a total of 500 mg of the omega-3 PUFAs.)

Vitamin B_{12}

Vitamin B_{12} is needed to make healthy blood cells and for optimal bone density. It is well known that neurologic dysfunction and chronic pain are consequences of deficiencies. Absorption from food sources depends on adequate stomach acid and drops with age. Vitamin B_{12} is currently being studied to evaluate the correlation of tissue levels (likely the more significant level) with the serum level markers that can readily be tested. Mauro and colleagues[44] found that vitamin B_{12} injections in patients with pain who were not B_{12} deficient resulted in reduced pain scores and analgesic use in both active treatment arms of a double-blind, placebo-controlled, crossover trial. In a British study, in 61- to 87-year-olds without cognitive impairment and with normal serum B_{12} serum levels, brain size correlated with the B_{12} level.[45] The normal values in Europe and Japan have a higher range than that in the United States.

A dose of 1000 μg/d taken sublingually may produce improved symptoms of pain, insomnia, and fatigue. The sublingual route avoids the need for injections while still bypassing any impairment in gastrointestinal tract absorption.

Vitamin C

Vitamin C is a powerful antioxidant and is needed for the production of collagen, some hormones, and neurotransmitters.[46] It is essential for tissue repair and adaptation to stress. Most animals can produce their own vitamin C, but humans cannot. The needs for vitamin C vary from day to day on the basis of the levels of stress, injury, or sickness. A moderate dose is 2000 mg/d. This dose is very modest when one considers that a 1.8-kg rat makes approximately 10 gm of vitamin C daily and can increase production 10-fold when stressed.

Magnesium

Magnesium is required for energy production and is used in more than 300 essential metabolic reactions.[47] (The most commonly available magnesium sulfate, oxide, and citrate [usually in a liquid form] designed for the treatment of constipation and colonoscopy preparation are not well suited for absorption through the bowel wall. For this reason I recommend magnesium glycinate, malate, and citrate [as powder or pills] and recommend it be purchased from a supplements or health store.) Magnesium is essential for optimal bone density and collagen production, helps regulate serum glucose levels,[48] controls the rate of nerve firing, and causes muscles to relax, making it the first choice for muscle cramps, spasms, myofascial tightness, and trigger points. Patients with Fibromyalgia are often magnesium deficient. Magnesium can improve blood pressure, palpitations,[49] migraine frequency,[50] and the cramping and pain of irritable bowel syndrome.[51] Magnesium can improve sleep[52] and is being studied for its role in neuropathic pain.[53,54]

Magnesium deficiency is one of the most common deficiencies seen with the American diet.[55] Magnesium is an intracellular mineral, and its serum levels, like those of calcium, are tightly regulated. Bones and muscles are reservoirs of magnesium, which may become depleted, even when the serum magnesium level is normal. The usefulness of red blood cell magnesium is not known because it is an anucleate cell and may also not reflect the sufficiency of intracellular stores.

Magnesium should be taken to bowel tolerance: one should take as much as tolerated on a daily basis to produce 1 to 2 easy-to-pass bowel movements. For some people this is 200 to 400 mg daily, and for others the doses is in thousands of milligrams. The result of overdose is diarrhea, which is remedied by lowering the daily dose of magnesium.

Turmeric and Ginger

Turmeric and ginger are related tubers, which have been extensively studied for their antiinflammatory properties. Terry and colleagues[56] in their systematic review of ginger for pain concluded that ginger was a powerful antiinflammatory useful in treating pain. Ginger functions as an antiinflammatory[57] by disrupting the cyclooxygenase 2 (COX-2) pathway at many points (ginger has 4 different ways to inhibit the enzyme COX-2, which promotes inflammation).[57]

Curcumin is the active component of the turmeric tuber. *Curcuma domestica* extracts were found to have similar effects to ibuprofen for OA of the knee.[58,59] Other studies have explored the antinflammatory properties of curcumin[60] and its usefulness for postoperative pain.[61] A review of hundreds of studies was published in *Alternative and Complementary Therapies* and concluded that "turmeric appears to outperform many pharmaceuticals in its effects against several chronic debilitating diseases, and does so with virtually no adverse side effects."[62]

Curcumin is best absorbed in the presence of oil and a small amount of black pepper. Heating also seems to activate the compound and make it more effective. (This is a personal observation and would be in keeping with the historical uses of turmeric as a spice used in cooking. The Ayurvedic preparation of Golden Milk involves heating the turmeric before use. Tablets of curcumin are convenient for travel and still are effective.)

Cinnamon does not have a known direct mechanism for affecting pain; however, it is being researched for its ability to reduce blood sugar levels and insulin resistance based on an insulinlike mechanism, which allows glucose to be absorbed into muscle cells bypassing the insulin receptor. This mechanism can indirectly affect pain by reducing inflammation and general health complications that accompany insulin resistance.[63–65]

SPECIAL DIETS

There are many different types of elimination diets that can be useful for patients to try. Here are a few examples of diets that can be helpful in a chronic pain practice.

- Gluten free: especially for migraine, fibromyalgia, brittle diabetes, irritable bowel, stiff person syndrome
- Grain free: especially for inflammatory bowel, autoimmune disorders
- Cow's dairy free: especially for diabetes, autoimmune disorders, eczema, asthma
- Vegetarian or vegan: for severe acne
- Nightshade vegetable elimination: nightshades are tomatoes, potatoes, peppers, eggplant and tobacco—especially for joint pains and arthritis
- Oxalate free: especially for interstitial cystitis

The gut is both a barrier and a pathway for molecules and other substances to be absorbed into the body. Recent research has demonstrated that an inflamed intestinal mucosa can lead to increased gut permeability and thereby allow entry of bacteria, toxics, and partially digested nutrients. Because of the close association of the immune system with the small intestine—80% of the immune system lies adjacent to the gut—there can be rapid reaction to immunogenic substances crossing the mucosal barrier. The microbiome is the mass of microorganisms that are mostly in the gut and also line all the mucous membranes and skin. The microbiome has 10 times as many cells as the number of cells in the body and 100 times the amount of DNA. The microbiome is affected by foods, and it has been shown that people and animals with ill health have different proportions and types of organisms than those who are in good health. The microbiome helps to digest and absorb nutrients, and it is affected by many of the drugs that are used in pain practice such as NSAIDs, biologics, and steroids as well as by the foods that one eats. Food elimination diets and leaky gut, which used to be the territory of only alternative practitioners, is now firmly established in mainstream science and medicine. NIH's, Human Microbiome Project Consortium[66] is a clearinghouse for the growing body of literature on the interface between diet, gut physiology and pathophysiology, the immune system, and health.

Some practitioners think that recommendations for diet restriction seem extreme, but the level of compliance I get with my patients often surprises me. It does require negotiation skills. It helps that I have seen this approach work in my own life, in my family, and in countless patients over many years. I usually start with the explanation that you "change your body chemistry every time you eat."[30] You increase or decrease inflammation with your food choices. I make it clear that the food restriction is recommended for a trial period, but during this time there needs to be strict adherence to the diet if we are to understand whether particular foods are causing negative effects. Then I negotiate an acceptable length of time. I like to get at least a month, but for some people it is no more than a day. After the first day, they get to decide if they can carry on for a second day. Patients get praised for whatever they were able to accomplish.

At the next follow-up, we analyze the results: how did they feel? Did they see any differences? Did they have better energy, did they sleep better, or did they have improved mood? Did they have easier bowel movements, fewer headaches, or less achy joints? Did they have less asthma or fewer rashes? Was their blood sugar better controlled if they are diabetic? Do they think it is worthwhile to continue on this path? Patients, of course are free to return to whatever diet they choose even if they get good results with the elimination of some foods. This aspect of choice is best laid out clearly, even though it is self-evident.

Anti Inflammatory Foods	Pro-inflammatory Foods
• All leafy green vegetables	• Sugar
• Avocados	• Bread
• Yams	• Pastries
• Berries	• Processed cereals
• Nuts and seeds	• White rice
• Lentils and beans	• White potatoes
• Quinoa	• Deep fried foods
• Buckwheat	• Red meat
• Whole grains	

EVALUATION OF OUTCOMES AND LONG-TERM RECOMMENDATIONS

Nutrition research is often criticized because it does not look more like drug research. Useful research into nutrients should not mirror the RCTs of drug research, because nutrients, which bodies are programmed to use, work more slowly and physiologically than do drugs, which are new-to-nature molecules that often have dramatic therapeutic effects and dramatic side effects. Nutrients work synergistically with each other, and studying them in isolation has provided some useful information but fails to show the bigger picture of how health can change when the overall nutritional status improves. The large-scale study reported by Ford and colleagues[2] in the EPIC study cited earlier is an example of an outcomes study that uses a whole systems approach.

With very few exceptions, people do not get drug deficiencies. There is compelling evidence that people regularly get nutritional deficiencies. "Poor diet and physical inactivity account for four hundred thousand deaths, or 16.6 percent of total deaths, per year in the United States."[67] It is becoming clear that the Standard American Diet is making us sick: that the epidemic of obesity and diabetes, with all the attendant health and pain complications, are food-borne illnesses, fostered by the heavily processed and sweetened diet. A quick search of PubMed shows that there is ample medical literature citing diabetes and obesity as risk factors for adverse outcomes for all other diseases and for medical interventions of all kinds.

The effect of a good diet is that patients may have more energy; lower levels of cholesterol, triglycerides, blood glucose, and insulin; and lower blood pressure. Patients may lose weight, especially the fat around their bellies; have less depression; and reduce their risk of a variety of lifestyle-related illnesses. They may be able to reduce their dependence on medications for their blood pressure, cholesterol, type II diabetes, pain, and inflammation.

Food and nutrition are foundational tools in the treatment of painful and inflammatory conditions. There is compelling evidence showing the benefits of a healthy diet composed mainly of unprocessed, plant-based foods.

REFERENCES

1. Hung HC, Joshipura KJ, Jiang R, et al. Fruit and vegetable intake and the risk of major chronic disease. J Natl Cancer Inst 2004;96(21):1577–84.
2. Ford ES, Bergmann MM, Kröger J, et al. Healthy living is the best revenge: findings from the European Prospective Investigation Into Cancer and Nutrition–Potsdam Study. Arch Intern Med 2009;169(15):1355–62.
3. Ng SW, Slining MM, Popkin BM. Use of caloric and noncaloric sweeteners in US consumer packaged foods, 2005–2009. J Acad Nutr Diet 2012;112(11):1828–34.
4. Barnard ND, Cohen J, Jenkins DJ, et al. A low-fat vegan diet and a conventional diabetes diet in the treatment of type 2 diabetes: a randomized, controlled, 74-Wk clinical trial. Am J Clin Nutr 2009;89(5):1588S–96S.
5. Berkow SE, Barnard ND, Saxe GA, et al. Diet and survival after prostate cancer diagnosis. Nutr Rev 2007;65(9):391–403.
6. Colantuoni C, Schwenker J, McCarthy J, et al. Excessive sugar intake alters binding to dopamine and mu-opioid receptors in the brain. Neuroreport 2001;12(16): 3549–52.
7. Drake VJ. Nutrition and inflammation. Oregon State University, Corvalis, OR: Linus Pauling Institute; 2010. Available at: http://lpi.oregonstate.edu/infocenter/inflammation.html. Accessed October 24, 2014.
8. Dietrich M, Jialal I. The effect of weight loss on a stable biomarker of inflammation, C-reactive protein. Nutr Rev 2005;63(1):22–8.
9. The Family Dinner Project. Available at: http://thefamilydinnerproject.org. Accessed October 24, 2014.
10. Slow Food International. Available at: http://www.slowfood.com. Accessed October 24, 2014.
11. Food Inc. Available at: http://www.takepart.com/foodinc. Accessed October 24, 2014.
12. Campbell TC. The mystique of protein and its implications. Ithaca, NY: T. Colin Campbell Center for Nutrition Studies; 2014. Available at: http://nutritionstudies.org/mystique-of-protein-implications/. Accessed October 24, 2014.
13. Block G. Foods contributing to energy intake in the US: data from NHANES III and NHANES 1999–2000. J Food Compost Anal 2004;17:439–47.
14. How much sugar do you eat? You may be surprised. New Hampshire Department of Health and Human Services. Available at: http://www.dhhs.nh.gov/dphs/nhp/documents/sugar.pdf. Accessed October 24, 2014.
15. de Punder K, Pruimboom L. The dietary intake of wheat and other cereal grains and their role in inflammation. Nutrients 2013;5(3):771–87.
16. Barclay AW, Petocz P, McMillan-Price J, et al. Glycemic index, glycemic load, and chronic disease risk — a meta-analysis of observational studies. Am J Clin Nutr 2008;87(3):627–37.
17. Schwalfenberg GK. The alkaline diet: is there evidence that an alkaline pH diet benefits health? J Environ Public Health 2012;2012:727630.
18. Willett W. Eat, drink and be healthy: the Harvard Medical School Guide to healthy eating. New York: Simon & Schuster; 2001.
19. Environmental Working Group. Available at: www.ewg.org. Accessed October 24, 2014.
20. The Glycemic Index. Available at: http://www.glycemicindex.com. Accessed October 24, 2014.
21. Institute of Medicine. To err is human. Washington, DC: National Academy of Sciences Press; 2000.

22. Institute of Medicine. Shorter lives poorer health: panel on understanding cross-national health differences among high-income countries. Washington, DC: National Academy of Sciences Press; 2013.
23. Starfield B. Is US health care really the best in the world? JAMA 2000;284(4): 483–5.
24. James JT. A new, evidence-based estimate of patient harms associated with hospital care. J Patient Saf 2013;9(3):122–8.
25. Volkow ND, Frieden TR, Hyde PS, et al. Medication-assisted therapies - tackling the opioid-overdose epidemic. N Engl J Med 2014;370:2063–6.
26. Bronstein AC, Spyker DA, Cantilena LR, et al. Annual report of the American Association of Poison Control Centers' National Poison Data System (NPDS): 28th annual report. Clin Toxicol 2011;49:910–41.
27. Singh G. Gastrointestinal complications of prescription and over-the-counter nonsteroidal anti-inflammatory drugs: a view from the ARAMIS database. Am J Ther 2000;7(2):115–21.
28. Wenner M. Humans carry more bacterial cells than human ones. New York: Nature Publishing Group; 2007. Available at: http://www.scientificamerican.com/article/strange-but-true-humans-carry-more-bacterial-cells-than-human-ones/. Accessed October 24, 2014.
29. King TS, Elia M, Hunter JO. Abnormal colonic fermentation in irritable bowel syndrome. Lancet 1998;352(9135):1187–9.
30. Tick H. Holistic pain relief. Novato (CA): New World Library; 2013.
31. Bethesda MD. Dietary and herbal supplements. National Center for Complementary and Alternative Medicine (NCCAM); 2013. Available at: http://nccam.nih.gov/health/supplements. Accessed October 24, 2014.
32. Holick MF. Vitamin D deficiency. N Engl J Med 2007;357(3):266–81.
33. Melamed ML, Michos ED, Post W, et al. 25-hydroxyvitamin D levels and the risk of mortality in the general population. Arch Intern Med 2008;168(15): 1629–37.
34. Plotnikoff GA, Quigley JM. Prevalence of severe hypovitaminosis D in patients with persistent, nonspecific musculoskeletal pain. Mayo Clin Proc 2003;78(12): 1463–70.
35. Macfarlane GJ, Palmer B, Roy D, et al. An excess of widespread pain among South Asians: are low levels of vitamin D implicated? Ann Rheum Dis 2005; 64(8):1217–9.
36. Al Faraj S, Al Mutairi K. Vitamin D deficiency and chronic low back pain in Saudi Arabia. Spine 2003;28(2):177–9.
37. de Torrente de la Jara G, Pecoud A, Favrat B. Musculoskeletal pain in female asylum seekers and hypovitaminosis D3. BMJ 2004;329(7458):156–7.
38. Grimaldi AS, Parker BA, Capizzi JA, et al. 25(OH) vitamin D is associated with greater muscle strength in healthy men and women. Med Sci Sports Exerc 2013;45(1):157–62.
39. Ramsden CE, Mann JD, Faurot KR, et al. Low omega-6 vs. low omega-6 plus high omega-3 dietary intervention for chronic daily headache: protocol for a randomized clinical trial. Trials 2011;12:97.
40. Ramsden CE, Faurot KR, Zamora D, et al. Targeted alteration of dietary n-3 and n-6 fatty acids for the treatment of chronic headaches: a randomized trial. Pain 2013;154(11):2441–51.
41. Lee YH, Bae SC, Song GG. Omega-3 polyunsaturated fatty acids and the treatment of rheumatoid arthritis: a meta-analysis. Arch Med Res 2012;43(5): 356–62.

42. Goldberg RJ, Katz J. A meta-analysis of the analgesic effects of omega-3 poly-unsaturated fatty acid supplementation for inflammatory joint pain. Pain 2007; 129(1–2):210–23.

43. Maroon JC, Bost JW. Omega-3 fatty acids (fish oil) as an anti-inflammatory: an alternative to nonsteroidal anti-inflammatory drugs for discogenic pain. Surg Neurol 2006;65(4):326–31.

44. Mauro GL, Martorana U, Cataldo P, et al. Vitamin B12 in low back pain: a randomised, double-blind, placebo-controlled study. Eur Rev Med Pharmacol Sci 2000;4(3):53–8.

45. Vogiatzoglou A, Refsum H, Johnston C, et al. Vitamin B12 status and rate of brain volume loss in community-dwelling elderly. Neurology 2008;71(11): 826–32.

46. Higdon J. Vitamin C. Oregon State University, Corvalis, OR: Linus Pauling Institute; 2013. Available at: http://lpi.oregonstate.edu/infocenter/vitamins/vitaminC/. Accessed October 24, 2014.

47. Higdon J. Magnesium. Linus Pauling Institute; 2013. Available at: http://lpi.oregonstate.edu/infocenter/minerals/magnesium/. Accessed October 24, 2014.

48. Kim DJ, Xun P, Liu K, et al. Magnesium intake in relation to systemic inflammation, insulin resistance, and the incidence of diabetes. Diabetes Care 2010;33(12): 2604–10.

49. Seelig M. Cardiovascular consequences of magnesium deficiency and loss: pathogenesis, prevalence and manifestations - magnesium and chloride loss in refractory potassium repletion. Am J Cardiol 1989;63(14):4G–21G.

50. Demirkaya S, Vural O, Dora B, et al. Efficacy of intravenous magnesium sulfate in the Treatment of acute migraine attacks. Headache 2001;41(2):171–7.

51. Murakami K, Sasaki S, Okubo H, et al. Association between dietary fiber, water and magnesium intake and functional constipation among young Japanese women. Eur J Clin Nutr 2007;61(5):616–22.

52. Nielsen FH, Johnson LK, Zeng H. Magnesium supplementation improves indicators of low magnesium status and inflammatory stress in adults older than 51 years with poor quality sleep. Magnes Res 2010;23(4):158–68.

53. Rondon LJ, Privat AM, Daulhac L, et al. Magnesium attenuates chronic hypersensitivity and spinal cord NMDA receptor phosphorylation in a rat model of diabetic neuropathic pain. J Physiol 2010;588:4205–15.

54. Brill S, Sedgwick PM, Hamann W, et al. Efficacy of intravenous magnesium in neuropathic pain. Br J Anaesth 2002;89(5):711–4.

55. Whang R. Magnesium deficiency: pathogenesis, prevalence, and clinical implications. Am J Med 1987;82:24–9.

56. Terry R, Posadzki P, Watson LK, et al. The use of ginger (*Zingiber officinale*) for the treatment of pain: a systematic review of clinical trials. Pain Med 2011; 12(12):1808–18.

57. Lantz RC, Chen GJ, Sarihan M, et al. The effect of extracts from ginger rhizome on inflammatory mediator production. Phytomedicine 2007;14(2–3):123–8.

58. Altman RD, Marcussen KC. Effects of a ginger extract on knee pain in patients with osteoarthritis. Arthritis Rheum 2001;44(11):2531–8.

59. Kuptniratsaikul V, Thanakhumtorn S, Chinswangwatanakul P, et al. Efficacy and safety of Curcuma domestic extracts in patients with knee osteoarthritis. J Altern Complement Med 2009;15(8):891–7.

60. Jurenka JS. Anti-inflammatory properties of curcumin, a major constituent of *Curcuma longa*: a review of preclinical and clinical research. Altern Med Rev 2009; 14(2):141–53.

61. Agarwal KA, Tripathi CD, Agarwal BB, et al. Efficacy of turmeric (curcumin) in pain and postoperative fatigue after laparoscopic cholecystectomy: a double-blind, randomized placebo controlled study. Surg Endosc 2011;25(12):3805–10.
62. Duke JA. The garden pharmacy: turmeric, the queen of COX-2-inhibitors. Alternative Compl Ther 2007;13(5):229–34.
63. Khan A, Safdar M, Aki Khan MM, et al. Cinnamon improves glucose and lipids of people with type 2 diabetes. Diabetes Care 2003;26(12):3215–8.
64. Roussel AM, Hininger I, Benaraba R, et al. Antioxidant effects of a cinnamon extract in people with impaired fasting glucose that are overweight or obese. J Am Coll Nutr 2009;28(1):16–21.
65. Solomon TP, Blannin AK. Changes in glucose tolerance and insulin sensitivity following 2 weeks of daily cinnamon ingestion in healthy humans. Eur J Appl Physiol 2009;105(6):969–76.
66. Bethesda MD. Human microbiome project. National Institutes of Health; 2013. Available at: http://commonfund.nih.gov/hmp/presentationpolicies. Accessed October 24, 2014.
67. Mokdad AH, Marks JS, Stroup DF, et al. Actual causes of death in the United States, 2000. JAMA 2004;291(10):1238–45.

Complementary Medicine in Chronic Pain Treatment

Charles A. Simpson, DC, DABCO

KEYWORDS

- Complementary and alternative medicine • Chronic pain • Therapies
- Evidence-based medicine

KEY POINTS

- Complementary therapies are widely used among chronic pain populations.
- Physicians and clinicians who treat chronic pain should inquire about and respect the use of complementary therapies.
- To enhance an effective therapeutic relationship, clinicians should be able to discuss complementary medicine use nonjudgmentally and in light of the scientific evidence regarding effectiveness and potential for complications.
- There is evidence that supports the effectiveness of many complementary therapies.

INTRODUCTION

This article discusses several issues related to therapies that are considered "complementary" or "alternative" to conventional medicine (CM). A definition of "complementary and alternative medicine" (CAM) is considered in the context of the evolving health care field of complementary medicine. A rationale for pain physicians and clinicians to understand these treatments of chronic pain is presented. The challenges of an evidence-based approach to incorporating CAM therapies are explored. Finally, a brief survey of the evidence that supports several widely available and commonly used complementary therapies for chronic pain is provided.

EMERGENCE OF COMPLEMENTARY AND ALTERNATIVE MEDICINE

Book One of Paul Starr's 1982 seminal work, *The Social Transformation of American Medicine,* documents the rise of organized medicine to a position of dominance and hegemony over health care.[1] Although this transformation depended on increased emphasis on education, science, and research, it also fostered an explicit proscription of traditions, histories, and practices of many competing health care disciplines.

At the turn of the twentieth century, American medical practice had just emerged from traditions of heroic medicine that had long coexisted with more moderate, less

3990 Southwest Lafollett Road, Cornelius, OR 97113, USA
E-mail address: casimpsondc@gmail.com

Phys Med Rehabil Clin N Am 26 (2015) 321–347
http://dx.doi.org/10.1016/j.pmr.2014.12.005
1047-9651/15/$ – see front matter © 2015 Elsevier Inc. All rights reserved.

invasive therapies promoted by William Buchan (domestic medicine), Samuel Hahnemann (homeopathy), Samuel Thompson (naturopathic medicine), and Daniel D. Palmer (chiropractic).

Seeing a challenge to medical dominance, organized medicine, through the agency of the American Medical Association (AMA), began a purge of homeopaths in their ranks, disparaged herbalists, midwives, chiropractors, and other nonmedical professionals. For example, AMA opposition to chiropractic care persisted well into the twentieth century until the final resolution of *Wilk v. American Medical Association* in 1990 that led to the disbanding of the AMA Committee on Quackery, which had the explicit purpose to "contain and eliminate" the chiropractic profession.

Despite ongoing efforts to marginalize these alternate and competitive healing traditions, many of them persisted and even flourished. For the most part, these streams of nonmedical practice went unnoticed by mainstream medicine until the Eisenberg[2] 1993 article in *New England Journal of Medicine*. In that survey study, Eisenberg observed that 34% of survey respondents reported using one or more "unconventional" therapies, and about one-third of those saw a provider of the therapy. He went on to extrapolate from the survey data to estimate that Americans made 425 million visits to unconventional medicine providers in 1990, a number that exceeded visits to all US primary care physicians at that time. Further estimates were of $13.7 billion spent on unconventional care. Eisenberg's "discovery" of the magnitude of health care occurring outside of the medical mainstream of physician offices, clinics, and hospitals caught the attention of many.

TERMINOLOGY: WHAT IS "COMPLEMENTARY AND ALTERNATIVE MEDICINE"?

Despite its prevalence, cost, and patterns of use, a definition of "complementary and alternative medicine" has been problematic. The Eisenberg[2] study used the term "unconventional medicine," which they defined as "medical interventions not taught widely at U.S. medical schools or generally available at U.S. hospitals. Examples include acupuncture, chiropractic, and massage therapy."

Although Eisenberg's definition was perhaps accurate in 1993, by 2003, 98 US medical schools included CAM-related curricula.[3] In the second decade of the 2000s, acupuncture, chiropractic therapy, and massage therapy can be found in hospitals across the United States. A 2010 survey of US hospitals found that 42% of respondents offered one or more CAM services, most commonly massage therapy and acupuncture. Chiropractic care is provided at 47 major Veterans Affairs (VA) facilities across the United States.[4] Chiropractic therapy is available in many US hospitals.

"Complementary" medicine and "alternative" medicine have different meanings. In addition to Eisenberg's "unconventional medicine," other terms are often applied to the field as well to integrative medicine, holistic medicine, and others. The National Center for Complementary and Alternative Medicine (NCCAM) is a center in the National Institutes of Health (NIH) that was created by Congress in 1998. The mission of the Center "is to define through rigorous scientific investigation, the usefulness and safety of complementary and alternative medicine interventions and their roles in improving health and health care."[5] NCCAM acknowledges the ambiguity surrounding the definitions of these diverse health care practices and offers a summary of the various terms presented in **Table 1**. NCCAM now endorses the use of "complementary health approaches" to define the field. All of these terms are contrasted with "conventional," "biomedical," "allopathic," and "mainstream" medicine as practiced by medical (MD)/osteopathic (DO) physicians and their allied professionals, such as nurses and physical therapists. This article uses the term "complementary medicine"

Table 1 Definitions	
Alternative medicine	Used in place of CM
Complementary medicine	Used together with CM
Integrative medicine	Usually practiced by conventionally trained physicians, integrative medicine combines mainstream medical therapies and CAM therapies
Integrated medicine	Typically provided by teams of conventional and CAM clinicians
Holistic medicine	Considers body, mind, and spirit in health and healing.

to refer to health care clinicians, practices, and interventions that are usually distinct from conventional medical care. Patients use these approaches along with, or complementary to, their conventional medical care.

HOW IS COMPLEMENTARY MEDICINE DIFFERENT?

There clearly are differences between health care available in physician offices, clinics, and hospitals and interventions provided by complementary medicine practitioners. There are 3 features of complementary medicine that distinguish it from CM. Complementary therapies are individualized to each patient. Complementary medicine providers almost universally incorporate a philosophy of health that emphasizes and leverages an innate capacity for healing in every individual. Finally, complementary medicine tends to acknowledge the existence of properties of living systems that are resistant to understanding by contemporary reductionist scientific methods of inquiry that inform CM.

These distinguishing features present significant challenges to research and assembling meaningful evidence. They also create opportunities to develop more effective, efficient, and humanizing care for a very difficult population of patients, such as those with chronic pain. A recent observation by Cicerone[6] on evidence-based practice and the limits of rational rehabilitation points out that "…we need to acknowledge the subjective meanings of illness and disability to the patients we serve. Any efforts to build our practice based on the best available systematic evidence are unlikely to succeed unless we include patients' values and beliefs and incorporate this perspective into our rehabilitation research. This aspect of evidence-based rehabilitation raises important questions about our fundamental roles and how we will choose to practice and define our field in the future."

Individualized treatment is a hallmark of most complementary therapies. For example, an acupuncture practitioner may evaluate 2 patients, both with the same CM diagnosis, but develop 2 radically different treatment plans based on the Oriental medicine examination findings and assessment. This approach seems to work well for patients. Studies of patients who obtain care from complementary medicine practitioners reveal high levels of satisfaction with the practitioners and the outcome of the therapies. These providers spend time with their patients; they are successful in endorsing patients' complaints and in explaining to patients the nature of their health problems. Treatment planning tends to be more of a collaboration between therapist and patient than is often experienced in CM practice. Interventions are developed that are consistent with each patient's expectations, needs, and preferences. Individualized treatments, however, pose significant threats to the validity of typical randomized controlled clinical trial methodology.

Philosophy of care is not something that most CM practitioners ponder extensively. Health care philosophic discourse underlies many CAM therapies. Chiropractic, for example, contains an extensive literature that can loosely be described as "philosophy." Beginning with the founder, D.D. Palmer, chiropractic thinkers have historically focused not so much on the rational scientific underpinnings of this healing art, but on the art itself. "Innate Intelligence" is posited by Palmer and his successors as a fundamental life force that, when fully expressed without interference, the ultimate expression of health occurs, naturally and without need of intrusion from outside agents. In this chiropractic philosophic world view, the aim of the chiropractor is to locate and correct interferences with this natural expression of the life force. Exclusive focus on this "philosophy" has largely been abandoned by modern evidence-based chiropractors. Other complementary medicine disciplines also have underlying philosophies of life force. It is identified as "chi" in Oriental medicine, "prana" in yoga, "doshas" in Aruvedic medicine, "vix medica naturae" in naturopathic medicine, and each discipline has elaborated some measure of a conceptual life force that guides and propels healing and health.

Conventional medicine with its intellectual traditions anchored in western scientific thought is understandably skeptical of notions of "innate intelligence," "chi," or other conceptualization of a putative life force. Finding no "testable hypotheses" to investigate a possible life force, convention has largely dismissed such philosophic musing. Oschman[7] provides a comprehensive review of this seeming "impenetrable intellectual barrier" between CAM and CM world views.

WHO USES COMPLEMENTARY MEDICINE…AND WHY?

Surveys conducted by the Centers for Disease Control and Prevention (CDC) have shown that complementary medicine users come from all demographics.[8] Nearly 40% of the adult population reports using some form of complementary medicine, wherein "complementary medicine" includes both practitioner-based therapies, such as massage and acupuncture, and self-administered treatments, such as deep breathing or nutritional supplements. More than 11% of children have used it as well. Users tend to be more likely female (women generally use more health care services of all types) and have higher levels of education and income. Some studies indicate that complementary medicine appeals to individuals with a heightened sense of self-efficacy and internal locus of control.[9] Complementary medicine use persists into old age. Roughly one-third of adults 70 to 84 years and one-fourth of elders 85 years of age and older use complementary medicine.[10]

Most people use nonmainstream health care along with CM.[11] Dissatisfaction with CM is not usually a motivator for complementary medicine use.[12,13] Complementary medicine users are likely to report poor health status, that they find symptomatic relief with complementary medicine, and that complementary medicine approaches are consistent with the value they place on the role of nonphysical factors of mind/body connections in health and disease. Users are also more likely to engage actively in their health care decisions rather than "simply to accept unquestionably the physician's knowledge and expertise."[14]

Patients use complementary medicine for a wide variety of clinical conditions. Adults most frequently use complementary medicine to treat disorders of the musculoskeletal system. Findings from the 2007 National Health Interview Survey were reported by Barnes and colleagues,[8] as summarized in **Fig. 1**.

Complementary medicine use by children also is focused on musculoskeletal problems, as shown in **Fig. 2**.

Complementary medicine use is common in many clinical populations. A survey of primary care patients at a VA facility found that about one-half of respondents used

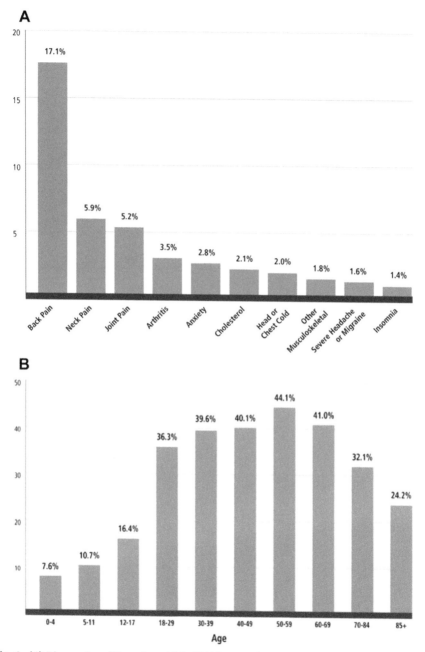

Fig. 1. (*A*) Diseases/conditions for which CAM is most frequently used among adults, 2007; (*B*) CAM use by Age, 2007; (*C*) CAM use by race/ethnicity among adults, 2007. (*From* Barnes PM, Bloom B, Nahin RL. CDC National Health Statistics Report #12. Complementary and alternative medicine use among adults and children: United States, 2007. Natl Health Stat Rep 2008;(12):1–23.)

C

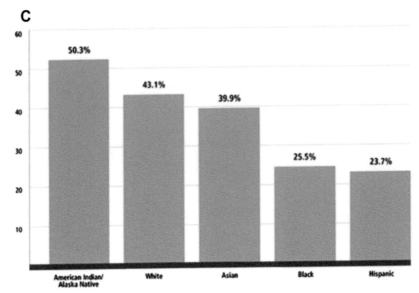

Fig. 1. (*continued*).

some form of complementary medicine for managing chronic pain and illness as well as for wellness and health promotion.[15] It is commonly used by patients with cancer along with conventional cancer care. For example, 80% of patients with thyroid cancer,[16] more than 70% of a sample of patients with colon, breast, and prostate

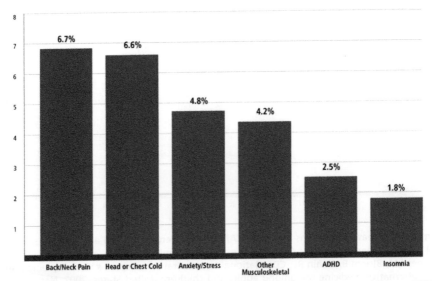

Fig. 2. Diseases/conditions for which CAM is most frequently used among children, 2007. ADHD, attention deficit hyperactivity disorder. (*From* Barnes PM, Bloom B, Nahin RL. CDC National Health Statistics Report #12. Complementary and alternative medicine use among adults and children: United States, 2007. Natl Health Stat Rep 2008;(12):1–23.)

cancer,[17] and from 6% to 91% of patients with pediatric cancer report using at least one form of complementary medicine.

COMPLEMENTARY MEDICINE USE IN CHRONIC PAIN

As noted in the CDC surveys, complementary medicine is used most commonly for pain problems of the back, neck, joints, arthritis, and other musculoskeletal disorders. Patients with chronic pain report an even higher frequency of complementary medicine use than in the general population.

In a survey of primary care patients on long-term opioid therapy, 44% reported at least one complementary medicine modality over the preceding 12 months.[18] Complementary medicine use has also been reported by more than 40% of patients with peripheral neuropathy,[19] 50% of chronic migraine sufferers,[20] and 52% of primary care patients with chronic pain.[21]

Assessing the efficacy and effectiveness of complementary therapies in chronic pain is problematic. The methodological challenges of efficacy studies in complementary medicine are discussed later. Patient surveys and pragmatic studies of effectiveness of these interventions suggest that most patients using complementary therapies find them helpful.

Chronic Pain

The study by Fleming and colleagues[18] of opioid-using patients with chronic pain in primary care looked at a broad sample of patients with chronic, noncancer pain. Complementary medicine users reported the therapy was "helpful" from 59% (for acupuncture) to 90% (for massage) of the time.

Cancer Pain

CAM use is widespread among patients with cancer. Up to about 60% of adult patients with cancer report using at least one nonconventional treatment for pain, nausea, fatigue, and other cancer-associated symptoms.[22] Forty-four percent of women with lung cancer report CAM use,[23] and 20% of patients at a private cancer clinic report receiving massage.[24] The National Cancer Institute booklet on "Pain Control" notes "other ways to control pain" that include massage, acupuncture, hypnosis, and imagery—biofeedback, meditation, and therapeutic touch (TT). The message to patients with cancer is, "Along with your pain medicine, your health care team may suggest you try other methods to control your pain. However, unlike pain medicine, some of these methods have not been tested in cancer pain studies. But they may help improve your quality of life by helping you with your pain, as well as stress, anxiety, and coping with cancer."[25]

Headache

An analysis of national health survey data indicated that 50% of US adults with migraines or severe headaches used at least one CAM over the past 12-month period.[26] Self-reported efficacy of complementary medicine approaches, while modest, is prevalent with 40% to 90% of chronic headache patients reporting use of at least one nonconventional therapy.[27]

Low-Back Pain

A *Consumer Reports* survey of patients intended to provide "real-life accounts" of patient experience with a variety of treatments for low-back pain. Fifty-nine percent of respondents who saw a chiropractor were "completely" or "very" satisfied with their treatment. This report compared with 44% for those who saw a physician specialist and 34% who saw a primary care provider for their back pain.[28] In a "systematic review of systematic reviews" for treatment of nonspecific low-back pain, Kumar and colleagues[29] observed that despite weaknesses in the research designs of the primary studies, "...massage may be an effective treatment option in the short term..."

Surveys of convenience samples of complementary medicine users show 98% of respondents replied "always" or "usually" to the question, "Has the treatment or recommendation you received from this provider helped you?" Eighty-two percent of patients answered "usually" or "always" to: "Has the treatment or recommendation you received reduced your use of prescription drugs?" Ninety-two percent of respondents answered "usually" or "always" to: "Has the treatment or recommendation you received reduced your use of other medical care for this problem?"[30]

EVIDENCE-BASED COMPLEMENTARY MEDICINE

Although patient surveys and pragmatic studies indicate that complementary medicine is helpful, these essentially anecdotal reports are not convincing for many observers. Critics of complementary medicine summarily dismiss it because it is unscientific and lacks a research evidence base. However, a recent search of the *Cochrane Collaboration* for the term "complementary and alternative medicine" returns 1000 results and 621 reviews. A search of PubMed returns 13,654 citations. A search on PubMed for "acupuncture" returned more than 9000 citations. Limiting the search term to "complementary and alternative medicine and chronic pain" returned 357 citations on PubMed and 107 results on the Cochrane database.

The research on complementary medicine is collated and reviewed in several other databases, as listed in **Table 2**. These resources assist researchers as well as clinicians at the bedside. There clearly is a growing body of research on CAM.

CHALLENGES OF EVIDENCE-BASED COMPLEMENTARY MEDICINE

Developing the evidence about complementary medicine therapies for chronic pain is problematic from several perspectives. There are problems with blinding of both subjects and clinicians, the confounding caused by expectations that subjects and therapists may bring to interventions involving complementary medicine such as acupuncture, subject allocation by complex clinical conditions that may have multifactorial origins and uncertain clinical end points and, finally, publication and editorial bias.

Complementary medicine therapies are often inherently resistant to analysis by commonly used clinical research methods. For example, in the hierarchy of evidence, the randomized controlled trial (RCT) is considered to be the gold standard. Nevertheless, many argue that this methodology, although well suited to the study of drugs, may not be the best research design to study complex, individualized treatments routinely offered by complementary medicine practitioners.[31,32] In a drug trial, the mechanism of action is usually well understood, whereas in complementary medicine, the interventions are often multipronged, such as manipulation and exercise in a neck pain trial. Isolating the "active ingredient" in this type of clinical intervention is difficult in the context of an RCT.

Blinding

Trials of manipulative therapy (spinal manipulative therapy [SMT]) and other manual therapies have been plagued by the difficulty in developing a "sham" treatment and concurrently controlling for the "nonspecific" effects of the hands-on practitioner-patient interaction with the sham treatment. Concealing active versus placebo

Table 2
Evidence based complementary medicine sources

Database	Description	Location
Natural Standard	Founded by health care providers and researchers to provide high-quality, evidence-based information about CAM including dietary supplements and integrative therapies. Grades reflect the level of available scientific data for or against the use of each therapy for a specific medical condition.	https://naturalmedicines.therapeuticresearch.com/
Natural Medicines Data Base	Has grown to be recognized as the scientific gold standard for evidence-based information on this topic. Leaders in CM as well as complementary, alternative, and integrative medicine recognize the Database as the go-to resource for the most complete and practical information.	http://naturaldatabase.therapeuticresearch.com/home.aspx?cs=&s=ND
Society for Acupuncture Research	Our Mission is to promote, advance, and disseminate scientific inquiry into Oriental medicine systems, which include acupuncture, herbal therapy, and other modalities. We value quantitative and qualitative research addressing clinical efficacy, physiologic mechanisms, patterns of use, and theoretic foundations.	http://www.acupunctureresearch.org/page-1160977
The MANTIS Database	MANTIS addresses all areas of alternative medical literature. It has also become the largest index of peer-reviewed articles for several disciplines, including chiropractic, osteopathy, homeopathy, and manual medicine.	http://www.healthindex.com/MANTIS.aspx
Dynamed	Our community of clinicians synthesizes the evidence and provide objective analysis in an easily-digestible format. We follow a strict evidence-based editorial process focused on providing unbiased information to help guide physicians in their decision-making process.	https://dynamed.ebscohost.com/
Trip Database	Trip is a clinical search engine designed to allow users to quickly and easily find and use high-quality research evidence to support their practice and/or care.	http://www.tripdatabase.com/

manipulation, for example, is challenging. SMT-naïve research subjects likely can detect genuine from placebo manipulations. SMT-experienced subjects certainly can tell the difference. Blinding the therapist in an SMT trial is similarly quite difficult, especially when compared with blinding of clinicians in a drug trial.

Acupuncture poses similar threats to methodological integrity.[33] Various sham acupuncture interventions have been proposed, including "minimal" needling to only a shallow, putatively nontherapeutic depth, needling at an "inert" acupuncture point, and using a placebo needle that does not penetrate the skin at all. However, these "placebo" procedures produce clinical and physiologic effects that are sometimes indistinguishable from genuine interventions. Acupuncture clinicians discount the existence on inert points, noting the "tree-and-branch" perspective of acupuncture meridians, which suggests that although the flow of chi is maximally affected at traditional acupuncture points, areas adjacent and remote from these points also produce an effect, negating the notion of an "inert" acupuncture point.

Expectations

Expectations by trial participants, patients, and clinicians can further confound the outcomes of all clinical trials. Subjects bring preconceptions, positive or negative, about the trial's interventions, as revealed in informed consent statements. Subjects biased favorably toward a "complementary medicine" intervention will likely report positive effects, regardless of whether the treatment is active or placebo. Haas and colleagues[34] note in their trial of manipulation that participant expectations and the therapist interaction with the subject "can have a relatively important effect on outcomes in open-label randomized trials of treatment efficacy. Therefore, attempts should be made to balance the DPE [doctor patient encounter] across treatment groups and report degree of success in study publications."

Allocation

Evidence about any treatment of chronic pain is further confounded by the complex nature of the condition itself. Patient selection is often a significant challenge to study validity. The wide variety of pathologic, functional, and behavioral disorders that are operant in chronic pain conditions defies the development of coherent and consistent diagnostic categories. Combining a wide variety of patients with "low-back pain," for example, into a conceptually uniform study group ignores the wide variety of conditions that may be classified into this category. It is no wonder that such trials frequently produce equivocal results for almost any intervention whether conventional or complementary and fail to reveal significant differences in effectiveness between treatment arms, between genuine treatment and sham or placebo, or between treatment and no treatment.

End Points

Problems associated with measuring the clinical effect of an intervention in chronic pain conditions are not unique to complementary medicine research. Pain is a subjective experience and has little in the way of an objective clinical finding, such as a laboratory value to evaluate clinical effectiveness. Several instruments are typically used to measure pain before intervention and after intervention, including a variety of pain scales (eg, visual analog pain scales), self-reported disability (Oswestry and neck disability index), and self-reported health (SF-36). Between-subject variability in how these instruments measure pain and changes in pain over time is problematic.[35] Other outcomes, such as return to work or cessation of medical care, have also been suggested. Deyo[36] discusses some approaches to this dilemma in the context of low-back pain research. The development of the PROMIS (Patient Reported Outcomes Measurement Information System) by the NIH offers measures of primary and secondary clinical endpoints that are reliable and meaningful to patients.[37]

Publication Bias

Finally, publication and indexing biases are obstacles to assembling and assessing reliable evidence about complementary medicine therapies.[38] As is often the case in CM research, studies with positive results are more likely to be submitted for publication. Many studies of CAM are in foreign language journals, thus limiting their exposure to English-speaking audiences. A more subtle bias also is observed in CM-published research on CAM. As one CAM researcher put it, "A negative study of acupuncture concludes that 'acupuncture doesn't work.' The analogue would be a negative drug trial that concluded 'medicine does not work'" (Hammarschlag R, personal communication, 2005).

The challenges of applying evidence of this nature to the practical realities of treating patients have been increasingly recognized.[6] Fortunately, researchers, particularly in the complementary medicine field, are actively developing research strategies that are more appropriate for both the individualized nature of complementary medicine interventions and the complex, multifactorial nature of chronic conditions, such as chronic pain.[39]

WHY SHOULD A PHYSIATRIST LEARN ABOUT COMPLEMENTARY AND ALTERNATIVE MEDICINE THERAPIES FOR CHRONIC PAIN?

There is a compelling case why CM physicians, especially in the challenging field of pain medicine, might want to better understand complementary medicine therapies.

- Because complementary medicine use is widespread, it is more likely than not that patients with chronic pain are already using at least one CAM therapy concurrently with conventional treatments.
- The evidence for some complementary therapies is equivalent to that which supports many commonly prescribed conventional treatments (**Table 3**).
- There are potential complications that arise with the combination of complementary and conventional therapies.
- Increasing public health concerns for the escalating use of opioid medication lobbies heavily for seeking other approaches to managing chronic pain.
- CAM therapies can improve the quality of care for patients with chronic pain.

At least 116 million American adults suffer from chronic pain.[40] It is estimated that 40% of them fail to achieve adequate relief.[41] Surveys of CAM users note a high prevalence of chronic conditions, including chronic pain. Anecdotal evidence suggests that patients find relief with complementary medicine interventions. Observers of complementary medicine note that "consumers will continue to use CAM, particularly in chronic conditions, in which patients struggle to find any treatment that may cure their condition or improve their quality of life."[42]

Current conventional medical treatments for chronic pain include a variety of approaches involving medication, surgery, and other interventions. Nevertheless, despite the cost of these treatments (up to $300 billion worth), the outcomes are often disappointing. Treatment of chronic low-back pain, for example, has seen a dramatic increase in resource use. Deyo and colleagues[43] reviewed experience in Medicare over the past decade and found "...a 629% increase in Medicare expenditures for

Table 3
Comparison of the evidence for conventional and complementary therapies for low-back pain

Therapy	Evidence as Summarized by *Cochrane Collaboration Reviews*
NSAIDs	The review authors conclude that NSAIDs are slightly effective for short-term symptomatic relief in patients with acute and chronic low-back pain without sciatica (pain and tingling radiating down the leg). In patients with acute sciatica, no difference in effect between NSAIDs and placebo was found. Only 42% of the studies were considered to be of high quality.
Opioids	In general, people that received opioids reported more pain relief and had less difficulty performing their daily activities in the short term than those who received a placebo. However, there are little data about the benefits of opioids based on objective measures of physical functioning. We have no information from RCTs supporting the efficacy and safety of opioids used for more than 4 mo. Furthermore, the current literature does not support that opioids are more effective than other groups of analgesics for low-back pain, such as anti-inflammatories or antidepressants. The quality of evidence in this review ranged between "very low" and "moderate." See more at: http://summaries.cochrane.org/CD004959/BACK_opioids-for-the-treatment-of-chronic-low-back-pain#sthash.axeqopHv.dpuf
Therapeutic ultrasound	We did not find any convincing evidence that ultrasound is an effective treatment of low-back pain. There was no high-quality evidence that ultrasound improves pain or quality of life. The quality of the evidence on ultrasound leaves much to be desired. In this review, we found "moderate" quality evidence regarding back-related function. The evidence on other outcomes was of "low" or "very-low" quality.
SMT	The results of this review demonstrate that SMT appears to be as effective as other common therapies prescribed for chronic low-back pain, such as exercise therapy, standard medical care, or physiotherapy.
Acupuncture	For chronic low-back pain, results show that acupuncture is more effective for pain relief than no treatment or sham treatment, in measurements taken up to 3 mo. The results also show that for chronic low-back pain, acupuncture is more effective for improving function than no treatment, in the short term. Acupuncture is not more effective than other conventional and "alternative" treatments. When acupuncture is added to other conventional therapies, it relieves pain and improves function better than the conventional therapies alone.
Massage therapy	Massage was more likely to work when combined with exercises (usually stretching) and education. The amount of benefit was more than that achieved by joint mobilization, relaxation, physical therapy, self-care education, or acupuncture. It seems that acupressure or pressure point massage techniques provide more relief than classic (Swedish) massage, although more research is needed to confirm this. In summary, massage might be beneficial for patients with subacute (lasting 4 to 12 wk) and chronic (lasting longer than 12 wk) nonspecific low-back pain, especially when combined with exercises and education.

Abbreviation: NSAIDs, nonsteroidal anti-inflammatory drugs.

epidural steroid injections; a 423% increase in expenditures for opioids for back pain; a 307% increase in the number of lumbar MRIs among Medicare beneficiaries; and a 220% increase in spinal fusion surgery rates...[however] The limited studies available suggest that these increases have not been accompanied by population-level improvements in patient outcomes or disability rates." As disturbing as it seems for adults suffering chronic pain, new research has disclosed an alarming increase in hospitalization of children for pain. An article in the July 2013 issue of the journal *Pediatrics* found an 831% increase in hospital admissions from 2004 through 2010.[44]

Most CAM interventions are "low tech-high touch" in nature. They are often perceived as inherently safe and natural by patients and practitioners. However, there is a growing body of evidence that illuminates adverse reactions to commonly used CAM therapies either by themselves or when combined with CM. Drug-herb interactions, for example, present potential challenges to patient safety and may compromise therapeutic effect. Eisenberg[2] noted that patients use CAM and CM concurrently for the same condition upward of 83% of the time. What is potentially more troublesome is that CAM users failed to disclose CAM use to CM physicians. Subsequent investigation indicates that this failure to disclose has not improved over time.[45] Better understanding by both CM and CAM practitioners of risks can modify the potential for adverse outcomes.

Avoiding adverse CM-CAM interactions can obviously improve patient care. Inquiring about CAM use, especially from an objective and evidence-based perspective, can enhance patient communication. The cultural competency of nonjudgmental acknowledgment of CAM use, particularly when reinforced by objective evidence of safety and effectiveness, can reinforce a productive therapeutic relationship between patient and physician. It is well recognized that effective physician-patient communication is a critical element predicting better patient satisfaction and compliance.[46] Moreover, as reliable evidence of CAM effectiveness emerges, CM physicians may be in a position to integrate evidence-based CAM approaches in an active manner rather than passively accepting what patients with chronic pain may already be attempting to integrate on their own.

CAM therapies are especially attractive when compared with the questionable efficacy and adverse effects of at least some CM therapies for pain. In particular, given the growing concern about mortality and morbidity associated with opioid therapy for chronic pain (discussed in the article by Ballantyne elsewhere in this issue), it is incumbent on practitioners who treat chronic pain to be aware of "opioid-sparing" therapies, including CAM therapies.

EVIDENCE REGARDING SELECTED COMPLEMENTARY MEDICINE THERAPIES

For purposes of discussion in this section, complementary medicine therapies will be limited to those commonly accessible in the community for patients with chronic pain and, for the most part, administered under the guidance of licensed health care professionals. Although this approach may exclude some valuable and frequently used therapies, it does encompass therapies that are in regular use by patients with chronic pain, are at least somewhat institutionalized, have been used or referred to by CM providers, and are capable of being integrated clinically and administratively into the care of patients with chronic pain. The array of complementary medicine therapies can be categorized further by their intellectual and philosophic nature as being either essentially biologically based or energy based.

- *Biologically based therapies* are explained and practiced fundamentally in ways that are familiar to practitioners trained in the conventional medical model of western scientific inquiry. Clinical conditions are mostly described in terms of disturbed anatomy and physiology. Treatment interventions are categorized by their physiologic effects. Outcomes are measured in objective terms. These disciplines, such as chiropractic and natural medicine, often view themselves as being within the context of orthodox scientific thought. Many of these therapies have been rigorously scrutinized through the lens of western medical scientific investigation. The disciplines themselves are developing intellectual, administrative, and physical infrastructure to conduct research.

- *Energy-based therapies* are most often founded on putative notions of natural systems of "invisible energetic relations and connections that govern living form and function."[7] Although some of these energy-based therapies have undergone scientific inquiry, most notably acupuncture, the fundamental world view of energy-based healers has not been altered to conform to the understandings offered by rational reductionistic methods. For example, science has attempted to understand the physiologic basis of acupuncture. However, few acupuncture practitioners endorse or, more importantly, practice within this intellectual context, preferring instead to explain what they do in the language of Oriental medicine, such as the flow of chi.

BIOLOGICALLY BASED THERAPIES
Spinal Manipulative Therapy

SMT is the most widely used complementary medicine therapy.[2] It is widely practiced by a variety of specialties including doctors of chiropractic (DCs), DOs, MDs, physical therapists, and some lay practitioners. It is estimated that DCs deliver more than 90% of all manipulative therapy.[47] Chiropractic training in manipulative techniques is arguably the most extensive among manipulation practitioners.

SMT is thought to improve pain by locating and treating disturbed joint and muscle function described as dysfunction, subluxation, fixation, and other terminology that may vary by discipline, training, and technique. Of the complementary medicine therapies, manipulation has been studied the most extensively. NCCAM has identified 537 clinical trials of manipulative and other bodywork therapies such as massage. Although the results are often ambiguous, there is clear evidence that manipulation is superior to sham treatment and equivalent to other conservative interventions for acute spinal pain problems.[48]

Recent investigations show long-term benefit for neck pain,[49] headaches,[50] and chronic mechanical spine pain.[51] *Cochrane Collaboration Reviews* of SMT for chronic low-back and neck pain found that these modalities are essentially equivalent to other therapies commonly prescribed for these conditions.[52,53]

Therapeutic Massage

Massage therapy encompasses more than 150 named body work systems and perhaps thousands of variations and individual techniques. Therapeutic, clinical, or medical massage is engaged to treat specific clinical conditions. The physiologic effects of massage are well documented, including muscular relaxation, improved blood and lymph circulation, and neuro-hormonal-immunologic effects. There are more than 20 clinical trials of massage for pain. *Physical Medicine and Rehabilitation Clinics of North America* reviewed therapeutic massage in 1999.[54] A more recent *Cochrane Review* of massage for low-back pain concluded, "Massage might be beneficial for patients with subacute and chronic non-specific low-back pain, especially when combined with exercises and education."[55]

Breath Pattern Retraining

In 1975, Lum[56] introduced the concept of disordered breathing patterns as the underlying cause of "a collection of bizarre and unrelated symptoms," including cardiovascular, neurologic, respiratory, gastrointestinal, musculoskeletal, psychological, and other syndromes. More recently, Chaitow[57] emphasized disturbed breathing patterns as the cause of chronic pain. Proposed mechanisms are summarized as "respiratory alkalosis, leading to reduced oxygenation of tissues (including the brain), smooth muscle constriction, heightened pain perception, speeding up of spinal reflexes, increased excitability of the corticospinal system, hyperirritability of motor and sensory axons, changes in serum calcium and magnesium levels, and encouragement of myofacsial trigger points..." Breath pattern retraining therapists note that the respiratory mechanism is the only physiologic function that is under both autonomic and voluntary control.

A recent RCT[58] revealed equivalent improvement from 12 sessions of breath therapy on visual analog scale, Roland Scale, and SF-36 when compared with high-quality, extended physical therapy. Breath therapy was found to be safe.

Natural Medicine Therapies

Several complementary medicine practices use nutritional supplements and herbs (known collectively as nutraceuticals) in the treatment of chronic pain. Although these natural medicine approaches are most commonly identified with doctors of naturopathic medicine (ND), herbs and supplements are frequently used by acupuncture/ Oriental medicine and chiropractic providers as well.

Natural medicine can be used directly for analgesia (white willow bark, for example) and antispasmodics (valerian and passiflora are examples). Nutritional and herbs interventions are most commonly applied to modify perceived underlying physiologic disturbances, such as fibromyalgia, depression, osteoarthritis (OA), and rheumatoid arthritis (RA). Of commonly used nutritional approaches, glucosamine and chondroitin sulfate have been most extensively studied. Glucosamine has been shown to slow cartilage deterioration and relieve the pain in knee OA. A 2011 *Cochrane Collaboration Review* found that standardized doses of white willow bark and devil's claw reduces back pain "about the same as" Vioxx.[59]

Many nutraceutical interventions are thought to modify disturbed metabolism that underlies chronic pain conditions such as fibromyalgia. Although much nutraceutical information on the Internet is proprietary and commercial in nature, there are several evidence-based sources of information such as the Natural Standard (https:// naturalmedicines.therapeuticresearch.com/) and Natural Medicines Comprehensive Database (http://naturaldatabase.therapeuticresearch.com/home.aspx?cs=&s=ND).

Body Awareness Therapy

Several approaches to chronic pain treatment involve the idea that improved postural coordination by using conscious processes alter automatic postural coordination and ongoing muscular activity. These "body awareness therapies" (BAT) may be practiced by physical and occupational therapists, massage therapists as well as nonlicensed body-work professionals. Two common BAT are described: Alexander technique (AT) and Feldenkrais.

AT is described as "... a method that works to change (movement) habits in our everyday activities. It is a simple and practical method for improving ease and freedom of movement, balance, support and coordination. The technique teaches the use of the appropriate amount of effort for a particular activity, giving you more energy for all your activities. It is not a series of treatments or exercises, but rather a reeducation of the mind and body."[60] A recent systematic review of AT found "strong evidence" for effectiveness in chronic low-back pain.[61]

Feldenkrais is said to improve function by "expanding the self-image through movement sequences that bring attention to the parts of the self that are out of awareness and uninvolved in functional actions. Better function is evoked by establishing an improved dynamic relationship between the individual, gravity, and society."[62] Jain and colleagues[63] provide a recent review of the method, its use, and the relevant research and research gaps concerning this BAT.

Prolotherapy

The use of proliferation therapy (prolotherapy) has waxed and waned for nearly a century. Often provided by CM practitioners, prolotherapy is also frequently in the therapeutic armamentarium of ND. Following an injury, failure of adequate tendon or ligament healing is thought to result in instability, connective tissue insufficiency, or lack of tensile strength. Normal use of these compromised structures causes pain. Prolotherapy consists of injections of an array of substances intended to trigger growth factors in local connective tissue and restart the repair sequence that results in more normal and functional tissue.

A 2005 critical review of prolotherapy[64] retrieved more than 30 studies of prolotherapy for spinal pain. These studies reflected wide variation in treatment protocols and concluded that, "… clinical studies published to date indicate that it may be effective at reducing spinal pain." An updated *Cochrane Review* concluded that when used alone, prolotherapy injections were not an effective treatment of chronic low-back pain, and when they are combined with exercise, manipulation, and other treatments, they can help chronic low-back pain and disability.[65]

Trigger Point Manipulation

Travell and Simons[66] offered an early treatise on myofascial trigger points (TrP) that was defined originally as, "a hyperirritable spot in skeletal muscle that is associated with a hypersensitive palpable nodule in a taut band. The spot is tender when pressed and can give rise to characteristic referred pain, motor dysfunction, and autonomic phenomena."

The understanding of the cause of TrPs has evolved. Current thinking has been summarized as, "TrPs are evoked by the abnormal depolarization of motor end plates… presynaptic, synaptic, and postsynaptic mechanisms of abnormal depolarization (ie, excessive release of acetycholine [ACh], defects of acetylcholinesterase, and upregulation of nicotinic ACh-receptor activity, respectively)."[67]

No objective diagnostic tests for TrPs are available. TrPs are diagnosed by manual palpation to identify a tender nodule, often at characteristic locations in muscle that produce characteristic radiating pain when stimulated. Despite this "low-tech" diagnostic method, TrP detection has good test-retest reliability.[68] Various approaches to treating TrPs have been elaborated, including manual compression, "spray and stretch," injection, dry needling, and modalities such as ultrasound, electric stimulation, low-level laser. TrP treatment is often rendered by certain CM physical medicine practitioners, but most frequently by chiropractors, acupuncturists, and massage practitioners.

ENERGY-BASED THERAPIES

Energy medicine is a domain in CAM that deals with energy fields of 2 types: veritable, which can be measured, and putative, which has yet to be measured.

The veritable energies include mechanical vibrations (such as sound) and electromagnetic forces, including visible light, magnetism, monochromatic radiation (such as laser beams), and rays from other parts of the electromagnetic spectrum. These veritable energy-based therapies involve the use of specific, measurable wavelengths and frequencies to treat patients.

In contrast, putative energy fields are based on the concept that human beings are infused with a subtle form of energy. This vital energy or life force is known under different names in different cultures and traditions, such as qi in traditional Chinese medicine (TCM), ki in the Japanese Kampo system, doshas in Ayurvedic medicine, and prana, etheric energy, fohat, orgone, odic force, mana, and homeopathic resonance elsewhere. Vital energy is thought to flow throughout the material human body, but it has not been unequivocally measured by means of conventional instrumentation. Nonetheless, therapists claim that they can work with this subtle energy, see it with their own eyes, and otherwise sense its presence and quality and then use it to effect changes in another's physical body to influence health.

VERITABLE ENERGY THERAPIES
Magnetic Therapy

Magnetic therapy has a long and controversial history in medicine. It has recently regained popularity in the marketplace. Application is by way of electromagnetic coils, in connection with acupuncture treatment and by way of static magnets. Magnetic therapy is typically applied to the skin overlying the affected area. The popular press indicates the use of magnets for treating a wide variety of chronic pain problems such as migraine, OA, and injury to muscles, ligaments, and tendons. Contraindications are few but do include pregnancy, pediatrics, and implantable electronic devices.

Contemporary clinical trials of magnet therapy have produced conflicting results. A study of carpal tunnel syndrome in 2002 found no statistically significant difference between magnets and placebo. However, the authors did note, "Although this study did not show magnets to be more effective than the placebo, the reduction in pain with this simple intervention was remarkable."[69] In a double-blind, placebo-controlled trial, static magnets produced statistically significant ($P<.05$) short-term pain relief in OA of the knee.[70] A Cochrane Review of various magnet therapies found low and very low levels of evidence such that for "all forms of [magnetic] stimulation the evidence is not conclusive and uncertainty remains."[71]

Microcurrent Stimulation

Microcurrent stimulation has been used in CM for the treatment of nonunion fracture and delayed healing. The exact mechanism of action is unknown but may involve intracellular regulation of Ca^+. Microcurrent stimulation has found application in the treatment of soft tissue disorders as well.

McMakin has published 3 studies of this modality, which is termed frequency-specific microcurrent (FSM), in patients with chronic pain. The studies are case series reports involving head, neck, and face pain,[72] chronic low-back pain,[73] and fibromyalgia associated with cervical spine trauma.[74] In the most recent study, Curtis and colleagues[75] began to explore the mechanisms of FSM. Their subjects revealed reductions in inflammatory cytokines, increase in β endorphins as well as subjective reports of pain relief in fibromyalgia. A recent study of FSM for delayed onset muscle soreness found significant differences at 24, 48, and 72 hours after exercise.

Low-Level Laser Therapy

Low-level laser therapy (LLLT) is a form of phototherapy that involves the application of low-power laser light to areas of the body to stimulate healing. It is also known as cold laser, soft laser, or low-intensity laser. It is hypothesized that photons are absorbed in the mitochondria. The light energy is converted to chemical energy within the cell that affects the permeability of the cell membrane, which in turn produces various physiologic effects. These physiologic changes affect a variety of cell types, including macrophages, fibroblasts, endothelial cells, and mast cells.

LLLT is widely used in physical therapy, chiropractic practice, and other physical medicine practice. Although reportedly safe, the modality is relatively new and is still controversial with respect to its effectiveness. A MedLine search retrieves more than 500 citations. A recent systematic review of the literature of LLLT for acute and chronic neck pain[76] concluded, "...Significant positive effects were reported in four of five trials..." *Cochrane Reviews* of LLLT used in OA and RA revealed, "Conflicting evidence of benefit...for the treatment of osteoarthritis."[77] LLLT for RA is somewhat more positive in that the therapy "...provides short-term pain relief for patients with rheumatoid arthritis."[78] Significantly, both reviews noted positive therapeutic results and called for more high-quality research on LLLT. A recent *Cochrane Review* of LLLT for nonspecific low-back pain was more reserved, concluding, "...that there are insufficient data to draw firm conclusions on the clinical effect of LLLT for low-back pain."[79]

PUTATIVE ENERGY THERAPIES
Acupuncture and Oriental Medicine

Among the "putative energy" therapies, none have received the notice and scrutiny of acupuncture. The practice of Oriental medicine itself includes a range of systems, interventions, schools of thought, and techniques. One such system, TCM, is widely taught and practiced in the United States. TCM encompasses herbs, massage, qigong, and acupuncture.

In the TCM view, the body is a delicate balance of 2 opposing and inseparable forces: yin and yang. Yin represents the cold, slow, or passive principle, while yang represents the hot, excited, or active principle. Among the major assumptions in TCM are that health is achieved by maintaining the body in a "balanced state" and that disease is due to an internal imbalance of yin and yang. This imbalance leads to blockage in the flow of qi (or vital energy) and of blood along pathways known as meridians. TCM practitioners typically use herbs, acupuncture, and massage to help unblock qi and blood in patients in an attempt to bring the body back into harmony and wellness.[80] These therapies are intended to balance the flow of qi and not to produce a specific physiologic effect.

Acupuncture describes a family of procedures involving stimulation of anatomic locations on the skin by a variety of techniques. There are several approaches to diagnosis and treatment in American acupuncture that incorporate medical traditions from China, Japan, Korea, and other countries. The most studied method of stimulation of acupuncture points uses penetration of the skin by thin, solid, metallic needles, which are manipulated manually or by electrical stimulation.[81]

The body of research literature on acupuncture is robust. A search on PubMed for "acupuncture" returned more than 21,000 citations. Limiting the search terms to "acupuncture and chronic pain" returned more than 1200 articles. The *Cochrane Collaboration* lists 479 results for "acupuncture" and 57 evidence-based medicine (EBM) reviews specifically for "acupuncture and chronic pain." A comprehensive review of this literature base is well beyond the scope of this article, but it is apparent that there is conclusive evidence of the effectiveness and safety of this therapy.

It is clear that acupuncture is widely used by patients with chronic pain. A telephone survey reported by Breivik and colleagues[82] found 13% of patients with chronic pain in Europe to be using acupuncture. Research methodology challenges in the investigation of acupuncture stubbornly persist. Meta-analyses frequently conclude that although acupuncture can be shown to be effective for pain relief, the therapy itself has not been shown to be superior to other therapies.[83] The most recent meta-analyses of acupuncture for neck and chronic low-back pain strengthen evidence for the effectiveness of this intervention.[84–87]

Craniosacral Therapy

Craniosacral therapy (CST) developed from the work of an American osteopath, Dr William Sutherland, in the early 1900s. It is founded on the notion of the primary respiratory mechanism that involves intrinsic motions of the cranial bones, the dura, and the flow of cerebrospinal fluid (CSF). Restricted motion of the cranial bones at the sutures is thought to impede CSF flow and lead to disordered function and disease. Rhythmic motions are said to be measurable with instruments, but in clinical practice, it is by palpation that a CST practitioner identifies disturbed cranial rhythms and applies corrective gentle manipulations.

CST is known in the osteopathic profession preferentially as cranial osteopathy. The chiropractic profession has a technique that encompasses much of CST, and others as well, known as the sacro-occipital technique. CST is also practiced by a variety of other hands-on practitioners, including physical and massage therapists, dentists, and lay practitioners.

CST is included under the "putative" energy category in that the motions of the primary respiratory mechanism have not been irrefutably demonstrated. Skeptics and critics inside[88] and out[89] of the osteopathic medicine profession have challenged the existence of these subtle rhythms. Reliability studies of the manual diagnosis of disturbed cranial rhythms have been disappointing.[90] The *Cochrane Collaboration* contains no EBM reviews of CST. A systematic review of CST "found insufficient evidence to support craniosacral therapy."[91]

Homeopathy

Homeopathy is a system of diagnosis and treatment founded by Samuel C. Hahnemann in Germany in the late eighteenth century. Homeopathy is currently practiced widely in Europe and Great Britain and by many practitioner types in the United States, including MD, DO, DC, ND, and lay providers. Clinical evaluations include detailed history interviews that lead to individualized treatment regimens, depending on a host of physical, emotional, and psychological factors. The therapies include the use of homeopathic remedies, which are derived from plant, mineral, and other extracts that have been serially diluted, often to the point where, statistically at least, no physical molecules of the original substance remain.

This fact of course challenges fundamentally the notions of science and the physical universe that underlie CM. Most CM practitioners simply cannot accept the idea that a substance that has nothing physically "there" can have any real effect beyond that attributable to placebo. Nonetheless, several studies in reliable scientific journals report the apparent effectiveness of homeopathic products.

There is an extensive literature on homeopathy. A PubMed search for "homeopathy" returned more than 4900 citations. Many of these are foreign language publications. A search of "homeopathy and chronic pain" returned 37 citations. A search of the British journal *Homeopathy* for "chronic pain" retrieved 145 articles. As with natural medicine approaches to pain treatment, a homeopathic practitioner is more likely to be evaluating and treating underlying causes of pain rather than treating pain itself. Critics of homeopathy observe that the effects of the modality rely largely on the process of the homeopathic practitioner-patient interaction and relationship (expectations, empathy, endorsement) rather than any physiologic mechanism.

Ayurvedic Medicine

"Ayurveda," which literally means "the science of life," is a natural healing system developed in India. Ayurvedic texts claim that the sages who developed India's original systems of meditation and yoga developed the foundations of this medical system. It has been described as follows: "In the prebiblical Ayurvedic origins, every creation inclusive of a human being is a model of the universe. In this model, the basic matter and the dynamic forces (Dosha) of the nature determine health and disease, and the medicinal value of any substance (plant and mineral). The Ayurvedic practices (chiefly that of diet, life style, and the Panchkarama) aim to maintain the Dosha equilibrium. Despite a holistic approach aimed to cure disease, therapy is customized to the individual's constitution (Prakruti). Numerous Ayurvedic medicines (plant derived in particular) have been tested for their biological (especially immunomodulation) and clinical potential using modern ethnovalidation, and thereby setting an interface with modern medicine."[92]

Ayurveda is a comprehensive system of medicine that places equal emphasis on the body, mind, and spirit and strives to restore the innate harmony of the individual. Some of the primary Ayurvedic treatments include diet, exercise, meditation, herbs, massage, exposure to sunlight, and controlled breathing. In India, Ayurvedic treatments have been developed for various diseases (eg, diabetes, cardiovascular conditions, and neurologic disorders). However, a survey of the Indian medical literature indicates that the quality of the published clinical trials generally falls short of contemporary methodological standards with regard to criteria for randomization, sample size, and adequate controls."[93]

A MedLine search for "Ayurvedic medicine" returned 66 results. A systematic review of ayurvedic medicine for treatment of RA concluded that, "There is a paucity of RCTs of Ayurvedic medicines for RA. The existing RCTs fail to show convincingly that such treatments are effective therapeutic options for RA."[94] However, as with other many CAM therapies, especially the energy-based modalities, the issues raised by double-blind methodologies and placebo effects have not been thoroughly accounted for. The "spiritual strength" of the Ayurvedic healer and the utility of the placebo effect are both acknowledged and considered significant in many non-western healing traditions.[95]

Touch Therapies

Touch is a fundamental human sense. The skin is arguably the largest sensory organ of the body. The power of human touch has been recognized throughout the history of medicine. TT and its derivatives are energy-based therapies that have become common in some hospitals and other clinical settings. An entry on the TT Web site describes the approach as follows: "Therapeutic Touch is a contemporary healing modality drawn from ancient practices and developed by Dora Kunz and Dolores Krieger. The practice is based on the assumptions that human beings are complex fields of energy, and that the ability to enhance healing in another is a natural potential.

Therapeutic Touch (TT) is used to balance and promote the flow of human energy. It is taught in colleges around the world and has a substantial base of formal and clinical research. This research has shown that TT is useful in reducing pain, improving wound healing, aiding relaxation, and easing the dying process. It can be learned by anyone with a sincere interest and motivation towards helping others."[96]

A Medline search for "therapeutic touch and pain" returned 3 citations. A *Cochrane Review* of TT for acute wound healing found insufficient evidence that TT enhances wound healing.[97] However, a pilot trial of TT in a cognitive behavioral therapy program found patients with chronic pain who received TT in addition to relaxation and cognitive behavioral therapy (CBT) fared better in terms of enhanced self-efficacy and unitary power as well as having lower attrition rates than patients who only received relaxation training and CBT.

A study at the University of Wisconsin-Eau Claire studied another touch therapy (Tellington Touch) in patients about to undergo venipuncture. The intervention is described as, "gentle physical touch and consisting of four components: a mental attitude of openness, use of the hands and fingers, breath awareness, and moderate finger/hand pressure." Analysis of qualitative descriptions by patients and the phlebotomist-nurse demonstrated that this massagelike, caring touch promoted relaxation and produced a helpful distraction in patients about to undergo a potentially painful procedure. Although further study is warranted, the implications for physicians and others who have hands-on contact with patients of any sort, and patients with chronic pain in particular, seem obvious. The development of these skills may be of significant benefit to patients.

Reiki and Energy Healing Therapies

Reiki (pronounced RAY-kee) is Japanese for a universal life energy. It is derived from rei, meaning "free passage" or "transcendental spirit," and ki, meaning "vital life force energy" or "universal life energy." Reiki is based on the belief that when spiritual energy is channeled through a Reiki practitioner, the patient's spirit is healed, which in turn heals the physical body.[98,99] Reiki practice usually involves no direct physical contact between practitioner and recipient. By the practitioner holding the hands over the patient's body, the recipient is said to draw energy from the universal life force through the practitioner.

In the late 1800s, Dr Mikao Usui developed modern reiki from ancient Asian healing traditions said to be thousands of years old. Introduced to the West in the 1970s, reiki has become a popular CAM therapy in the United States. Reiki and other energy healing (EH) therapies have also attracted the attention of CM practitioners and researchers.[100] A recent review noted, "The National Institutes of Health is funding numerous EH studies that are examining its effects on a variety of conditions, including temporomandibular joint disorders, wrist fractures, cardiovascular health, cancer, wound healing, neonatal stress, pain, fibromyalgia, and AIDS. Several well-designed studies to date show significant outcomes for such conditions as wound healing and advanced AIDS, and positive results for pain and anxiety, among others. It is also suggested that EH may have positive effects on various orthopaedic conditions, including fracture healing, arthritis, and muscle and connective tissue. Because negative outcomes risk is at or near zero throughout the literature, EH is a candidate for use on many medical conditions."[101]

Reiki is practiced by a variety of licensed health care practitioners, including CM and CAM physicians, allied health care providers (registered nurses, physical therapists, occupational therapists), psychotherapists, massage practitioners as well as nonlicensed reiki "masters." Although reiki and other EH therapies are not without their critics,[102] these high-touch, low-tech interventions are being adopted by hospitals, clinics, and physician offices as useful adjuncts to patient care.[103,104] Higher patient satisfaction, improved clinical outcomes, and lower costs are ascribed to implementing reiki and other EH therapies.

SUMMARY

Far from being on the fringes of modern health care, many complementary therapies are in regular and frequent use by many patients with chronic pain. Increasingly, these unconventional therapies are subjected to the same rigorous investigation that is expected of all contemporary EBM practices. Arguably, many complementary therapies hold up very well to this scrutiny and certainly as well as many commonly prescribed conventional medical therapies.

The fact that they are in common use by patients with chronic pain suggests the need for pain physicians and clinicians to understand them. The emerging evidence that they are safe, clinically effective, and cost-effective when appropriately rendered further recommends them. That these therapies explicitly incorporate the power of intention, awareness, and intentions in the human interaction of the healing encounter may well be the key in achieving a more individualized, sensitive, and humanized approach to the treatment of a most difficult and challenging patient population—those with chronic pain.

REFERENCES

1. Starr P. The social transformation of American medicine. New York: Basic Books; 1982.
2. Eisenberg D. Unconventional medicine in the United States—prevalence, cost, and patterns of use. N Engl J Med 1993;328:426–525.
3. Institute of Medicine (US) Committee on the Use of Complementary and Alternative Medicine by the American Public. Complementary and Alternative Medicine in the United States. Washington, DC: National Academies Press (US); 2005. 8, Educational Programs in CAM. Available at: http://www.ncbi.nlm.nih.gov/books/NBK83809/.
4. American Chiropractic Association. ACA Today. Available at: http://www.acatoday.org/level2_css.cfm?T1ID=14&T2ID=36. Accessed October 15, 2014.
5. NCCAM website. Available at: http://nccam.nih.gov/about/ataglance. Accessed October 15, 2014.
6. Cicerone KD. Evidence-based practice and the limits of rational rehabilitation. Arch Phys Med Rehabil 2005;86:1073–4.
7. Oschman J. Energy medicine in therapeutics and human performance. Edinburgh (Scotland): Butterworth-Heinman; 2003.
8. Barnes PM, Bloom B, Nahin R. CDC National Health Statistics Report #12. Complementary and alternative medicine use among adults and children: United States, 2007. Natl Health Stat Rep 2008;(12):1–23.
9. Schützler L, Witt CM. Internal health locus of control in users of complementary and alternative medicine: a cross-sectional survey. Berlin (Germany): Institute for Social Medicine, Epidemiology and Health Economics, Charité Universitätsmedizin Berlin; 2014.
10. AARP, NCCAM. Complementary and alternative medicine: what people aged 50 and older discuss with their health care providers. Consumer Survey Report; April 13, 2010.
11. National Center for Complementary and Alternative Medicine (NCCAM). Complementary, alternative, or integrative health: what's in a name? Available at: http://nccam.nih.gov/health/whatiscam.Accessed September 16, 2014.

12. Bishop FL, Yardley L, Lewith GT. Why consumers maintain complementary and alternative medicine use: a qualitative study. J Altern Complement Med 2010; 16(2):175–82. http://dx.doi.org/10.1089/acm.2009.0292.
13. Sirois FM. Motivations for consulting complementary and alternative medicine practitioners: a comparison of consumers from 1997-8 and 2005. BMC Complement Altern Med 2008;8:16. http://dx.doi.org/10.1186/1472-6882-8-1.
14. Astin J. Why patients use alternative medicine results of a national study. JAMA 1998;279(19):1548–53. http://dx.doi.org/10.1001/jama.279.19.1548.
15. Healthcare Analysis & Information Group (HAIG). 2011 Complementary and alternative medicine. Department of Veterans Affairs, Veterans Health Administration. Available at: http://shfwire.com/files/pdfs/2011CAM_FinalReport.pdf. Accessed September 16, 2014.
16. Rosen JE, Saper RB, Gardiner P, et al. What are your patients using and are they telling you about it? Complementary and alternative medicine use among patients with thyroid cancer: 2010. Presented at the 14th International Thyroid Congress. Paris, September 11–16, 2010. Abstract OC-149. Available at: http://news.cancerconnect.com/high-prevalence-of-cam-use-among-thyroid-cancer-patients/ . Accessed September 16, 2014.
17. Molassiotis A, Fernadez-Ortega P, Pud D, et al. Use of complementary and alternative medicine in cancer patients: a European survey. Ann Oncol 2005;16: 655–63. http://dx.doi.org/10.1093/annonc/mdi110. Available at: http://annonc.oxfordjournals.org/content/16/4/655.full.pdf. Accessed September 16, 2014.
18. Fleming S, Rabago DP, Mundt MP, et al. CAM therapies among primary care patients using opioid therapy for chronic pain. BMC Complement Altern Med 2007; 7:15.
19. Brunelli B, Gorson KC. The use of complementary and alternative medicines by patients with peripheral neuropathy. J Neurol Sci 2004;218:59–66.
20. Adams J, Barbery G, Lui CW, et al. Complementary and alternative medicine use for headache and migraine a critical review of the literature. Headache 2013;53(3):459–73.
21. Rosenberg EI, Genao I, Chen I, et al. Complementary and alternative medicine use by primary care patients with chronic pain. Pain Med 2008;9:1065–72.
22. Ernst E. The prevalence of complementary/alternative medicine in cancer. Cancer 1998;83:777–82 [pii:10.1002/(SICI)1097-0142(19980815)83:4<777:: AID-CNCR22>3.0.CO;2-O].
23. Wells M, Sarna L, Cooley ME, et al. Use of complementary and alternative medicine therapies to control symptoms in women living with lung cancer. Cancer Nurs 2007;30(1):45–55.
24. Bernstein BJ, Grasso T. Prevalence of complementary and alternative medicine use in cancer patients. Oncology (Williston Park) 2001;15(10):1267–72 [discussion: 1272–8, 1283].
25. NIH National Cancer Institute. Pain control. NIH Publication No. 14-6287. Revised May 2014. Available at: http://www.cancer.gov/cancertopics/coping/paincontrol.pdf.Accessed September 22, 2014.
26. Wells RE, Bertisch SM, Buettner C, et al. Complementary and alternative medicine use among adults with migraines/severe headaches. Headache 2011;51: 1087–97.
27. Kristoffersen ES, Aaseth K, Grande RB, et al. Self-reported efficacy of complementary and alternative medicine; the Akershus study of chronic headache. J Headache Pain 2013;36:14. Available at: http://www.thejournalofheadacheandpain.com/content/14/1/36. Accessed September 22, 2014.

28. Consumer Reports.org. Relief for your aching back. What worked for our readers. Available at: http://www.consumerreports.org/cro/2013/01/relief-for-your-aching-back/index.htm. Accessed September 22, 2014.

29. Kumar S, Beaton K, Hughes T, et al. The effectiveness of massage therapy for the treatment of nonspecific low back pain: a systematic review of systematic reviews. Int J Gen Med 2013;6:733–41. http://dx.doi.org/10.2147/IJGM.S50243. Available at: http://www.ncbi.nlm.nih.gov/pmc/articles/PMC3772691/#__ffn_sectitle. Accessed September 17, 2014.

30. Weeks J. The integrator blog. March 29, 2012. Available at: http://theintegratorblog.com/index.php?option=com_content&task=view&id=816&Itemid=93.   Accessed October 16, 2014.

31. Paterson C, Dieppe P. Characteristic and incidental (placebo) effects in complex interventions such as acupuncture. BMJ 2005;330:1202–5.

32. Sullivan MD. Placebo controls and epistemic control in orthodox medicine. J Med Philos 1993;18(2):213–31.

33. Linde K, Jonas WB, Melchart D, et al. The methodological quality of randomized controlled trials of homeopathy, herbal medicines and acupuncture. Int J Epidemiol 2001;30:526–31.

34. Haas M, Vavrek D, Neradilek MB, et al. A path analysis of the effects of the doctor-patient encounter and expectancy in an open-label randomized trial of spinal manipulation for the care of low back pain. BMC Complement Altern Med 2014;16:14. Available at: http://www.biomedcentral.com/1472-6882/14/16.

35. Farrar J, Young JP Jr, LaMoreaux L, et al. Clinical importance of changes in chronic pain intensity measured on an 11-point numerical pain rating scale. Pain 2001;94:149–58.

36. Deyo R. Report of the NIH Task Force on research standards for chronic low back pain. J Pain 2014;15(6):569–85.

37. NIH PROMIS®. Available at: http://www.nihpromis.org/default#2. Accessed October 16, 2014.

38. Shekell P, Morton SC, Suttorp MJ, et al. Challenges in systematic reviews of complementary and alternative medicine topics. Ann Intern Med 2005;142(12 (Pt 2)):1042–7.

39. Langevin HM, Wayne PM, MacPherson H, et al. Paradoxes in acupuncture research: strategies for moving forward. Evid Based Complement Alternat Med 2011;2011:180805.

40. Committee on Advancing Pain Research, Care and Education. Relieving pain in America. Washington, DC: National Academies Press; 2011.

41. Whitten CE, Evans CM, Cristobal K. Pain management doesn't have to be a pain: working and communicating effectively with patients who have chronic pain. Perm J 2005;5(2):41–8.

42. Lundgren J, Ugalde V. The demographics and economics of complementary alternative medicine. Phys Med Rehabil Clin N Am 2004;15(4):955–61.

43. Deyo RA, Mirza SK, Turner JA, et al. Overtreating chronic back pain: time to back off? J Am Board Fam Med 2009;22:62–8.

44. Coffelt TA, Bauer BD, Carroll AE. Inpatient characteristics of the child admitted with chronic pain. Pediatrics 2013. http://dx.doi.org/10.1542/peds.2012-1739.

45. Eisenberg DM, Davis RB, Ettner SL, et al. Trends in alternative medicine use in the united States, 1990-1997. Results of a follow-up national survey. JAMA 1998; 280(18):1569–75.

46. Hirsh AT, Atchison JW, Berger JJ, et al. Patient satisfaction with treatment for chronic pain: predictors and relationship to compliance. Clin J Pain 2005; 21(4):302–10.

47. Shekelle PG, Adams AH, Chassin MR, et al. Spinal manipulation for low back pain. Ann Intern Med 1992;117:590–8.

48. Chou R, Huffman L. Nonpharmacologic therapies for acute and chronic low back pain: A review of the evidence for an American Pain Society/American College of Physicians clinical practice guideline. October 2, 2007.

49. Bronfort G. The effectiveness of cervical adjustment for acute and chronic neck pain: excerpts from a systematic review and best evidence synthesis. J Amer Chiro 2003;40(7):42.

50. McCrory DC, Penzien DB, Hasselblad V, et al. Evidence report: behavioral and physical treatments for tension-type and cervicogenic headache. Des Moines (IA): Foundation for Chiropractic Education and Research; 2001.

51. Muller R, Giles LG. Long-term follow-up of a randomized clinical trial assessing the efficacy of medication, acupuncture, and spinal manipulation for chronic mechanical spinal pain syndromes. J Manipulative Physiol Ther 2005;29(1):3–11.

52. Rubinstein SM, van Middlekoop M, Assendelft WJ, et al. Spinal manipulative therapy for chronic low-back pain. Cochrane Database Syst Rev 2013;(2). CD008112. Available at: http://summaries.cochrane.org/CD008112/BACK_spinal-manipulative-therapy-for-chronic-low-back-pain. Accessed September 30, 2014.

53. Gross A, Miller J, D'Sylva J, et al. Manipulation or mobilisation for neck pain. Cochrane Database Syst Rev 2010;(1):CD004249. http://dx.doi.org/10.1002/14651858.CD004249.pub3.

54. Braverman DL, Schulman RA. Massage techniques in rehabilitation medicine. Phys Med Rehabil Clin N Am 1999;10(3):631–49, ix.

55. Available at: http://www.cochrane.org/reviews/en/ab001929.html. Accessed October 16, 2014.

56. Lum LC. Hyperventilation: the tip of the iceberg. J Psychosom Res 1975;19: 375–83.

57. Chaitow L. Breathing pattern disorders, motor control and low back pain. J Osteo Med 2004;7(1):34–41.

58. Mehling WE, Hamel KA, Acree M, et al. Randomized, controlled trial of breath therapy for patients with chronic low back pain. Altern Ther Health Med 2005; 11(4):44–52.

59. Gagnier J, van Tulder M, Berman B, et al. Herbal medicine for low-back pain. 2011. Available at: http://summaries.cochrane.org/CD004504/BACK_herbal-medicine-for-low-back-pain. Accessed September 30, 2014.

60. Available at: http://www.alexandertechnique.com/at.htm. Accessed October 20, 2014.

61. Woodman JP, Moore NR. Evidence for the effectiveness of Alexander Technique lessons in medical and health-related conditions: a systematic review. Int J Clin Pract 2012;66(1):98–112.

62. Available at: http://www.feldenkrais.com/method/standards/index.html#what.

63. Jain S, Janssen K, DeCelle S, et al. Alexander technique and Feldenkrais method: a critical overview. Phys Med Rehabil Clin N Am 2004;15(4):811–25 vi. Review.

64. Dagenais S, Haldeman S, Wooley JR. Intraligamentous injection of sclerosing solutions (prolotherapy) for spinal pain: a critical review of the literature. Spine J 2005;5(3):310–28.

65. Simon D, Yelland MJ, Mar CD, et al. Prolotherapy injections for chronic low-back pain. Cochrane Database Syst Rev 2007. Available at: http://onlinelibrary.wiley.com/doi/10.1002/14651858.CD004059.pub3/abstract. Accessed September 30, 2014

66. Travell JG, Simons DG. Myofascial pain and dysfunction: the trigger point manual: the upper extremities, vol. 1. Baltimore (MD): Williams & Wilkins; 1983.

67. McPartland J. Travell trigger points–molecular and osteopathic perspectives. J Am Osteopath Assoc 2004;104(6):244–9.

68. Al-Shenqiti AM, Oldham JA. Test-retest reliability of myofascial trigger point detection in patients with rotator cuff tendonitis. Clin Rehabil 2005;19(5):482–7.

69. Carter R, Hall T, Aspy CB, et al. The effectiveness of magnet therapy for treatment of wrist pain attributed to carpal tunnel syndrome. Fam Pract 2002;51(1):38–40.

70. Wolsko PM, Eisenberg DM, Simon LS, et al. Double-blind placebo-controlled trial of static magnets for the treatment of osteoarthritis of the knee: results of a pilot study. Altern Ther Health Med 2004;10(2):36–43.

71. O'Connell NE, Wand BM, Marston L, et al. Non-invasive brain stimulation techniques for chronic pain. Cochrane Database Syst Rev 2014;(4):CD008208. http://dx.doi.org/10.1002/14651858.CD008208.pub3.

72. McMakin C. Microcurrent treatment of myofascial pain in the head, neck and face. Topics Clin Chiro 1998;5(1):29–35.

73. McMakin C. Microcurrent therapy:a novel treatment for chronic low back myofascial pain. J Bodyw Mov Ther 2004;8:143–53.

74. McMakin C, Gregoryb WM, Phillips TS. Cytokine changes with microcurrent treatment of fibromyalgia associated with cervical spine trauma. Journal of Bodywork and Movement Therapies 2005;9(3):169–76.

75. Curtis D, Fallows S, Morris M, et al. The efficacy of frequency specific microcurrent therapy on delayed onset muscle soreness. J Bodyw Mov Ther 2010;14(3):272–9.

76. Chow RT, Barnsley L. Systematic review of the literature of low-level laser therapy (LLLT) in the management of neck pain. Lasers Surg Med 2005;37(1):46–52.

77. Available at: http://www.cochrane.org/reviews/en/ab002046.html. Accessed October 20, 2014.

78. Available at: http://www.cochrane.org/reviews/en/ab002049.html. Accessed October 20, 2014.

79. Yousefi-Nooraie R, Schonstein E, Heidari K, et al. Low level laser therapy for nonspecific low-back pain. Cochrane Database Syst Rev 2008;(2):CD005107. http://dx.doi.org/10.1002/14651858.CD005107.pub4.

80. Available at: http://nccam.nih.gov/health/backgrounds/wholemed.htm#tcm. Accessed October 22, 2014.

81. Acupuncture. NIH Consens Statement 1997;15(5):1–34.

82. Breivik H, Collett B, Ventafridda V, et al. Survey of chronic pain in Europe: prevalence, impact on daily life, and treatment. Eur J Pain 2005;10(4):287–333.

83. Manheimer E, White A, Berman B, et al. Meta-analysis: acupuncture for low back pain. Ann Intern Med 2005;142(8):651–63.

84. Fu LM, Li JT, Wu WS. Randomized controlled trials of acupuncture for neck pain: systematic review and meta-analysis. J Altern Complement Med 2009;15(2):133–45.

85. Trinh K, Graham N, Gross A, et al. Acupuncture for neck disorders. Spine (Phila Pa 1976) 2007;32(2):236–43.
86. Yuan J, Purepong N, Kerr DP, et al. Effectiveness of acupuncture for low back pain: a systematic review. Spine 2008;33(23):E887–900.
87. Trigkilidas D. Acupuncture therapy for chronic lower back pain: a systematic review. Ann R Coll Surg Engl 2010;92(7):595–8.
88. Bledsoe BE, Licciardone JC. The elephant in the room: does OMT have proved benefit? J Am Osteopath Assoc 2004;104:405–6.
89. Available at: http://www.canoe.ca/HealthAlternativeColumns/010816.html. Accessed October 22, 2014.
90. Moran RW, Gibbons P. Intraexaminer and interexaminer reliability for palpation of the cranial rhythmic impulse at the head and sacrum. J Manipulative Physiol Ther 2001;24:183–90.
91. Green C, Martin CW, Bassett K, et al. A systematic review of craniosacral therapy: biological plausibility, assessment reliability and clinical effectiveness. Complement Ther Med 1999;7(4):199–270.
92. Chopra A, Doiphole VV. Ayurvedic medicine. Core concept, therapeutic principles, and current relevance. Med Clin North Am 2002;86(1):75–89, vii.
93. Available at: http://nccam.nih.gov/health/backgrounds/wholemed.htm#am. Accessed October 23, 2014.
94. Park J, Ernst E. Ayurvedic medicine for rheumatoid arthritis: a systematic review. Semin Arthritis Rheum 2005;34(5):705–13.
95. Jonas WB, Levin JS. Essentials of complementary and alternative medicine. Baltimore (MD): Lippencott, Williams and Wilkins; 1999. p. 210.
96. Available at: http://www.therapeutictouch.org/. Accessed October 23, 2014.
97. O'Mathuna DP, Ashford RL. Therapeutic touch for healing acute wounds. Cochrane Database Syst Rev 2003;(4):CD002766. http://dx.doi.org/10.1002/14651858.CD002766.
98. Available at: http://nccam.nih.gov/health/whatiscam/index.htm#d11. Accessed October 23, 2014.
99. Available at: http://www.holistic-online.com/Reiki/hol_reiki_introduction.htm. Accessed October 25, 2014.
100. Chu DA. Tai Chi, Qi Gong and Reiki. Phys Med Rehabil Clin N Am 2004;15(4):773–81, vi.
101. Dinucci EM. Energy healing: a complementary treatment for orthopaedic and other conditions. Orthop Nurs 2005;24(4):259–69.
102. Available at: http://www.ncahf.org/articles/o-r/reiki.html. Accessed October 25, 2014.
103. Sawyer J. The first Reiki practitioner in our OR. AORN J 1998;67(3):674.
104. Available at: http://www.reiki.org/reikinews/reiki_in_hospitals.html. Accessed October 25, 2014.

Interdisciplinary Rehabilitation

Niriksha Malladi, MD

KEYWORDS

• Multidisciplinary • Interdisciplinary • Pain rehabilitation • Chronic pain • Pain clinic

KEY POINTS

• Interdisciplinary pain rehabilitation programs are infrequently used in the United States in the treatment of chronic pain.
• Comprehensively addressing the contributors to chronic pain, which include behavioral, psychological and physical dimensions, has shown evidence-based efficacy in improving functioning and reducing pain-related distress.
• This approach also holds the potential for reducing the escalating costs of chronic pain care.

Interdisciplinary pain rehabilitation programs for the management of chronic pain remain underused in the United States. The reasons for their limited use are numerous, starting with restricted health care coverage for such programs. However, it is worthwhile to revisit a model that has consistently shown evidence-based benefit for patients, and that focuses on the achievable goals of improvement in both function and pain as well as decreased medical and societal costs. It is apparent that traditional medical interventions are not effectively tackling the problem of chronic nonmalignant pain. Deaths from pain-related opioid use are one concern stemming from the present approach. As the prevalence of chronic pain grows, patients increasingly require treatments to reduce their pain, suffering, and disability. Multiple analyses of the most effective ways of reducing chronic nonmalignant pain identify the need for coordinated, comprehensive care, including addressing physical and psychological complications associated with chronic pain syndrome.[1,2]

An interdisciplinary treatment approach applies to the millions of patients with chronic pain generating nearly 70 million physician office visits annually, and the 130 million outpatient, hospital, and emergency room visits.[3,4] There are also indirect costs, including employers dealing with absenteeism and disability costs. The US military, which faces back-related pain as the leading cause of disability, has found a use for this model with veterans.[5,6] Despite the different cultural contexts of patients

Pacific Rehabilitation Centers, 2515 140th Avenue Northeast, Suite 110, Bellevue, WA 98005, USA
E-mail address: nmalladi@pacificrehabilitation.com

Phys Med Rehabil Clin N Am 26 (2015) 349–358
http://dx.doi.org/10.1016/j.pmr.2014.12.008
1047-9651/15/$ – see front matter

living with chronic pain, which are influenced in large part by the patients' developmental, social, and psychological histories, comprehensive pain programs have shown efficacy for providing pain relief and improving physical limitations throughout the industrialized world, possibly because common human factors such as development of maladaptive coping skills, fear of movement, and mood disorders play a large role in development and perpetuation of pain disorders.[1]

The precursor of pain rehabilitation using an interdisciplinary approach has been credited to John Bonica, M.D. He recognized the need for coordinated pain services in injured World War II soldiers who needed specialized care.[7] Chronic pain rehabilitation programs were first formed in the United States in the 1970s, and functional restoration approaches emerged in the 1980s.[7] The alternatives available to patients for chronic pain treatment have typically been exhausted before patients are referred to interdisciplinary programs. These treatments include opioid and analgesic medications; targeted injections; ablation procedures; surgeries; chiropractic care; massage; physical therapy; and complementary alternative treatments, including acupuncture. Many of these treatments lack long-term efficacy for chronic pain, can expose the patient to risk, and rely on passive management of pain (relief provided by biomedical or manual treatments done by providers). Although effective for acute pain conditions, these treatments do not have a curative or a significant rehabilitative effect for patients with chronic pain. In contrast, interdisciplinary pain programs are designed to decrease medical use by improving patients' ability to independently manage their pain, improve functional and physical endurance, pain severity, quality of life, and employment capacity.

The distinction between an evidence-based interdisciplinary model and the frequently used, but less intensive, multidisciplinary approach is important. The terms are frequently used interchangeably in the literature but have distinct meanings. An interdisciplinary team is based in the same facility and works toward the same goals developed after a comprehensive evaluation. The treatment approach allows for functional recovery through musculoskeletal conditioning, cognitive-behavior therapy (CBT), relaxation techniques, and pain medication tapering. Vocational education is a component of many programs. The interdisciplinary approach stresses seamless communication between team members, daily communication, and weekly team meetings to discuss progress and barriers to recovery. It is time intensive and requires a high level of staffing for the brief period (minimum of 3 weeks) that patients participate in the program.

Multidisciplinary treatment involves multiple clinicians who are concurrently treating the patient, but often without a coordinated discussion of the treatment plan, and may not have similar treatment philosophies. There is limited opportunity for integrated communication with this approach. Multidisciplinary treatment does not tend to involve a brief, intense period of treatment, and may go on indefinitely with variable levels of treatment and support provided to the patient.

STRUCTURE OF A PAIN MANAGEMENT PROGRAM

The core of an interdisciplinary program is a skilled team of clinicians. This team typically includes a physician educated in pain rehabilitation, a psychologist trained in CBT, counselors, case managers, and physical and occupational therapists. Additional team members can include nurses, psychiatrists, and biofeedback specialists. Vocational rehabilitation counselors, particularly for programs designed to assist with return to work following an industrial injury, are an integral part of the team. There are a small number of inpatient programs throughout the United States, but a larger number is outpatient based. Literature shows many variations of multidisciplinary or interdisciplinary care. A systematic review showed that daily intensive programs with more than 100 hours of therapy were superior in showing improvements in pain, function, and vocational outcomes compared with less intensive programs.[8]

The typical interdisciplinary pain rehabilitation program includes 3 to 4 weeks of treatment lasting 4 to 8 h/d, 5 d/wk. Because many patients have musculoskeletal impairments and have limited ability to be fully functional, patients are guided individually or in a group setting through progressive exercises to reverse the effects of deconditioning. Using the principles of CBT to learn adaptive pain coping strategies, they are taught self-management skills to manage any concomitant mood disorders that may be present, as well as decreasing avoidant behaviors secondary to fear of pain. Decreasing dependence on habit-forming medications such as opioids and benzodiazepines is another key feature of such programs. Patients typically taper use of medications while they gain self-management skills, enhancing their confidence that they can cope with increased activity with less use and without a significant worsening of their symptoms.

The average patient usually presents to an interdisciplinary pain clinic years after being diagnosed with chronic pain. Multiple efforts at managing their pain have been attempted, including medications, surgeries, physical therapy, aquatic therapy, spinal and joint steroid injections, nerve ablation procedures, dorsal column stimulator placement, intrathecal pump placement, chiropractic care, massage therapy, and acupuncture. For many, it is the patient and the referring provider's last effort to improve the patient's quality of life. Understandably, the patient's perception of disability is highly entrenched at this juncture, and represents a formidable challenge when trying to restore the patient to an improved state. Although the question of secondary gain from remaining disabled in a financial-legal setting, such as with workers compensation or personal injury, is important to consider with some patients, most have gradually slid into a level of comfort with their disabilities. This level of comfort may also have been reinforced by well-meaning providers who instruct the patient that they will always be in pain, will always need opioids, or have the back of a 70-year-old (when the patient is decades younger). More concerning is reinforcement of pain behaviors by providers who perform increasingly interventional procedures on patients targeting a pain generator but without having a clear understanding of the multiple contributors to chronic pain, which include distress, somatization, and depressed mood.[9]

Evaluating a new patient for the program involves taking a detailed history of the pain complaints, activity tolerances, prior diagnostic work-up, medication usage, prior treatments, social history, personal and family history of substance use, and psychological history.[3] Patients tend to give a history replete with passive attempts at managing their pain, including surgeries and procedures, but few are able to recount active self-management techniques.

An initial evaluation should include the domains of physical, emotional, cognitive, and behavioral functioning, along with assessing the patient's individual factors, clinical history of treatment, and impact on their daily living and quality of life.

Self-assessment and validated measurement tools are used during evaluations to identify the patients' major concerns and areas of dysfunction in their lives, including life activities such as work, recreation, and abilities for daily living. It also includes evaluating for comorbid conditions of depression, anxiety, posttraumatic stress disorder, and somatoform disorders. A history of prior medication use, including opiates, psychotropic medications, anticonvulsants, nonsteroidal antiinflammatories, muscle relaxants, and sleep medications, is obtained to identify opportunities for reducing polypharmacy, assessing safety, and determining when adjuvant medications may be useful.

Patients who are not appropriate for participation include those unable to learn for cognitive or psychopathologic reasons. Patients who are poorly motivated to participate because of a disability mindset are challenging candidates for such a program, but, if there are no objective physical or psychiatric restrictions inhibiting participation, it is reasonable to offer them the option of treatment, because empiric data indicate that they are usually able to make improvements in physical and emotional functioning.

CBT is used in interdisciplinary pain programs to bring to the forefront the maladaptive cognitions patients hold surrounding their pain, and use behaviors that augment the benefits of physical conditioning. Thoughts secondary to catastrophizing, kinesophobia, and fear of injury are challenged and restructured. Psychologists train patients in the acquisition of skills related to relaxation training and managing activities through pacing. Multiple psychosocial domains of pain respond positively to this mode of therapy, including disability and depression, cognitive coping, interference of pain on function, perceived control of pain, behavioral expression of pain, and social role functioning.[2,7,10] The efficacy of CBT-based treatment within chronic pain programs has been shown in multiple clinical controlled trials.[7,10–13] Compared with usual rehabilitative treatment, the expense of adding CBT is offset by fewer work days lost, and therefore lower indirect costs.[3,14]

PEDIATRIC PAIN MANAGEMENT

The prevalence of chronic pain in children is being increasingly recognized, and interdisciplinary approaches to treatment are being used nationally in tertiary care settings. Epidemiologic studies of chronic pain in children estimate that 30% of children and adolescents experience pain that lasts for longer than 3 months.[15] Generalized musculoskeletal pain, including extremity and back pain, is a common complaint,[15] along with chronic abdominal pain and headaches. With children, the effects are seen with school attendance, social involvement, reduced extracurricular participation and quality of life, and increased use of health care resources. Several academic centers have developed multidisciplinary approaches that coordinate teams of physicians in medicine and psychiatry, psychologists, physical and occupational therapists, nursing, and occasionally alternative medicine providers (eg, acupuncture, massage therapy). A high level of anxiety and depression has been linked with chronic pain and disability in children and adolescents.[16] Patients participating in pain rehabilitation programs instead of standard outpatient treatment had significantly larger improvements in functional disability, pain-related fear, and willingness to adopt a self-management approach to treating pain, with 88% of patients reporting being symptom free after 2 years,[17] likely reflecting greater neuroplasticity in children.

Similar to outpatient adult chronic pain programs, one of the primary obstacles to admission into multidisciplinary pediatric pain rehabilitation programs is insurance approval or reimbursement. Proponents of the approach have argued for the cost-effectiveness of the approach compared with years of medical use and suffering from chronic pain as reasons to allow access, particularly in the United States.[18]

EVIDENCE BASIS OF CARE

A 2014 Cochrane Review on multidisciplinary biopsychosocial rehabilitation for chronic low back pain evaluating 41 randomized controlled trials concluded that patients with chronic low back pain receiving this type of rehabilitation are likely to experience less pain and disability than those receiving usual care (ie, a physical treatment). The

Cochrane Review also concluded that multidisciplinary biopsychosocial rehabilitation had a positive influence on work status compared with physical treatment. There was moderate evidence that multidisciplinary treatment doubled the likelihood that people were able to work in the next 6 to 12 months compared with treatments designed to address physical factors.[18] This finding is similar to other systematic reviews showing that interdisciplinary interventions may have positive effects on work participation outcomes in the long term.[19] Return-to-work rates following a chronic pain program ranged from 29% to 86%, with a mean of 66%, whereas conventional medical treatments yielded lower rates, from 0% to 42% with a mean rate of 27%.[20]

Long-term effectiveness of interdisciplinary pain management programs has been studied and reported in the medical literature. Patients reporting improved outcomes in pain severity, interference of pain, perceived control of pain, treatment helpfulness, and reduced number of hours spent resting was seen at 6-month and 1-year follow-up in a United States–based study.[2] A Danish multidisciplinary pain center in a randomized controlled trial determined that treatment outcomes showed a significant reduction in pain intensity and improved health-related quality of life at 6 months after the program.[21] Chronic back pain has been well studied as one of the leading causes of chronic pain. Pain management programs have been found to be superior to exercise programs in reducing disability, fear-avoidance beliefs, and pain, and in enhancing the quality of life of patients with chronic low back pain. The effects are sustained, because benefits of participation were present at least 1 year after the intervention as well.[1]

Evidence-based clinical practice guidelines by the American Pain Society list the following recommendation for management of chronic low back pain: in patients with non-radicular low back pain who do not respond to usual, noninterdisciplinary interventions, it is recommended that clinicians consider intensive interdisciplinary rehabilitation with a cognitive/behavioral emphasis (strong recommendation, high-quality evidence).[22]

There are few studies evaluating long-term (>10 years) follow-up. A smaller sample (n = 26) evaluated at 13-year follow-up showed maintenance of treatment gains in pain intensity and interference, and mood disturbance.[23] Demonstration of maintained gains is notable given that the primary individual treated in interdisciplinary pain programs had treatment-resistant pain before participation.

Interdisciplinary pain management has also been found to have greater overall effectiveness compared with other common pain management interventions, including medication and CBT.[7,24] Standard medical treatment and less integrated multidisciplinary care were less effective than interdisciplinary pain programs.[7,8,25]

Interdisciplinary treatment programs can also be used for treatment of chronic daily headaches, improving average pain, mood, disability, and quality of life.[26] Other chronic pain disorders reported in the medical literature to response to interdisciplinary management include whiplash and neck pain, fibromyalgia, headaches, and repetitive strain disorders.[20]

Patients with comorbid pain disorders, such as fibromyalgia, as well as occupational musculoskeletal disorders, show benefit for both painful conditions after participating in an exercise and cognitive therapy–based program. One study has shown that 41% of patients no longer met the fibromyalgia diagnosis at discharge.[27]

REDUCING OPIOID DEPENDENCY WITH A PAIN REHABILITATION APPROACH

One of the major criteria for providers to refer patients to the pain management program is lack of effective pain relief despite chronic opioid therapy. The efficacy of chronic opioid therapy for painful conditions, such as back pain, is in dispute.[7,28,29] Opiates have been associated with increased psychological distress and use of health care resources.[7,30] Patients typically undertake opioid reduction or elimination as part of the program. The prevalence of opioid use disorder among patients with chronic pain undergoing chronic opioid therapy is as much as 35%.[31]

For patients on higher doses, usually exceeding morphine equivalent daily dosage of 120 mg/d, inpatient medical detoxification may be used before participation in the program. Patients on lower doses are gradually weaned off during the course of the program. Huffman and colleagues[32] reported that, following participation in a chronic pain rehabilitation program that incorporated opioid tapering, only posttreatment depression increased the probability of resumption of opioid use 12 months later.

The approach taken in an interdisciplinary model is to enhance patients' physical conditioning and cognitive education with information about the risks of chronic opioid therapy, which include opioid-induced hyperalgesia, neuroendocrine effects such as testosterone deficiency, dependence and tolerance, immune effects, risks of sedation, and respiratory depression. Side-effects such as constipation may have led to daily use of laxatives and stool softeners. Weight gain is seen commonly. Chronic use of prescription opioids for pain is increasing in patients with codiagnoses of mental health and substance abuse disorders.[33] Despite opioid tapering, patients typically report the same or improved levels of pain and significantly improved physical function by the end of interdisciplinary pain program treatment.[34] There are direct cost savings and reduced polypharmacy following completion of the pain program. Medication costs following completion of a 3-week intensive program resulted in $2404.80 annual medication savings per patient.[35]

INTERDISCIPLINARY PAIN MANAGEMENT AS AN ALTERNATIVE TO SURGERY FOR LUMBAR DISCOGENIC PAIN

Certain diagnoses and their surgical treatments, such as lumbar fusion for degenerative disc disease, have come under scrutiny for suboptimal outcomes and high disability rates.[7,36] Pursuing the elusive pain generator for surgical correction is problematic when the experience of chronic pain is contributed to by well-recognized biopsychosocial factors and complex interactions with the environment. The patient's psychological history and social circumstances affect and change the contribution of any illness or injury to the pain experience. Identifying that pathways other than surgery, injections, and medications can make substantial improvements to the management of chronic pain has widened the scope of treatment to a team approach. The cost of treatment of spinal disorders in industrialized countries is widely regarded as excessive, particularly for pain disorders and degenerative disc conditions. Lumbar spine fusion procedures have been increasing for occupation-related conditions, and the literature shows debate on the efficacy of fusion procedures for degenerative disc conditions.[37] Data from randomized trials have not shown benefits of spinal fusion compared with intensive interdisciplinary rehabilitation for chronic low back pain without instability or nerve root impingement, as shown in an average of 11 years' follow-up.[38] Lumbar fusions in the workers' compensation setting have low return-to-work rates, ranging from 26% to 36%, reoperation rates of 22% to 27%, and high rates of chronic opioid therapy 2 years after surgery.[37] Interdisciplinary rehabilitation for patients with delayed recovery after spine surgery improved their outcomes, showing a role for continuum of care that includes intensive rehabilitation after surgery. Preventing a prolonged period of disability and postoperative opioid dependence also improved outcomes.[37]

An 8 to 15 years' follow-up study on patients with chronic low back pain who underwent randomization with either spinal fusion or multidisciplinary cognitive-behavior and exercise rehabilitation found no difference in patient self-rated outcomes between surgical and nonoperative treatment. Given the risks of surgery and need for reoperation in a significant number of patients, having access to nonsurgical care should be an option for patients.[38] Significant cost savings are expected in the long term, in addition to minimizing risks of additional surgery.

ECONOMICS OF INTERDISCIPLINARY TREATMENT

The financial benefits of undertaking interdisciplinary rehabilitation are evident in the long-term decrease in the use of medications, unnecessary procedures, diagnostic studies, surgeries, and doctor visits. Although the average monthly cost of treatment was similar in both primary care and pain clinics, the patients undergoing comprehensive treatment had significantly fewer emergency room visits and primary care visits, and less medication use for pain management.[7,39] Patients who received a team-based CBT program took fewer days of sick leave, and the number likely to go on medical leave 1 year after treatment was half that of the comparison treatment group.[7,40]

The primary concern surrounding expanding use of interdisciplinary pain programs has been the high level of staffing and cost of running such programs. Cost savings for persons who had received pain program treatment over the course of their lifetimes for health care and disability costs has been calculated at $356,288 savings each compared with conventional medical therapy.[20] However, the costs of administering the program range from $14,000 to $30,000 for a 3-week to 4-week outpatient program. Hospital-based programs offering inpatient medical detoxification from opioids and benzodiazepines have additional costs depending on length of stay.

SUMMARY

Chronic pain is a complex problem that has been poorly addressed with the present biomedical model for treatment. The costs of health care are increasing, and treating chronic pain with escalating opioid use and aggressive procedures targeting short-term improvement has proved to be ineffective and unsustainable.

The type of treatment that has shown effectiveness and cost-efficacy has been a structured approach to pain management that incorporates the various dimensions and contributors to chronic pain, addressing the physical, psychological, and social dysfunction present with chronic pain syndromes. Using a framework of CBT, physical conditioning, education, and an appropriate framework for medication use, a safe and effective model needs to be available to patients to manage their painful conditions. Interdisciplinary pain programs can fill that role.

Despite the demonstrated utility of pain programs in the last 2 decades, the number of Commission on Accreditation of Rehabilitation Facilities (CARF)-accredited pain clinics has declined from 210 in 1998 to 58 in 2011.[7] Largely because of concerns about up-front costs of the programs, the insurance industry has declined health coverage for interdisciplinary pain treatment. Given its abilities beyond standard medical care to return injured workers with chronic pain to gainful employment, the remaining pain programs are largely serving patients with industrial injuries. There is a mandate for improving the standard of pain care in the United States in the Affordable Care Act, which calls for interdisciplinary specialty centers for pain treatment,[7] and the future may see a call for the growth of such clinics again. There remains a need for knowledge of appropriate management of chronic pain among providers. Public policy and clinical practice require innovative, evidence-based approaches to sustainably support patients with chronic pain needs.

REFERENCES

1. Monticone M, Ferrante S, Rocca B, et al. Effect of a long-lasting multidisciplinary program on disability and fear-avoidance behaviors in patients with chronic low back pain. Clin J Pain 2013;29(11):929–38.
2. Oslund S, Robinson RC, Clark TC, et al. Long-term effectiveness of a comprehensive pain management program: strengthening the case for interdisciplinary care. Proc (Bayl Univ Med Cent) 2009;22(3):211–4.
3. Malaty A, Sabharwal J, Lirette LS, et al. How to assess a new patient for a multidisciplinary chronic pain rehabilitation program: a review article. Ochsner J 2014; 14:96–100.
4. Johannes CB, Le TK, Zhou X, et al. The prevalence of chronic pain in United States adults: results of an Internet-based survey. J Pain 2010;11(11):1230–9.
5. Murphy JL, Clark ME, Banou E. Opioid cessation and multidimensional outcomes after interdisciplinary chronic pain treatment. Clin J Pain 2013;29(2):109–17.
6. Clark ME, Scholten JD, Walker RL, et al. Assessment and treatment of pain associated with combat-related polytrauma. Pain Med 2009;10(3):456–69.
7. Gatchel RJ, McGeary DD, McGeary CA, et al. Interdisciplinary chronic pain management: past, present and future. Am Psychol 2014;69(2):119–30.
8. Guzman J, Esmail R, Karjalainen K, et al. Multidisciplinary rehabilitation for chronic low back pain: systemic review. BMJ 2001;322(23):1511–6.
9. Pincus T, Burton AK, Vogel S, et al. A systematic review of psychological factors as predictors of chronicity/disability in prospective cohorts of low back pain. Spine 2002;27(5):E109–20.
10. Morley S, Williams A, Eccleston C. Examining the evidence about psychological treatments for chronic pain: time for a paradigm shift? Pain 2013;154(10): 1929–31.
11. Molton IR, Graham C, Stoelb BL, et al. Current psychological approaches to the management of chronic pain. Curr Opin Anaesthesiol 2007;20(5):485–9.
12. Turk DC, Swanson KS, Tunks ER. Psychological approaches in the treatment of chronic pain patients–when pills, scalpels, and needles are not enough. Can J Psychiatry 2008;53(4):213–23.
13. McCracken LM, Turk DC. Behavioral and cognitive-behavioral treatment for chronic pain: outcome, predictors of outcome, and treatment process. Spine 2002;27(22):2564–73.
14. Schweikert B, Jacobi E, Seitz R, et al. Effectiveness and cost-effectiveness of adding a cognitive behavioral treatment to the rehabilitation of chronic low back pain. J Rheumatol 2006;33(12):2519–26.
15. King S, Chambers CT, Huguet A, et al. The epidemiology of chronic pain in children and adolescents revisited: a systematic review. Pain 2011;152(12):2729–38.
16. Odell S, Logan DE. Pediatric pain management: the multidisciplinary approach. J Pain Res 2013;6:785–90.
17. Simons LE, Sieberg CB, Pielech M, et al. What does it take? Comparing intensive rehabilitation to outpatient treatment for children with significant pain related disability. J Pediatr Psychol 2013;38(2):213–23.
18. Kamper SJ, Apeldoorn AT, Chiarotto A, et al. Multidisciplinary biopsychosocial rehabilitation for chronic low back pain. Cochrane Database Syst Rev 2014;(9):CD000963.
19. Norlund A, Ropponen A, Alexanderson K. Multidisciplinary intentions: review of studies of return to work after rehabilitation for low back pain. J Rehabil Med 2009;41:115–21.

20. Gatchel RJ, Okifuji A. Evidence-based scientific data documenting the treatment and cost-effectiveness of comprehensive pain programs for chronic nonmalignant pain. J Pain 2007;7(11):779–93.
21. Becker N, Sjogren P, Bech P, et al. Treatment outcome of chronic non-malignant pain patients managed in a Danish multidisciplinary pain center compared to general practice: a randomized controlled trial. Pain 2000;84(2–3):203–11.
22. Chou R, Loeser JD, Owens DK, et al. Interventional therapies, surgery, and interdisciplinary rehabilitation for low back pain: an evidence-based clinical practice guideline from the American pain society. Spine 2009;34(10):1066–77.
23. Patrick LE, Altmaier EM, Found EM. Long-term outcomes in multidisciplinary treatment of chronic low back pain: results of a 13-year followup. Spine 2004; 29(8):850–5.
24. Weiner SS, Nordin M. Prevention and management of chronic back pain. Best Pract Res Clin Rheumatol 2010;24(2):267–79.
25. Scascighini L, Toma V, Dober-Spielmann S, et al. Multidisciplinary treatment for chronic pain: a systematic review of interventions and outcomes. Rheumatology (Oxford) 2008;47(5):670–8.
26. Barton PM, Schultz GR, Jarrell JF, et al. A flexible format interdisciplinary treatment and rehabilitation program for chronic daily headache: patient clinical features resource utilization and outcomes. Headache 2014;54(8):1320–36.
27. Hartzell MM, Neblett R, Perez Y, et al. Do comorbid fibromyalgia diagnoses change after a functional restoration program in patients with chronic disabling occupational musculoskeletal disorders? Spine 2014;39(17):1393–400.
28. Von Korff M, Kolodny A, Deyo RA, et al. Long-term opioid therapy reconsidered. Ann Intern Med 2011;155:325–8.
29. Chou R. Steering patients to relief from chronic low back pain: Opioids' role. J Fam Pract 2013;62(3 Suppl):S8–13.
30. Deyo RA, Smith DH, Johnson ES, et al. Opioids for back pain patients: primary care prescribing patterns and use of services. J Am Board Fam Med 2011; 24(6):717–27.
31. Boscarino JA, Rukstalis MR, Hoffman SN, et al. Prevalence of prescription opioid use disorder among chronic pain patients: comparison of the DSM-5 vs DSM-4 diagnostic criteria. J Addict Dis 2011;30(3):185–94.
32. Huffman KL, Sweis GW, Gase A, et al. Opioid use 12 months following interdisciplinary pain rehabilitation with weaning. Pain Med 2013;14(12):1908–17.
33. Edlund MJ, Martin BC, Devries A, et al. Trends in use of opioids for chronic noncancer pain among individuals with mental health and substance use disorders: the TROUP study. Clin J Pain 2010;26(1):1–8.
34. Townsend CO, Kerkvliet JL, Bruce BK, et al. A longitudinal study of the efficacy of a comprehensive pain rehabilitation program with opioid withdrawal: Comparison of treatment outcomes based on opioid use status at admission. Pain 2008; 140(1):177–89.
35. Cunningham JL, Rome JD, Kerkvliet JL, et al. Reduction in medication costs for patients with chronic nonmalignant pain completing a pain rehabilitation program: a prospective analysis of admission, discharge, and 6 month follow-up medication costs. Pain Med 2009;10(5):787–96.
36. Tarnanen S, Neva MH, Dekker J, et al. Randomized controlled trial of postoperative exercise rehabilitation program after lumbar spine fusion: Study protocol. BMC Musculoskelet Disord 2012;13:123.
37. Mayer TG, Gatchel RJ, Brede E, et al. Lumbar surgery in work-related chronic low back pain: can a continuum of care enhance outcomes? Spine J 2014;14(2):263–73.

38. Mannion AF, Brox JI, Fairbank JC. Comparison of spinal fusion and nonoperative treatment in patients with chronic low back pain: long-term follow-up of three randomized controlled trials. Spine J 2013;13(11):1438–48.
39. Rodriguez MJ, Garcia AJ. A registry of the aetiology and costs of neuropathic pain in pain clinics: results of the registry of aetiologies and costs (REC) in neuropathic pain disorders study. Clin Drug Investig 2007;27(11):771–82.
40. Ektor-Andersen J, Ingvarsson E, Kullendorff M, et al. High cost-benefit of early team-based biomedical and cognitive-behaviour intervention for long-term pain-related sickness absence. J Rehabil Med 2008;40(1):1–8.

Chronic Whiplash Pain

Richard Seroussi, MD, MSc (Engin)[a,b,*], Virtaj Singh, MD[a,b],
Adrielle Fry, MD[a]

KEYWORDS

- Chronic pain • Whiplash • Review • Musculoskeletal • Neurologic • Physiatry

KEY POINTS

- Physiatrists are ideally suited to diagnose and treat whiplash injuries, provided they appreciate the sources of chronic pain for this patient population.
- Although most medical providers take the view that whiplash is a self-limited neck sprain/strain, peer-reviewed literature over the past 20 years gives more accurate data regarding why 20% to 30% of patients transition to chronic whiplash syndrome.
- Researchers have implicated the cervical facet joint as a primary pain generator in chronic whiplash. However, they continue to examine other anatomic causes, including the cervical intervertebral disc, spinal ligaments, temporomandibular joint, and paraspinal muscles, to improve clinical management of whiplash injuries.

INTRODUCTION

Whiplash injuries are common sources of chronic pain diagnosed and treated within a physiatry practice. These injuries are caused by sudden acceleration-deceleration events to the human body, most often caused by rear-end motor vehicle accidents but also by other types of collisions, slip and fall events, and sports-related injuries. An epidemiologic study in the United States in 2000 estimated that 901,442 emergency department visits in that year were for neck sprain/strain.[1] In addition, about 28% of motor vehicle accident emergency department visits had neck sprain/strain as the predominant injury.[1]

Following whiplash injuries, patients may have a variety of symptoms collectively known as whiplash-associated disorders (WADs).[2,3] For many patients, symptoms resolve from within a few days up to 3 months. However, more than a third of patients who have a whiplash-type injury develop chronic pain, which is pain lasting for longer than 3 to 6 months.[4–7] Radanov and colleagues[6] published a study based on a cohort of 117 patients with WAD whom they followed from approximately 7 days after the

[a] Department of Rehabilitation Medicine, University of Washington, 1959 Northeast Pacific Street, Box 356490, Seattle, WA 98195, USA; [b] Seattle Spine & Sports Medicine, 3213 Eastlake Avenue East, Suite A, Seattle, WA 98102, USA
* Corresponding author.
E-mail address: res@seattlespine.com

Phys Med Rehabil Clin N Am 26 (2015) 359–373
http://dx.doi.org/10.1016/j.pmr.2015.01.003
1047-9651/15/$ – see front matter © 2015 Elsevier Inc. All rights reserved.

injury until 2 years after initial injury. As shown in **Fig. 1**, this analysis found that 44% of patients remained symptomatic at 3 months, 30% remained symptomatic at 6 months, 24% remained symptomatic at 1 year, and 18% remained symptomatic 2 years after the whiplash-type injury. These percentages are conservative estimates of the long-term morbidity after WAD compared with other studies.

As another example, a British study dating back to the 1980s found that more than 40% of patients were symptomatic from whiplash injuries 2 years after the date of injury. This same cohort was tracked for several years and found to have, on balance, permanent injuries.[4,5,8] In our clinical practices, we find this 2-year mark to be a fairly accurate average time interval for patients with WAD to reach maximum medical improvement, among those who have not recovered from their injuries.

Given the prevalence of whiplash injuries and their impact on patient function, this topic warrants the attention of both specialist and primary care providers who treat patients with whiplash. This article describes the current understanding of the pain mechanisms behind common whiplash symptoms, including neck pain, headaches, back pain, upper extremity symptoms, jaw pain, and widespread pain or central sensitization. Effective treatment of these injuries is a large subject, beyond the scope of this article, which limits the focus to pain mechanisms associated with whiplash.

Although whiplash is commonly associated with neck pain, the second or third most common chronic injury among patients with WAD is lower back pain,[3,7–11] which is sometimes called lumbar whiplash. Despite the major incidence of lumbar whiplash, this article focuses on neck and upper body symptoms and does not emphasize lower back injuries, which have received only passing epidemiologic interest without extensive research regarding the clinical biomechanics or the pathophysiology of injury.

On a final introductory note, many medical providers, including most primary care providers and surgical specialists, mistakenly assume that patients with WAD have simple neck sprains/strains and that these injuries always heal within 3 months. This

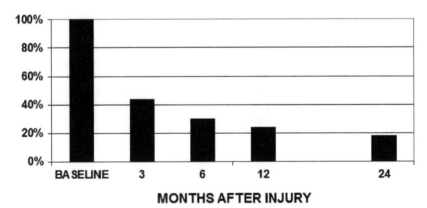

PERCENTAGE OF PATIENTS WITH ONGOING SYMPTOMS AFTER WHIPLASH INJURY

MONTHS AFTER INJURY

Fig. 1. Time course of recovery for patients with acute whiplash over 2 years, based on the prospective study by Radanov and colleagues.[6] (*Data from* Radanov BP, Sturzenegger M, Di Stefano G. Long-term outcome after whiplash injury. A 2-year follow-up considering features of injury mechanism and somatic, radiologic, and psychosocial findings. Medicine (Baltimore) 1995;74:281–97.)

assumption contrasts with research that has been done over the past 20 years examining WAD sources of pain, including the cervical facet (zygapophyseal) joints, cervical discs, paracervical muscles, and cervical spinal ligaments. Biomechanical and clinical researchers have identified specific structures—most notably the cervical facet joints—as sources of chronic neck pain after whiplash injuries, often in the setting of normal or ambiguous MRI scans.[12–14]

Thus there is a large gap between the common clinical understanding of whiplash and the more accurate and specialized research dedicated to this disorder. Physiatrists are often called on to fill this gap between a cursory understanding of whiplash among other health care providers and cutting edge concepts from the pain literature.

CERVICOTHORACIC PAIN AND POSTTRAUMATIC HEADACHE

The most common complaint following a whiplash-type injury is neck pain. Patients often present with nonradicular neck pain and stiffness, which on careful physical examination is documented as decreased and painful cervical range of motion as well as paracervical tenderness to palpation.[15] Loss of range of motion is commonly thought to be caused by muscle guarding. However, patients with chronic WAD generally have decreased cervical range of motion,[15–18] well beyond the expected time for muscle injury recovery, and there are likely other factors involved—including injury to the cervical facet joints, cervical intervertebral discs, and central (nervous system) amplification of pain—that contribute to chronic neck stiffness in this population.

Associated Thoracic Pain and Posttraumatic Headache

Neck pain from WAD is often accompanied by mid to upper thoracic pain and/or posttraumatic headache. Although it is probable that the thoracic region can undergo primary joint and muscle injury, this pain source has not received much attention in the WAD literature. By contrast, it is well established that lower cervical facet joint or discogenic injury cause pain referral patterns into the thoracic region (eg, Refs.[19–21]). Based on our clinical experiences and the current literature, a great portion of mid to upper thoracic pain among patients with WAD likely represents referred pain from the neck area.

Posttraumatic headache is often experienced in the occipital region with frontal and retro-orbital radiation. This headache usually arises from injury to the upper cervical facet joints, with the C2-3 facet joint in particular as a likely cause.[19,22] However, astute clinicians should remember that there can be other causes for chronic posttraumatic headache in this population, including (but not limited to):

1. Postconcussive headache, which often has migrainous features
2. Headache associated with posttraumatic temporomandibular joint (TMJ) disorder
3. Headache caused by injury of structures above the C2-3 facet joint, including the atlantoaxial (C1-2) joint and the greater or lesser occipital nerves
4. Headache caused by internal disruption of the cervical intervertebral discs, most notably at the C2-3 level
5. Headache associated with thoracic outlet syndrome (TOS), possibly caused by vertebral attachments of hypertonic scalene muscles causing abnormal forces on the facet joints

This article discusses thoracic pain and headache within the broad category of neck pain but these other potential sources should be kept within the differential diagnosis, especially among patients recalcitrant to treatment. One author (RS) in particular repeatedly humbled to finds that his patients with whiplash have headache resolution with treatment of posttraumatic TOS or TMJ disorder. Regarding postconcussive syndrome, clinicians who have a core practice treating whiplash understand that some patients have varying degrees of concomitant concussion. This subject is not covered here, but it should be considered within the differential diagnosis for posttraumatic headache.

Facet Injury

According to peer-reviewed research, the main cause of neck pain and headache among patients with chronic motor vehicle crash–related injuries is injury to the cervical facet joint.[12,13,19,22–27] As an example of this literature, a strict double-blinded, randomized controlled trial using diagnostic cervical spinal injections (so-called medial branch blocks) was published in 1996. The investigators reported that 60% of chronic nonradicular neck pain after motor vehicle crash–related injuries was caused by cervical facet joint injury, most commonly the C2-C3 facet joint level but also throughout other levels of the cervical spine.[19] Biomechanical and postmortem (ie, cadaveric) studies also clearly document facet injuries after simulated or actual motor vehicle crash exposure (eg, Refs.[14,28–33]).

The biomechanical basis for facet joint injury began to emerge about 20 years ago in experiments that used high-speed digital image processing to detail the kinematics, or observed motion, of simulated rear-impact collisions. Using cadaveric cervical specimens subjected to laboratory motor vehicle crashes, researchers found a so-called S-shaped curve in response to rear impact for the human neck in the sagittal plane. This S-shaped curve is illustrated in **Fig. 2**, which is derived from one of the first landmark studies by Grauer and colleagues[34] in 1997.

Fig. 2 shows that, within a fraction of a second after rear impact, the upper part of the neck goes into flexion and retraction; the chin goes toward the chest and the occiput moves posteriorly with respect to the trunk. This movement creates an S shape to the neck when viewed in the sagittal plane. This finding challenged a conventional view that the neck moved into a uniform hyperextension after rear impact. Multiple investigators since this early study have verified the presence of

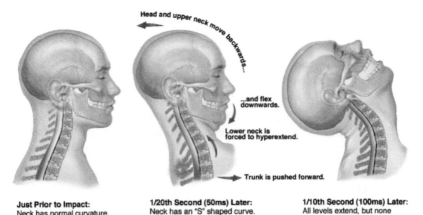

Just Prior to Impact:	1/20th Second (50ms) Later:	1/10th Second (100ms) Later:
Neck has normal curvature.	Neck has an "S" shaped curve. Lower neck with possible facet injury.	All levels extend, but none excessively. Likely after the moment of injury.

Fig. 2. The S-shaped curve of the cervical spine in response to rear-impact collision, derived from the work of Grauer and colleagues,[34] as well as the work of other investigators. (*Courtesy of* Nucleus Medical Media, Kennesaw, GA; with permission. Images © 2002 Nucleus Communications. Available at: www.nucleusinc.com.)

the S-shaped curve, using postmortem biomechanical data as well as limited in vivo data with human volunteers.[30,31,35–38] This response to rear impact is thought to put both abnormal compressive and tensile forces on the facet joints, providing a biomechanical basis for what is observed clinically as facet joint injury (eg, Refs.[29,30,32,38]).

There are even animal models for WAD facet joint injury.[39–43] One animal model using rats has documented that carefully controlled distention of the facet joint causes central nervous system (CNS), or centrally mediated, increases in pain, consistent with clinical findings and other research discussed later.[43]

Disc Injury

A less common source of neck pain and cervicogenic headache seen in our clinical practices and documented in the WAD literature is internal disruption to the intervertebral disc.[33,37,44–47] Most patients with cervical discogenic pain do not present with radiculopathy but with axial pain and pain referral patterns either above the neck as headache or below the neck as upper back pain. Patients rarely present with radiculopathy, but much more frequently cervicobrachial symptoms are caused by TOS or other factors, as discussed later.

The scope of research to support cervical discogenic pain, in contrast with facet injury, is limited, as noted in reviews on anatomic pain generators for WAD.[12,14] One reason for this decreased evidence is the inability to use noninvasive imaging or diagnostic spinal injections to provide anesthetic blockade of cervical intervertebral discs. Schellhas and colleagues[21] in 1996 carefully correlated cervical discography with cervical MRI for patients with axial neck pain versus a control group and showed that most discogenic findings on MRI are not predictive of the cause of the pain. In the absence of cervical radiculopathy, fracture, or spinal cord injury, MRI is generally neither sensitive nor specific for pinpointing the source of pain after cervical trauma.

In a 1993 landmark postmortem study titled "Acute Injuries to Cervical Joints. An Autopsy Study of Neck Sprain," Taylor and Twomey[44] demonstrated contained disc protrusions and so-called rim lesions among patients who died in motor vehicle crashes of traumatic brain injuries but who had normal neck radiographs at the time of autopsy. One key feature of their study was to provide cadaveric specimens from a control group who died of nontraumatic causes, with the study pathologists blinded to the cause of death. Rim lesions were uniquely posttraumatic findings involving a hemorrhagic tear of the disc annulus from the adjacent vertebral endplate, likely caused by excessive tensile forces, which is thought to be one basis of discogenic injury from WAD. **Fig. 3** shows the findings from this study. On a separate continent, Jonsson and colleagues[46] published a similar study, without a control group and with more emphasis on findings at the facet joints and at the craniocervical junction.

These and other studies with cadaveric histology also help show the inadequacy of current imaging technologies (including MRI and computed tomography) for detecting these pathoanatomic lesions.[33,35,48–52]

Other Sources of Cervicothoracic Pain

Cervicothoracic pain after whiplash is also hypothesized to come from primary muscle injury, spinal ligamentous injuries, and centrally mediated pain. A brief note is given to injury to the dorsal root ganglion, given an intriguing pig model that showed pressure gradients within the cervical spinal canal that might cause tissue damage at the level of the dorsal root ganglia during a simulated whiplash event.[53] This pressure gradient decreased with the use of a head restraint mechanism in pigs, consistent with effective whiplash prevention.[53] Centrally mediated pain is discussed later. All of this research

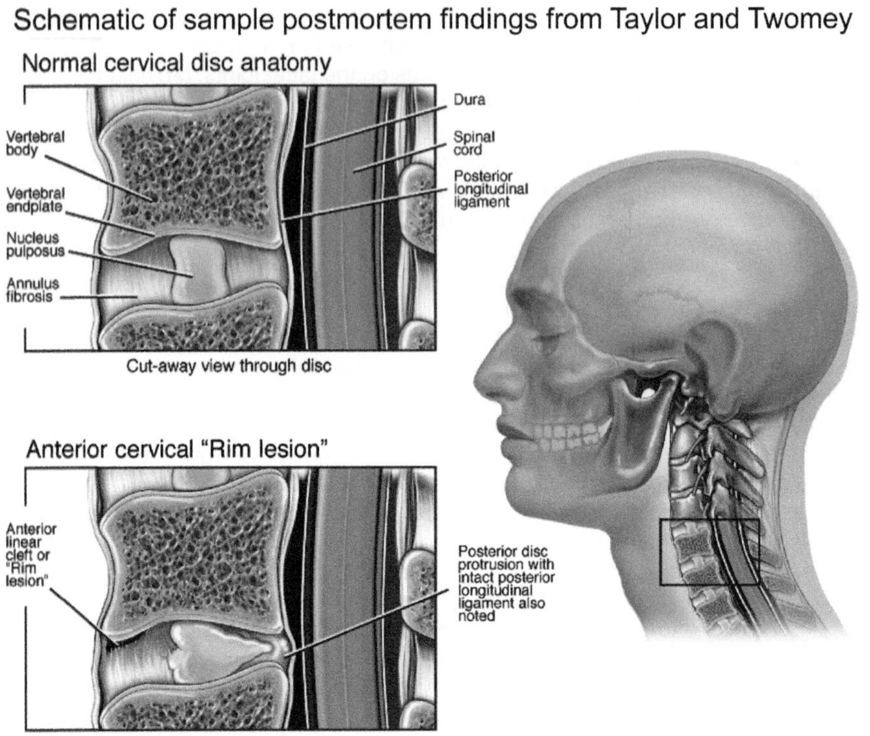

Schematic of sample postmortem findings from Taylor and Twomey

Normal cervical disc anatomy

Fig. 3. Sample postmortem findings from Taylor and Twomey,[44] documenting anterior cervical rim lesions and contained disc protrusions as posttraumatic findings. (*Courtesy of Nucleus Medical Media, Kennesaw, GA; with permission.*)

is still in progress, and throughout readers are referred to a few recent reviews regarding anatomic pain generators in the setting of chronic whiplash injury.[12,14]

Although muscle injury is not thought to be a source of chronic pain among patients with whiplash, it may indirectly influence chronic pain patterns through a variety of mechanisms, including the direct pull of muscle attachments on the facet joint capsule, chronic muscle atrophy after whiplash causing decreased neck strength and function, alterations in proprioception caused by muscle spindle injury, and other sources of aberrant neuromuscular control. Muscle injury is hypothesized to stem from the abrupt lengthening that occurs during the rapid movement of the head and neck despite reflex or active paracervical muscle activation.[12,14]

As treatment providers who recognize that published research does not always reflect practice in the clinic setting, we have assisted several patients with whiplash at a plateau in their recovery by applying trigger point needling to paraspinal and periscapular muscles. However, patients with years of injury generally do not respond to this type of muscle-focused therapy. In addition, we have developed an increased respect for the role of muscle with chronic injury, given our experience with TOS, as discussed later.

Another postulated mechanism of neck pain after whiplash injury is damage to cervical spinous ligamentous structures, as discussed in several recent reviews and sample postmortem and animal studies.[12,14,28,33,54,55] A 2001 cadaveric study by Yoganandan and colleagues[33] documented injuries to the ligamenta flava and anterior longitudinal ligaments, in addition to injury to the facet joints and cervical disc annuli for whole human cadavers subjected to laboratory rear-impact collisions. The postmortem study by Jonsson and colleagues[46] in 1991 (mentioned earlier) documented extensive spinal ligamentous injuries, in addition to facet joint and intradiscal injuries.

CERVICOBRACHIAL PAIN AND NEUROLOGIC SYNDROMES

Patients with WAD often have symptoms radiating from the cervicothoracic area into 1 or both shoulders and at times into the upper extremities. For most patients, if symptoms radiate below the level of the elbow, there are associated neurologic signs and symptoms into the forearm, wrist, and hand. As discussed earlier, cervical radiculopathy should be in the differential diagnosis, although in practice it is rare compared with other cervicobrachial syndromes. Cervical myelopathy is extremely rare, often associated with a history of transient quadriparesis and long tract signs and symptoms. Nonetheless, myelopathy should be kept within the distant differential diagnosis and should not be missed.

By contrast, posttraumatic TOS is common in the setting of whiplash. Posttraumatic shoulder injury and upper extremity peripheral nerve injury, most commonly involving the median nerve at the wrist, a form of posttraumatic carpal tunnel syndrome, also occur among patients with WAD and may coexist with or mimic TOS. These syndromes are discussed here.

Thoracic Outlet Syndrome

TOS is most commonly caused by compression of the lower trunk of the brachial plexus within the scalene muscles. This compression is hypothesized to result from eccentric injury to the scalene muscles following whiplash injuries. The TOS diagnosis is often missed because it is not detected by advanced imaging or electrodiagnostic testing.[56–58] Instead, the diagnosis is made clinically, specifically by a history of patient intolerance to overhead and reaching activities, which cause tingling, heaviness, and pain into the affected upper extremity, with dysesthesias most often in an ulnar distribution. Physical examination reveals tenderness of the scalene muscles and less commonly along more distal sites of the brachial plexus. Neurologic examination often detects subtle weakness of the intrinsic muscles, consistent with dysfunction of the lower trunk of the brachial plexus.

Further detailed diagnostic work-up for TOS is beyond the scope of this article. However, rather than relying on imaging such as brachial plexus MRI or electrodiagnostic studies, searching for the extremely rare variant of neurogenic TOS showing intrinsic muscle motor axon loss, practitioners are encouraged to make the diagnosis clinically and to confirm their diagnostic suspicions with the use of the scalene motor block, which is an anesthetic blockade of the scalene muscle, most often done with ultrasonography and/or electromyographic guidance. The muscle is injected with local anesthetic and the practitioner gauges the patient's response with a symptom diary, similar to medial branch diagnostic blocks performed for the work-up of facet joint injury. This temporary muscle paralysis presumably alleviates TOS symptoms by decreasing pressure on the adjacent brachial plexus.

Detailed discussion of the treatment of TOS is outside the scope of this article but, as with other protocols, time to heal; noninvasive manual therapy such as chiropractic, massage, or physical therapy; restorative sleep; and accommodation to injury should be the mainstays of early treatment. More advanced treatments include muscle trigger point therapy, muscle chemodenervation of the scalene muscles, and surgical consultation for recalcitrant TOS. Practitioners should remember that numerous patients with acute whiplash injuries present with milder forms of TOS, but improve or resolve their upper extremity symptoms over weeks or months, without the need for diagnostic intervention.

A final note about TOS and whiplash injury: TOS gets scant attention in the research literature as an established cause of pain for patients with whiplash. However, the senior authors in this review (RS and VS) treat whiplash-associated TOS as core parts of their clinical practice. Our observations over the years have included:

1. For affected patients, the correct diagnosis and treatment are especially gratifying because they have often progressed from one practitioner to the next without an understanding of their symptoms. It is common for patients to have years between symptom onset and the TOS diagnosis in our clinical practices.
2. Women are much more affected than men, and astute practitioners document tenderness in the scalene muscle area among female patients far in excess of what is observed among male patients. This finding may have to do with the increased vulnerability of women to muscle injury and cervical retraction from whiplash,[32,59–61] although to our knowledge this has not been specifically studied for the scalene muscles.
3. Patients with hypermobility (most often female patients) seem more vulnerable to TOS and other more serious presentations of whiplash injury.
4. Without support from formal research, we believe that a greater proportion of patients with whiplash with TOS have left-sided findings, which we presume to be related to increased tethering of the left upper torso caused by the shoulder restraint for motor vehicle drivers.
5. The mechanism of TOS, which is thought to involve an initial eccentric injury to the scalene muscle followed by fibrotic changes and type II muscle atrophy,[58] challenges our assumption that muscle injury rarely causes major long-term functional loss. Given their ability to compress the brachial plexus, the scalene muscles are well selected to cause a syndrome with potentially severe and chronic consequences.

Shoulder Injury

Primary shoulder injury is less common after whiplash, compared with referred pain from the cervicothoracic region and TOS as causes of shoulder pain. Nonetheless, intrinsic shoulder injury should be part of the differential diagnosis for patients with whiplash. There is again scant literature regarding primary shoulder injury after whiplash (eg, Refs.[62–64]). In our clinical experience, patients often have an outstretched shoulder as part of the mechanism of injury or direct blunt trauma to the left shoulder against the car door for drivers involved in left-sided frontal or broadside collisions.

Shoulder injury is included in this article to remind readers that a careful examination of the shoulder needs to be done as part of any comprehensive assessment, and shoulder pain should be kept within the differential diagnosis for patients presenting with cervicobrachial symptoms. Patients can develop posttraumatic shoulder impingement syndromes with an associated bursitis, as well as labral tears of the glenohumeral joint. The risk of intrinsic shoulder injury is likely correlated with increased levels of shoulder abduction or forward flexion and with a stiffer closed kinetic chain between the torso, shoulder, and steering wheel at the time of impact.

In practice, intrinsic shoulder injury combined with upper extremity peripheral nerve injury can mimic TOS. Secondary shoulder problems can also occur among patients with decreased chronic mobility or usage of their shoulders, leading to varying degrees of adhesive capsulitis, scapular dysfunction including weakness of the scapular muscles, and secondary subacromial impingement from the poor posture associated with cervicothoracic trauma. When patients have intrinsic shoulder injury from whiplash, history and physical examination are the mainstays for forming a cogent differential diagnosis. Diagnostic shoulder injections and advanced imaging, such as magnetic resonance arthrogram, help confirm the diagnosis and allow a more detailed treatment plan for patients with recalcitrant injuries.

Posttraumatic Peripheral Nerve and Other Upper Extremity Injuries

Peripheral nerve entrapment should be considered when patients with whiplash present with upper extremity dysesthesias.[65] The focus here is mainly on posttraumatic carpal tunnel syndrome (CTS), but other potential peripheral nerve injuries are discusses. Posttraumatic CTS has been documented in only a few studies.[65,66] It is noted more frequently to occur to the driver as opposed to other passengers in the vehicle, presumably because of a close kinetic chain between the steering wheel, the upper extremity, and the upper torso at the time of impact. Note that Alpar and colleagues[67] in 2002 proposed carpal tunnel decompression for patients with whiplash with electrodiagnostically negative atypical CTS. However, to our knowledge, this has not been studied by other groups.

The proposed mechanisms for injury to the median nerve are blunt trauma of the palmar aspect of the wrist on the steering wheel with direct nerve compression or stretch from forced extension or flexion of the wrist, or a combination of these mechanisms.[65,66] In reality, this process may be more complex, because a single neuron spans from the cervical nerve root across the wrist: at the moment of rear impact, it may dramatically lengthen, given the fixed position of the steering wheel compared with the neck and torso, which recede into the car seat.

Greening and colleagues[68] used high-frequency ultrasonography to document an approximate 70% decrease in longitudinal median nerve movement, measured at the forearm, during a deep inspiration maneuver for patients with whiplash versus a control group. They also documented signs of neural mechanosensitivity for these patients, referring to increased pain with nerve trunk stretching and brachial plexus pressure maneuvers compared with controls. This finding may suggest a mechanism of double crush between TOS and posttraumatic CTS, an observation we have made in our clinical practices. For example, we use a brachial plexus stretch test, as described by Sanders and colleagues,[58] to help document the clinical presence of TOS, recognizing that this also causes increased pressure on the median nerve within the carpal tunnel.

A few retrospective studies establish a probable causal relationship between CTS and prior motor vehicle trauma, although these studies are not able to predict the incidence of this peripheral nerve injury.[65,66] Timing of onset of symptoms after the accident was addressed in 2 studies. The study by Coert and Dellon[65] found that 43 out of 44 cases of CTS had onset of symptoms in the first 6 months, with most patients experiencing symptoms in less than 1 month after the collision. A study by Ames[66] showed that all CTS cases had onset of symptoms within 2 months of impact.

The Coert and Dellon[65] study also retrospectively studied the incidence of ulnar neuropathy at the elbow and radial sensory neuropathy after a motor vehicle collision[65] and found ulnar neuropathy at the elbow to be common. However, this was not reported in the study by Ames[66] and has not been observed in our own clinical practices, where motor vehicle crash–related ulnar nerve injury has been rare. We also note that patients who are predisposed to developing CTS, such as those in the building trades or diabetics, seem to be at increased risk for developing posttraumatic CTS, even in the absence of preexisting symptoms. This observation suggests that there may be less of a safety factor with respect to injury threshold for blunt trauma at the wrist.

JAW PAIN

Another source of pain following whiplash injury is jaw pain. Although this complaint is typically evaluated and treated by dentists, it is important for physicians to recognize this symptom following whiplash injuries. Most postwhiplash jaw pain is caused by injury to the TMJ, which has been called temporomandibular disorder (TMD). A study of 400 patients with TMD showed that approximately 25% of those subjects had onset of pain and dysfunction after trauma, which was mainly a whiplash injury.[69]

A 2004 Swedish study showed that TMD had a higher occurrence in those patients with chronic WAD as opposed to matched controls, with similar findings reported elsewhere[70,71] and supported by a recent meta-analysis.[72] The exact mechanism of injury to the TMJ is not known but it is suspected that the rapid extension and flexion of the head combined with the inertia of the jaw causes the mandibular condyles to subluxate, resulting in disc displacement and sprain of the capsular ligaments of the TMJ. Patients present clinically with clicking of the jaw and jaw pain, most notably with chewing activities. As noted earlier, patients can develop posttraumatic headache associated with TMD,[72–74] which is often more treatable than that from upper cervical facet joint injury. In addition, some patients with TMD present with other neuromuscular abnormalities, including posttraumatic tinnitus and balance deficits.[75,76]

CENTRALLY MEDIATED PAIN

Researchers and clinicians have identified the presence of centrally mediated pain or CNS sensitization among patients with chronic WAD. Caused by CNS factors, this condition refers to a sensory hypersensitivity throughout the body to potentially noxious stimuli, such as deep pressure applied to muscles distant from the patient's region of pain. Among patients who develop chronic pain after acute tissue injury, it may be experienced clinically as a gain in both the spatial distribution and intensity of regional pain.

Koelbaek Johansen and colleagues[77] first established the presence of centrally mediated pain in the setting of chronic whiplash with an elegant experiment published in 1999. The researchers compared the pain response of 11 patients with chronic whiplash with a pain-free control group for 4 potentially noxious stimuli. Each stimulus was applied to 3 areas of the body: (1) the infraspinatus muscle (a painful region for all of these patients), (2) the brachioradialis muscle (painful for some patients), and (3) the tibialis anterior muscle area (not identified as painful for these patients). The potentially noxious stimuli were (1) light touch, (2) pinprick, (3) algometry (quantifiable blunt pressure to the skin), and (4) hypertonic computer-controlled intramuscular saline injection, a known noxious stimulus based on other research (saline injection was not applied to the brachioradialis). This comparison is shown in **Fig. 4**.

The patients with chronic WAD showed marked hyperalgesia for the tibialis anterior muscle compared with controls, despite their absence of lower extremity symptoms. The theoretic implication was that patients with chronic whiplash have CNS sensitization, or what is also called centrally mediated pain; patients with chronic WAD have amplification in their pain response at the CNS level, and do not simply have muscle strains, ligament sprains, or even local joint injuries to

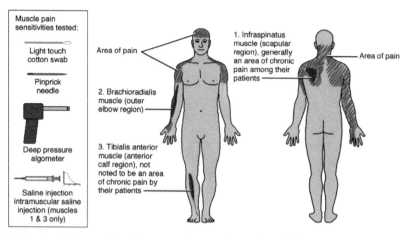

Fig. 4. The shaded areas show the approximate pain regions of the patients with whiplash. Note that patients did not identify tibialis anterior as painful, although this muscle showed marked hyperalgesia for deep pressure algometry and the hypertonic saline injection for patients with WAD versus controls. The muscles tested by Koelbaek Johansen and colleagues[77] are also shown. (*Data from* Koelbaek Johansen M, Graven-Nielsen T, Schou Olesen A, et al. Generalised muscular hyperalgesia in chronic whiplash syndrome. Pain 1999;83:229–34; and *Courtesy of* Nucleus Medical Media, Kennesaw, GA; with permission. Images © 2002 Nucleus Communications. Available at: www.nucleusinc.com.)

explain their overall clinical picture. This phenomenon has been verified repeatedly and continues to be extensively studied among patients who do not recover from whiplash injuries.[12,15,77–84]

A series of Australian studies by Sterling and colleagues[82] extensively assessed CNS sensitization among patients with whiplash, and found signs of mechanical hyperalgesia at the tibialis anterior region within 1 month after patients sustained whiplash injury, compared with a control group. Those who recovered within 2 months after injury had resolved this hyperalgesia and those who failed to recover continued to have this sign of centrally mediated pain. In addition, signs of psychological distress remained associated with lack of recovery and presumably with ongoing hyperalgesia among these patients.[80]

A key question that pain researchers are trying to answer is whether focal nociception, such as injury to a facet joint, leads to the state of CNS sensitization, and whether CNS sensitization resolves with adequate analgesia of the painful facet joint. This possibility seems intuitive, but the basic mechanisms of how this might or might not evolve is an active subject of ongoing research,[79,84] including with an animal model for facet joint injury.[43,85]

Centrally mediated pain, or CNS sensitization, is discussed elsewhere in this issue by Dr Michele Curatolo, a world-renowned expert on this research, and readers are referred to that article for a more detailed discussion of this evolving subject. Suffice to say that, for chronic whiplash, centrally mediated pain is a major factor contributing to pain severity and functional loss.

REFERENCES

1. Quinlan KP, Annest JL, Myers B, et al. Neck strains and sprains among motor vehicle occupants-United States, 2000. Accid Anal Prev 2004;36:21–7.

2. Spitzer WO, Skovron ML, Salmi LR, et al. Scientific monograph of the Quebec Task Force on Whiplash-Associated Disorders: redefining "whiplash" and its management [see comments]. Spine (Phila Pa 1976) 1995;20:1S–73S.

3. Berglund A, Alfredsson L, Jensen I, et al. The association between exposure to a rear-end collision and future health complaints. J Clin Epidemiol 2001;54:851–6.

4. Norris SH, Watt I. The prognosis of neck injuries resulting from rear-end vehicle collisions. J Bone Joint Surg Br 1983;65:608–11.

5. Gargan MF, Bannister GC. Long-term prognosis of soft-tissue injuries of the neck. J Bone Joint Surg Br 1990;72:901–3.

6. Radanov BP, Sturzenegger M, Di Stefano G. Long-term outcome after whiplash injury. A 2-year follow-up considering features of injury mechanism and somatic, radiologic, and psychosocial findings. Medicine (Baltimore) 1995;74:281–97.

7. Bannister G, Amirfeyz R, Kelley S, et al. Whiplash injury. J Bone Joint Surg Br 2009;91:845–50.

8. Squires B, Gargan MF, Bannister GC. Soft-tissue injuries of the cervical spine. 15-year follow-up. J Bone Joint Surg Br 1996;78:955–7.

9. Fast A, Sosner J, Begeman P, et al. Lumbar spinal strains associated with whiplash injury: a cadaveric study. Am J Phys Med Rehabil 2002;81:645–50.

10. Seroussi R. Lumbar whiplash. In: Cole AJ, Herring SA, editors. The low back pain handbook: a practical guide for the primary care clinician. 2nd edition. Philadelphia: Hanley & Belfus; 2003. p. 475–83.

11. DePalma M, Ketchum J, Saullo T, et al. Structural etiology of chronic low back pain due to motor vehicle collision. Pain Med 2011;12:1622–7.

12. Curatolo M, Bogduk N, Ivancic PC, et al. The role of tissue damage in whiplash associated disorders: discussion paper 1. Spine (Phila Pa 1976) 2011;36:S309–15.

13. Gellhorn AC. Cervical facet-mediated pain. Phys Med Rehabil Clin North Am 2011;22:447–58, viii.

14. Siegmund GP, Winkelstein BA, Ivancic PC, et al. The anatomy and biomechanics of acute and chronic whiplash injury. Traffic Inj Prev 2009;10:101–12.

15. Sterling M, Jull G, Vicenzino B, et al. Characterization of acute whiplash-associated disorders. Spine (Phila Pa 1976) 2004;29:182–8.

16. Dall'Alba PT, Sterling MM, Treleaven JM, et al. Cervical range of motion discriminates between asymptomatic persons and those with whiplash. Spine (Phila Pa 1976) 2001;26:2090–4.

17. Rosenfeld M, Seferiadis A, Carlsson J, et al. Active intervention in patients with whiplash-associated disorders improves long-term prognosis: a randomized controlled clinical trial. Spine (Phila Pa 1976) 2003;28:2491–8.

18. Vassiliou T, Kaluza G, Putzke C, et al. Physical therapy and active exercises–an adequate treatment for prevention of late whiplash syndrome? Randomized controlled trial in 200 patients. Pain 2006;124:69–76.

19. Lord SM, Barnsley L, Wallis BJ, et al. Chronic cervical zygapophysial joint pain after whiplash. A placebo-controlled prevalence study [see comments]. Spine 1996;21:1737–44 [discussion: 44–5].

20. Dwyer A, Aprill C, Bogduk N. Cervical zygapophyseal joint pain patterns. I: A study in normal volunteers. Spine 1990;15:453–7.

21. Schellhas KP, Smith MD, Gundry CR, et al. Cervical discogenic pain. Prospective correlation of magnetic resonance imaging and discography in asymptomatic subjects and pain sufferers. Spine 1996;21:300–11 [discussion: 11–2].

22. Lord SM, Barnsley L, Wallis BJ, et al. Third occipital nerve headache: a prevalence study. J Neurol Neurosurg Psychiatry 1994;57:1187–90.

23. Barnsley L, Lord SM, Wallis BJ, et al. The prevalence of chronic cervical zygapo-physial joint pain after whiplash. Spine 1995;20:20–5 [discussion: 6].
24. Lord SM, Barnsley L, Wallis BJ, et al. Percutaneous radio-frequency neurotomy for chronic cervical zygapophyseal-joint pain [see comments]. N Engl J Med 1996;335:1721–6.
25. Sapir DA, Gorup JM. Radiofrequency medial branch neurotomy in litigant and nonlitigant patients with cervical whiplash: a prospective study. Spine 2001;26: E268–73.
26. Speldewinde GC, Bashford GM, Davidson IR. Diagnostic cervical zygapophy-seal joint blocks for chronic cervical pain. Med J Aust 2001;174:174–6.
27. Schofferman J, Bogduk N, Slosar P. Chronic whiplash and whiplash-associated dis-orders: an evidence-based approach. J Am Acad Orthop Surg 2007;15:596–606.
28. Ivancic PC. Facet joint and disc kinematics during simulated rear crashes with active injury prevention systems. Spine (Phila Pa 1976) 2011;36:E1215–24.
29. Siegmund GP, Davis MB, Quinn KP, et al. Head-turned postures increase the risk of cervical facet capsule injury during whiplash. Spine (Phila Pa 1976) 2008;33: 1643–9.
30. Ivancic PC, Ito S, Tominaga Y, et al. Whiplash causes increased laxity of cervical capsular ligament. Clin Biomech (Bristol, Avon) 2008;23:159–65.
31. Stemper BD, Yoganandan N, Cusick JF, et al. Stabilizing effect of precontracted neck musculature in whiplash. Spine 2006;31:E733–8.
32. Stemper BD, Yoganandan N, Pintar FA. Gender- and region-dependent local facet joint kinematics in rear impact: implications in whiplash injury. Spine 2004;29:1764–71.
33. Yoganandan N, Cusick JF, Pintar FA, et al. Whiplash injury determination with conventional spine imaging and cryomicrotomy. Spine 2001;26:2443–8.
34. Grauer JN, Panjabi MM, Cholewicki J, et al. Whiplash produces an S-shaped curvature of the neck with hyperextension at lower levels. Spine 1997;22:2489–94.
35. Cusick JF, Pintar FA, Yoganandan N. Whiplash syndrome: kinematic factors influ-encing pain patterns. Spine 2001;26:1252–8.
36. Kaneoka K, Ono K, Inami S, et al. Motion analysis of cervical vertebrae during whiplash loading. Spine 1999;24:763–9 [discussion: 70].
37. Panjabi MM, Ito S, Pearson AM, et al. Injury mechanisms of the cervical interver-tebral disc during simulated whiplash. Spine 2004;29:1217–25.
38. Pearson AM, Ivancic PC, Ito S, et al. Facet joint kinematics and injury mechanisms during simulated whiplash. Spine 2004;29:390–7.
39. Chen C, Lu Y, Kallakuri S, et al. Distribution of A-delta and C-fiber receptors in the cervical facet joint capsule and their response to stretch. J Bone Joint Surg Am 2006;88:1807–16.
40. Kallakuri S, Singh A, Lu Y, et al. Tensile stretching of cervical facet joint capsule and related axonal changes. Eur Spine J 2008;17:556–63.
41. Lee KE, Davis MB, Mejilla RM, et al. In vivo cervical facet capsule distraction: mechanical implications for whiplash and neck pain. Stapp Car Crash J 2004; 48:373–95.
42. Lee KE, Franklin AN, Davis MB, et al. Tensile cervical facet capsule ligament mechanics: failure and subfailure responses in the rat. J Biomech 2006;39:1256–64.
43. Lee KE, Thinnes JH, Gokhin DS, et al. A novel rodent neck pain model of facet-mediated behavioral hypersensitivity: implications for persistent pain and whiplash injury. J Neurosci Methods 2004;137:151–9.
44. Taylor JR, Twomey LT. Acute injuries to cervical joints. An autopsy study of neck sprain. Spine 1993;18:1115–22.

45. Pettersson K, Hildingsson C, Toolanen G, et al. Disc pathology after whiplash injury. A prospective magnetic resonance imaging and clinical investigation. Spine 1997;22:283–7 [discussion: 8].
46. Jonsson H Jr, Bring G, Rauschning W, et al. Hidden cervical spine injuries in traffic accident victims with skull fractures. J Spinal Disord 1991;4:251–63.
47. Schofferman J, Garges K, Goldthwaite N, et al. Upper cervical anterior diskectomy and fusion improves discogenic cervical headaches. Spine 2002;27:2240–4.
48. Winkelstein BA, Nightingale RW, Richardson WJ, et al. The cervical facet capsule and its role in whiplash injury: a biomechanical investigation. Spine 2000;25:1238–46.
49. Siegmund GP, Myers BS, Davis MB, et al. Mechanical evidence of cervical facet capsule injury during whiplash: a cadaveric study using combined shear, compression, and extension loading. Spine 2001;26:2095–101.
50. Uhrenholt L, Charles AV, Hauge E, et al. Pathoanatomy of the lower cervical spine facet joints in motor vehicle crash fatalities. J Forensic Leg Med 2009;16:253–60.
51. Uhrenholt L, Nielsen E, Charles AV, et al. Non-fatal injuries to the cervical spine facet joints after a fatal motor vehicle crash: a case report. Med Sci Law 2009;49:218–21.
52. Uhrenholt L, Nielsen E, Charles AV, et al. Imaging occult lesions in the cervical spine facet joints. Am J Forensic Med Pathol 2009;30:142–7.
53. Svensson MY, Bostrom O, Davidsson J, et al. Neck injuries in car collisions–a review covering a possible injury mechanism and the development of a new rear-impact dummy. Accid Anal Prev 2000;32:167–75.
54. Tominaga Y, Ndu AB, Coe MP, et al. Neck ligament strength is decreased following whiplash trauma. BMC Musculoskelet Disord 2006;7:103.
55. Quinn KP, Winkelstein BA. Cervical facet capsular ligament yield defines the threshold for injury and persistent joint-mediated neck pain. J Biomech 2007;40:2299–306.
56. Crotti FM, Carai A, Carai M, et al. Post-traumatic thoracic outlet syndrome (TOS). Acta Neurochir Suppl 2005;92:13–5.
57. Kai Y, Oyama M, Kurose S, et al. Neurogenic thoracic outlet syndrome in whiplash injury. J Spinal Disord 2001;14:487–93.
58. Sanders RJ, Hammond SL, Rao NM. Thoracic outlet syndrome: a review. Neurologist 2008;14:365–73.
59. Brault JR, Siegmund GP, Wheeler JB. Cervical muscle response during whiplash: evidence of a lengthening muscle contraction. Clin Biomech (Bristol, Avon) 2000;15:426–35.
60. Siegmund GP, Sanderson DJ, Myers BS, et al. Awareness affects the response of human subjects exposed to a single whiplash-like perturbation. Spine 2003;28:671–9.
61. Carlsson A, Linder A, Davidsson J, et al. Dynamic kinematic responses of female volunteers in rear impacts and comparison to previous male volunteer tests. Traffic Inj Prev 2011;12:347–57.
62. Muddu BN, Umaar R, Kim WY, et al. Whiplash injury of the shoulder: is it a distinct clinical entity? Acta Orthop Belg 2005;71:385–7.
63. Chauhan SK, Peckham T, Turner R. Impingement syndrome associated with whiplash injury. J Bone Joint Surg Br 2003;85:408–10.
64. Berglund A, Alfredsson L, Cassidy JD, et al. The association between exposure to a rear-end collision and future neck or shoulder pain: a cohort study. J Clin Epidemiol 2000;53:1089–94.

65. Coert JH, Dellon AL. Peripheral nerve entrapment caused by motor vehicle crashes [see comments]. J Trauma 1994;37:191–4.
66. Ames EL. Carpal tunnel syndrome and motor vehicle accidents. J Am Osteopath Assoc 1996;96:223–6.
67. Alpar EK, Onuoha G, Killampalli VV, et al. Management of chronic pain in whiplash injury. J Bone Joint Surg Br 2002;84:807–11.
68. Greening J, Dilley A, Lynn B. In vivo study of nerve movement and mechanosensitivity of the median nerve in whiplash and non-specific arm pain patients. Pain 2005;115:248–53.
69. De Boever JA, Keersmaekers K. Trauma in patients with temporomandibular disorders: frequency and treatment outcome. J Oral Rehabil 1996;23:91–6.
70. Klobas L, Tegelberg A, Axelsson S. Symptoms and signs of temporomandibular disorders in individuals with chronic whiplash-associated disorders. Swed Dent J 2004;28:29–36.
71. Carroll LJ, Ferrari R, Cassidy JD. Reduced or painful jaw movement after collision-related injuries: a population-based study. J Am Dent Assoc 2007;138:86–93.
72. Haggman-Henrikson B, Rezvani M, List T. Prevalence of whiplash trauma in TMD patients: a systematic review. J Oral Rehabil 2014;41:59–68.
73. Friedman MH, Weisberg J. The craniocervical connection: a retrospective analysis of 300 whiplash patients with cervical and temporomandibular disorders. Cranio 2000;18:163–7.
74. Kolbinson DA, Epstein JB, Burgess JA. Temporomandibular disorders, headaches, and neck pain following motor vehicle accidents and the effect of litigation: review of the literature. J Orofac Pain 1996;10:101–25.
75. Boniver R. Temporomandibular joint dysfunction in whiplash injuries: association with tinnitus and vertigo. Int Tinnitus J 2002;8:129–31.
76. Steigerwald DP, Verne SV, Young D. A retrospective evaluation of the impact of temporomandibular joint arthroscopy on the symptoms of headache, neck pain, shoulder pain, dizziness, and tinnitus. Cranio 1996;14:46–54.
77. Koelbaek Johansen M, Graven-Nielsen T, Schou Olesen A, et al. Generalised muscular hyperalgesia in chronic whiplash syndrome. Pain 1999;83:229–34.
78. Stone AM, Vicenzino B, Lim EC, et al. Measures of central hyperexcitability in chronic whiplash associated disorder–a systematic review and meta-analysis. Man Ther 2013;18:111–7.
79. Smith AD, Jull G, Schneider G, et al. A comparison of physical and psychological features of responders and non-responders to cervical facet blocks in chronic whiplash. BMC Musculoskelet Disord 2013;14:313.
80. Sterling M, Kenardy J, Jull G, et al. The development of psychological changes following whiplash injury. Pain 2003;106:481–9.
81. Sterling M, Jull G, Vicenzino B, et al. Development of motor system dysfunction following whiplash injury. Pain 2003;103:65–73.
82. Sterling M, Jull G, Vicenzino B, et al. Sensory hypersensitivity occurs soon after whiplash injury and is associated with poor recovery. Pain 2003;104:509–17.
83. Sterling M, Treleaven J, Jull G. Responses to a clinical test of mechanical provocation of nerve tissue in whiplash associated disorder. Man Ther 2002;7:89–94.
84. Curatolo M, Petersen-Felix S, Arendt-Nielsen L, et al. Central hypersensitivity in chronic pain after whiplash injury. Clin J Pain 2001;17:306–15.
85. Winkelstein BA, Santos DG. An intact facet capsular ligament modulates behavioral sensitivity and spinal glial activation produced by cervical facet joint tension. Spine (Phila Pa 1976) 2008;33:856–62.

Chronic Daily Headache

Natalia Murinova, MD, MHA[a],*, Daniel Krashin, MD[b]

KEYWORDS

- Chronic daily headache • Chronic migraine • Chronic tension-type headache
- Chronic posttraumatic headache • Medication overuse headache

KEY POINTS

- The term chronic daily headache (CDH) is used when patients present with 15 or more headache attacks per month for 3 or more months.
- The International Headache Society Criteria should be used to diagnose specific CDH disorder. CDH is a symptom diagnosis that does not reflect the underlying cause of the headache.
- Secondary causes need to be ruled out before CDH is diagnosed as a primary headache syndrome.
- Medication overuse, comorbid psychiatric disease, physical deconditioning, and obesity complicate CDH.
- Effective treatment involves multimodal therapy, including education; pharmacologic intervention; nonpharmacologic, appropriate procedural intervention; and lifestyle changes.
- Treatments need to focus on improving function and well-being.

INTRODUCTION

In 1672, physician Thomas Willis described CDHs of the philosopher Viscountess Anne Conway.[1–3] Dr Harvey recommended mercury treatments, whereas Dr Willis recorded a long list of attempted treatments, attesting to the patient's determination to try every possible medical cure.[4] Dr Willis suggested treatment of refractory headaches with trepanation and poultices of millipedes and wood lice. Despite her willingness to engage in multiple treatments, she continued to suffer from severe headaches until her death.[4,5] Two hundred years later, Dr Liveing noted valerian as a possible treatment of frequent headaches, and Doctor Gowers described bromide and India hemp as headache treatments. However, the perfect cure for CDHs has not yet been found.

[a] Headache Clinic, Department of Neurology, University of Washington, 1959 Northeast Pacific Street, Seattle, WA, USA; [b] Chronic Fatigue Clinic UW, Department of Psychiatry, Anesthesiology and Pain Medicine, University of Washington, 1959 Northeast Pacific Street, Seattle, WA, USA
* Corresponding author.
E-mail address: nataliam@u.washington.edu

Phys Med Rehabil Clin N Am 26 (2015) 375–389
http://dx.doi.org/10.1016/j.pmr.2015.01.001
1047-9651/15/$ – see front matter © 2015 Elsevier Inc. All rights reserved.
pmr.theclinics.com

The International Headache Society defines CDH as a headache disorder whereby patients suffer 15 or more headache attacks per month for 3 or more months. Patients who have more than 4 headache days per month, have some associated disability, or report significant suffering might be at risk of progressing to CDH and may need preventive treatment.

PATIENT EVALUATION OVERVIEW

The specific diagnosis of CDH is key for properly managing patients. When counseling patients, it is helpful to explain that headache can be caused by either a structural problem or medication overuse (called secondary headache), by a change in the functioning of the brain (called primary headache), or by a combination of both. Asking the right questions can establish a specific diagnosis without further tests, so it is important to learn to use precise questions (**Table 1**).

After establishing that CDH is primary, not secondary, the primary CDH is further subdivided into primary headache subtypes of short duration, which is less than 4 hours, and long duration, which is 4 hours or greater. The 2 most common long-duration subtypes are chronic migraine (CM) and chronic tension-type headache. The short-duration headache disorders include hemicrania continua, new daily persistent headache, and chronic cluster headache. Most patients with CDH who present to specialists have either chronic tension-type headache or CM.

Asking the right questions
- What is the goal of your visit today?
- Do you have questions regarding your diagnosis?
- Is your main goal of visit pain relief?
- Are you seeking further testing?
- What are you worried about?
- What is the number of headache days per month that you are having? If your headaches last multiple days, count each day.
- Do you have any headache-free days?
- What is the duration of each individual headache?

Table 1
Questions for headache diagnosis

History of Headaches	Possible Answers and Their Implications
Do you have more than 15 headache days per month?	Diagnosis of CDH with >15 d of headaches per month If answer is no: diagnosis of episodic headaches
Are your headaches nonstop?	If yes, further workup needs to rule out a secondary headache diagnosis
Is the headache duration longer than 4 h?	4 h/d: likely chronic migraine or chronic tension-type headache <4 h: Trigeminal autonomic cephalalgia, such as cluster or hemicrania
Do you use abortive medications more than 10 d/mo?	Consider medication overuse headaches
What are the associated symptoms?	Nausea, light and sound sensitivity go along with chronic migraine phenotype Autonomic symptoms are often associated with trigeminal autonomic cephalalgia

- What medications do you use? (Ask specifically about the frequency of use of medications that can be associated with overuse, such as acetaminophen, ibuprofen, opioids, and triptans.)
- Do your headaches have any associated symptoms?
- Do you have any trouble with sleep?
- How much caffeine do you consume?
- Did you have recent changes in your weight?
- Do you also have anxiety and/or depression?
- Have you recently perceived increased stress in your life?
- What is your understating of the reason behind your headaches?
- What is your understanding of the medications that were prescribed to you?
- Are you okay with taking daily preventive medications?

RISK FACTORS FOR MIGRAINE PROGRESSION

A combination of many different factors can cause headaches in susceptible individuals, and chronic medication administration can cause long-term unexpected consequences (**Table 2**).[6] The most significant risk factors for headache progression are cumulative and include medication overuse, increased caffeine use, stress, anxiety, depression, high attack frequency, and obesity. Other factors include lower education level and lower socioeconomic status, trauma to the head or neck, and problems with insomnia and sleep apnea.[7,8]

Modifiable Risk Factors

Several modifiable risk factors have been identified[6]:

Frequency of headache attacks at baseline[6]
- Three or more headaches per month elevates risk for developing CDH.

Obesity[6]
- Obesity is associated with worsening pain intensity.
- Patients with obesity are often more difficult to treat and unresponsive to usual treatment.
- CDH is 3 times more likely with body mass index (BMI) 25 to 29 (overweight).
- CDH is 5 times more with BMI greater than or equal to 30 (obese).

MEDICATION OVERUSE

"Overuse of abortive medication can contribute to the transformation of episodic into transformed migraine."[6,9] High doses of certain medications can change the function

Table 2 Risk factors for headache	
Not-Readily-Modifiable Risk Factors	**Modifiable Risk Factors**
Age	Baseline high headache attack frequency with more than 3 headache days per month
Low education	Obesity
Socioeconomic status	Medication overuse
Head injury	Ongoing life stress
Female gender	High caffeine use
	Snoring

of the pain control mechanism in genetically predisposed patients. The mechanism is not fully understood, but it is thought that this phenomenon includes combination of many different mechanisms such as increased central sensitization via N-methyl-d-aspartate receptors and decreased antinociceptive mechanisms.[10] Chronic opioid use can further increase pain perception via rostral ventromedial medulla activation. Inhibitory γ-aminobutyric acid interneurons that modulate pain perception can be damaged by opioid-induced neurotoxicity.[10]

Highlights of medication overuse
- About 80% of patients with CM seen by headache specialists exhibit medication overuse.
- Medication overuse decreases the effectiveness of short-term and preventive treatment.
- Abortive medication use is more likely to cause CDH in patients who have a biologic predisposition to headaches.
- Medications used for other conditions, such as other chronic pain conditions, may induce CDH in genetically susceptible individuals.
- Even after medication overuse stops, CDH may continue.

Caffeine[6]
- Caffeine withdrawal can manifest as headache.
- Consumption of as little as 1 cup of coffee per day can worsen headaches in some patients.

Snoring/sleep apnea
- Sleep-disordered breathing is associated with cluster headache.
- Sleep apnea can present as daily headaches in the morning.
- Insomnia and CDH are often comorbid.

Depression and stressful life events[6,11]
- Major depression was present in 58.7% of patients with CM.[11] The prevalence of "some depression" was 85.8% in patients with CM, whereas it was only 28.1% in patients with episodic migraine.[11]
- Stressful life event is also a risk factor for CDH.

Subtypes of chronic daily headaches
- Chronic tension-type headache is defined as headaches occurring more than 15 days a month with no specific significant associated feature.
- CM is defined as having more than half of headache days with migraine features, such as unilateral pain, nausea, and light and sound sensitivity.
- Hemicrania continua is a unilateral headache associated with autonomic features.
- Chronic cluster headache is an excruciating unilateral headache associated with autonomic features (eg, tearing in the ipsilateral eye, runny nose, droopy eye, miosis, ptosis, restlessness).

Chronic Migraine

About 35 million people in the United States experience migraines annually. CM is estimated to be present in about 2% of the adult population (about 6 million Americans), with only 20% of these individuals having received formal diagnosis.[12] The International Classification of Headache Disorders 3 (beta) 2013 defines CM as "Headache occurring on 15 or more days per month for more than three months, with features of migraine on at least eight days per month."[13] CM is considered a complication of episodic migraine; each year, in approximately 2.5% of patients, episodic migraine transforms to CM. This transformation may occur with or without medication overuse. Patients meeting criteria for both CM and medication-overuse headache should be given both diagnoses.[13]

Approach to patients presenting with chronic headaches
1. Exclude secondary headache disorders.
2. Make a diagnosis of the specific primary headache disorder type (CM, chronic tension-type headache, hemicrania continua, or new daily persistent headache) using International Headache Society Criteria.[13]
3. Identify comorbid medical and psychiatric conditions and address as necessary.
4. Exclude medication overuse.
5. Limit all abortive medication use to less than 4 to 6 days per month in most patients with CDH (with the exception of long-acting nonsteroidal anti-inflammatory medications, which can be used for up to 10 days per month).
6. Start administration of preventive medication with the goal of decreasing use of abortive medications. Preventive medications are not fully therapeutic until overuse of abortive medications is addressed, and it can take months for them to be significantly effective.
7. Consider termination of headache cycle with dihydroergotamine (DHE) therapy.

Indications for neuroimaging[14]
1. Acute worsening in frequency and intensity of headaches
2. New or changed headaches present after age 50 years
3. History of sudden headache onset in someone who has never experienced headaches
4. New neurologic symptoms (eg, vision loss)
5. Focal or lateralizing neurologic signs
6. Papilledema
7. Headaches that worsen or improve with postural change (eg, upright vs supine)
8. Headaches provoked by a Valsalva maneuver (eg, a cough or sneeze)
9. Systemic symptoms (eg, fever)
10. Immunosuppression
11. History of cancer or other neoplastic disease
12. History of human immunodeficiency virus infection

PHARMACOLOGIC TREATMENT OPTIONS
Short-term Pharmacotherapy

The choice of short-term pharmacotherapy depends on the specific headache diagnosis. Patients with CM who are not overusing short-term drugs can treat headache exacerbations with migraine-specific drugs such as triptans, DHE-45, or long-acting nonsteroidal anti-inflammatory drugs (NSAIDs) (**Tables 3** and **4**). The use of these drugs must be limited to prevent medication overuse headache (MOH), which complicates treatment.

Table 3
Available triptans for occasional (not daily) use

Generic Name	Trade Name	Forms	Dose (mg)	MR in HR	Max Dose in 24 h (mg)	Year FDA Approved
Sumatriptan	Imitrex	Inj	4; 6	1	12	1992
Sumatriptan	Imitrex	Tab	50, 100	2	200	1995
Sumatriptan	Imitrex	NS	20	2	40	1997
Sumatriptan	Zecuity	TD	6.5 over 4 h			2013
Naratriptan	Amerge	Tab	2.5	4	5	1998
Rizatriptan	Maxalt	Tab	5; 10	2	20	1998
Rizatriptan	Maxalt-MLT	ODT	5; 10	2	20	1998
Zolmitriptan	Zomig	Tab	2.5; 5	2	10	2003
Zolmitriptan	Zomig-ZMT	ODT	2.5; 5	2	10	2003
Almotriptan	Axert	Tab	12.5	2	25	2001
Frovatriptan	Frova	Tab	2.5	2	5	2001
Eletriptan	Relpax	Tab	40	2	80	2002
Zolmitriptan	Zomig-NS	NS	5	2	10	2003
Sumatriptan Naproxen	Treximet	Tab	85 500	2	170 1000	2008

Abbreviations: Inj, injection; MR in HR, may repeat in x hours; NS, nasal spray; ODT, orally dissolving tablet; Tab, tablet; TD, transdermal.

Medication overuse, or rebound, can occur with the use of any abortive medications and is defined by the International Headache Society as the use the of[13]

1. "One or more triptans, on 10 days per month for >3 months"[13]
2. "Acetylsalicylic acid on 15 days per month for >3 months"[13]

Table 4
Nontriptan abortive treatment of migraines medications that provide quick pain relief when attacks occur

Generic Name	Trade Name	Forms	Dose (mg)	MR in HR	Max Dose in 24 h	Year FDA Approved
Dihydroergotamine	DHE 45	Inj	1	8	3 mg	1946
Dihydroergotamine	Migranal NS	NS	4	8	12 mg	1997
Isometheptene Dichloralphenazone Acetaminophen	Midrin	Tab	65 100 325	1	5 tabs	Never FDA approved; not recommended
Butalbital Acetaminophen Caffeine	Fioricet	Tab	50 325 40	4	4 tabs	1985; not recommended
Butalbital Aspirin Caffeine	Fiorinal	Tab	50 325 40	4	4 tabs	1976; not recommended

Abbreviations: Inj, injection; NS, nasal spray; Tab, tablet.

| Randomized controlled trials for chronic headaches (most trials conducted with patients with CM) | | | | |
Medication, Trial Year, Study	Number Treated	Dose of Medication	Primary End point/Results	Reported Side Effects
OnabotulinumtoxinA (2010)[15]		155 units		Neck pain, muscle weakness, eyelid ptosis
Topiramate (2007)[21]	N = 153[21] N = 35	100–200 mg	Frequency of migraine/migrainous days (37.3 vs 28.8%) (−6.4 vs −4.7, $P = .010$)	Paresthesias, upper respiratory tract infection and fatigue
Divalproex sodium (2008)[19]	N = 29	500 mg bid 250 mg bid; after the first week to 500 mg bid	Number of headache days at 3 mo (−6.85 ± 1.72; $P = .0105$), 6 mo (−7.49 ± 1.60; $P = .0055$), and 9 mo (−7.40 ± 1.75; $P = .0082$)	Side effects: somnolence, tremor, impotence; hair loss
Gabapentin (2003)[18]	N = 133 (95 sufficient treatment)	800 mg tid	9.1% in headache-free rates ($P = .0005$); ↓ headache-free days/month ($P = .0005$)	Adverse events: 39% of patients on gabapentin: dizziness, somnolence, ataxia and nausea
Tizanidine (2002)[17]	N = 45	8 mg tid Tizanidine was slowly titrated over 4 wk up to 24 mg or maximum tolerated dose (mean 18 mg)	Headache index ($P = .0025$), headache days per week ($P = .0193$), severe headache days per week ($P = .0211$)	Adverse effects in more than 10% of patients: somnolence, dizziness, dry mouth, and asthenia
Amitriptyline (2010)[22]	N = 23	25–50 mg/day	Decrease >50% in the number of days of pain in 72% ($P = .78$) (n.s.)	Dry mouth, weight gain and somnolence
Fluoxetine (1994)[23]	CDH = 64	20–40 mg po q day	Visual analog scale after 3 mo 50% vs 11% placebo ($P = .029$), 47% vs 23% improving at least 50% ($P = .097$, n.s.); significant improvement in monthly mood ratings; headache only during the third month ($P = .001$)	Sleep disturbance, and minor stomach pain

Abbreviations: N, number treated; n.s., not statistically significant.

3. "One or more NSAIDs other than acetylsalicylic acid on 15 days per month for >3 months"[13]
4. "Ergotamine on 10 days per month for >3 months"[13]
5. "One or more opioids on 10 days per month for >3 months"[13]

MOH is more likely when patients are taking multiple classes of short-term therapies (ie, the risk of rebound is cumulative).

Preventive Pharmacotherapy

Preventive therapy should be considered when patients experience 4 to 5 migraine days per month in the setting of normal function or when patients present with 2 to 3 migraine days per month with impaired function. Although preventive pharmacotherapy is often effective, only 33% of those with CM are using preventive medications. One example of a US Food and Drug Administration (FDA)-approved preventive treatment of CM is onabotulinumtoxinA. The FDA approved this treatment in 2010 based on phase III research studies evaluating migraine prophylaxis therapy (PREEMPT).[15] At 24-week follow-up, researchers assessed whether patients had experienced at least a 50% decrease in headache day frequency. About 47.1% of onabotulinumtoxinA-treated patients experienced at least this degree of improvement, whereas only 35.1% of placebo-treated patients had achieved this degree of improvement.[15]

According to Diener and colleagues,[16] the use of topiramate and local injection of onabotulinumtoxin are the only treatments of CM supported by adequately powered placebo-controlled randomized trials. Several medication trials have been underpowered, and/or the follow-up period is too short to be clinically relevant in patients with chronic headaches.[16] The use of tizanidine,[17] gabapentin,[18] and sodium valproate[19,20] has some empirical support.

There are many other medications that are used off label for the treatment of CM. **Table 5** summarizes several of these options.

Use of preventive medications in patients with obesity and weight concerns
- Topiramate, FDA-approved for CM, is the only medication associated with weight loss.
- β-Blockers and calcium channel blockers do not cause significant weight gain in most patients.
- Divalproex sodium and tricyclic antidepressants can lead to significant weight gain.

Major trial issues
- Different methodologies used in different studies
- Presence of medication overuse not well delineated
- Disparate outcome measures
- Different trial duration

According to D'Amico,[20] further large multicenter controlled trials with standardized outcome measures are needed. At present, there are few medications for which high-quality empirical support is available.[20]

OTHER MEDICATIONS

Open-label studies of CM medications suggest that the following medications may be efficacious: pregabalin, gabapentin, zonisamide, atenolol, olanzapine, and possibly memantine.

Open-Label Trials for Chronic Migraine

Preventive medications for chronic migraine with target dose
Open-Label Studies/Case Studies for CM
Pregabalin: 150 mg bid[24] N = 30; ↓ headache frequency ($P<.0001$) and ↓ severity ($P = .0005$)
Zonisamide: 100–400 mg/d[25] N=34; Headache severity and headache duration were decreased
Olanzapine: 2.5–35 mg/d[26] N = 50: reviewed records × 3 mo   2.5–35 mg; most patients (n = 19) received 5 or 10 mg/d (n = 17); significant ↓ in headache days, from 27.5 ± 4.9 before treatment to 21.1 ± 10.7 after treatment ($P<.001$, Student t test); ↓ headache severity before treatment (8.7 ± 1.6) and after treatment (2.2 ± 2.1) was also statistically significant ($P<.001$)
Memantine: 10–20 mg/d[27]   Case study "woman with chronic migraine who unexpectedly reported full remission of headache after memantine"

Abbreviation: N, number of patients.

Nonpharmacologic Treatment Options

Nonpharmacologic treatment options for chronic migraine	
Nonpharmacologic Treatment	**Notes**
Acupuncture: helpful for CM N = 33 patients 24 sessions over 12 wk	Moderate/severe headache days decreased from 20.2 to 9.8[28]
Biofeedback: helpful for CM N = 19 patients 8 sessions over 8 wk × 20 min Audiocassette tape daily at home	Helpful for CM as adjunctive treatment[29] Progressive muscle relaxation training, method by Bernstein and Borkovec
Physical exercise 40 min 3 times a week	Helpful for EM, no study in CM[30] CDH are less prevalent in subjects who exercise 3–7 d/wk (50% ↓ CDH)[31]
Relaxation therapy	Helpful for EM, no data in CM[30]

Abbreviation: EM, episodic migraine.

Alternative supplements have been studied more often in episodic migraine than in CM.

Findings from several studies in CDH are summarized in the following table.[32,33]

Other Alternative Agents	Notes
Melatonin, 9 mg[32]	Report of 2 patients with cluster headaches who became headache free
Magnesium[33]	Satisfaction in 40% of patients taking magnesium. Well tolerated[33]
Feverfew[33]	Satisfaction in 58% patients taking feverfew. Well tolerated[33]

Table 5
Prophylactic treatment of migraine

Generic Name and Class of Drugs	Trade Name	Dose (mg)	Possible Side Effects	Contraindications	FDA Approved
β-Blockers class of drugs			Fatigue, ⇩BP, ⇩HR, ⇧weight	Asthma depression	
Propranolol	Inderal	20–360	"	"	Yes
Metoprolol	Toprol	50–100	"	"	
Nadolol	Corgard	10–160	"	"	
Timolol	Blocadren	10–40	"	"	Yes
Atenolol	Tenormin	25–100	"	"	
Calcium channel blockers class			⇩BP, ⇩HR, constipation, arrhythmia		
Verapamil	Calan	80–480			
Diltiazem	Cardizem	60–360			
Amlodipine	Norvasc	2.5–10			
Antiepileptic class of drugs					
Divalproex	Depakote	250–1500	Drowsiness, ⇩hair, ⇧⇧⇧weight, ⇧LFTs, bone marrow Δ		Yes
Gabapentin	Neurontin	300–3600	Dizziness, ⇧⇧weight		
Pregabalin	Lyrica	25–600			
Topiramate	Topamax	25–400	⇩⇩Weight, cognitive Δ memory problems	Kidney stones	Yes
Zonisamide	Zonegran	25–400	⇩⇩Weight		
Lamotrigine	Lamictal	25–100	Stevens-Johnson syndrome		
Levatiracetam	Keppra				
Tricyclic antidepressants			⇧⇧Weight, dry mouth, QTC prolongation		
Amitriptyline	Elavil	10–50	⇧⇧Weight		
Nortriptyline	Pamelor	10–50	"		
Imipramine	Tofranil	25–50	"		
SSRIs class			Nausea, fatigue, serotonin syndrome		
Citalopram	Celexa	10–40	Sexual dysfunction		
Escitalopram	Lexapro	5–20			
SNRIs class					
Duloxetine	Cymbalta	20–60			
Milnacipram	Savella	12.5–200			
Venlafaxine	Exxefor	75–225			
Onabotulinum	Botox	155 units			Yes

Abbreviations: Δ, changes; ⇩⇩, decreases; ⇧⇧, increases; BP, blood pressure; HR, heart rate; SNRI, serotonin-norepinephrine reuptake inhibitor; SSRI, selective serotonin reuptake inhibitor; QTc, corrected QT interval on the EKG.

COMBINATION THERAPIES

Combining medications from different classes in the treatment of CDH is common practice by headache specialists; there is, however, a dearth of evidence supporting the effectiveness of combination medication therapies. For example, 191 patients with CM whose pain was inadequately controlled with topiramate were randomized to receive additional propranolol or placebo. No evidence of benefit was found from the addition of propranolol to topiramate.[34]

The Role of Nerve Blocks

When unilateral or bilateral occipital nerve blocks with local anesthetic and steroid were used in patients with CM with a prominent cervicogenic element, 52% experienced a 50% or greater reduction in headache days during the month following the procedure.[35] Another study of 37 patients with CM found that greater occipital nerve blocks and trigger point injections are equally effective.[36]

Surgical Treatment Options

Obesity is associated with increased migraine frequency and severity.[37] Two studies have shown reduction in episodic migraine after bariatric surgery, but no such data exist in CM.[38,39] Bariatric surgery studies need to include subjects with CM to determine the potential benefits of bariatric surgery.

The American Headache Society concludes, "Surgery for migraine is a last-resort option and is probably not appropriate for most sufferers. To date, there are no convincing or definitive data that show its long-term value."[40]

TREATMENT RESISTANCE/COMPLICATIONS

If CDH is resistant to treatment, it is important to establish that the original headache diagnosis is accurate and that the diagnosis has not changed. It is also helpful to evaluate patients' understanding of their diagnosis and their compliance with treatment. Many patients are noncompliant with their treatment or have relapse with medication overuse. The exact extent of noncompliance or nonadherence is not known for patients with chronic headache; however, in chronic fibromyalgia the studies show that up to two-thirds of patients are noncompliant with their treatment and these patients have much higher health care costs. (Zhao, 2011)[41] In a study of patients treated in a headache clinic, only 35% were compliant with preventive medication treatment. (Gaul, 2011)[42] It is important to foster realistic expectations regarding the outcome of treatment. If patients continue to overuse abortive medication and take preventive medication for only a short period, it is unlikely that they will succeed. In the authors' headache practice, they often encounter patients who have "tried all preventive medication" within a short period. Many patients with CDH try a new preventive medication only for a few days and discontinue this because they do not perceive an immediate benefit or take the preventive medication without addressing medication overuse. Often, there are other modifiable health factors that need to be addressed to achieve success.

ADDRESSING MODIFIABLE RISK FACTORS

Addressing increased frequency of headaches
- Use pharmacologic and nonpharmacologic treatment strategies (sleep, hygiene, exercise, nutrition, relaxation, and others) for patients with more than 4 headache days per month.

Addressing obesity in patients with daily headaches
- Migraineurs should be encouraged to maintain optimal weight and decrease weight if overweight or obese.
- The treatment plan should include diet modification, exercise, and behavioral support.

Medication treatment
- Medication noncompliance is a significant issue for CDH; it may occur if patients are unable to tolerate the initial dose of medication, if patients sense little to no effect from the prescribed medication, or if they are against medication treatment. Patients may be noncompliant with treatment for numerous reasons.
- Many patients are unaware that preventive medications must be used daily for 6 months and that abortive medication overuse decreases its success.
- Patients often believe that, in order for medications to be considered effective, they must lead to complete symptom relief.

Adapted from Lipton RB, et al.[43]

THE PROGNOSIS OF CHRONIC MIGRAINE

In a study of 383 self-reported patients with CM, only 26% reported fewer than 10 headache days per month during 2 years.[44] A study of 136 subjects with CM who presented to a specialty headache clinic found that 70% of patients had reverted to episodic migraine at 1-year follow-up, having less than 15 days per month.[45]

Predictors of remission include the following:

- Lower baseline headache frequency (fewer headache days per month)
- Complete withdrawal of overused medications
- Compliance with preventive medication regimen
- Regular physical exercise

SUMMARY/DISCUSSION

Establishing a correct diagnosis is merely the beginning of the treatment in CDH. Showing a caring attitude and empathy can strengthen trust between the patient and health care provider. This trusting rapport is crucial because CDH often requires long-term management and treatment compliance. It is not uncommon for patients to experience CDH recurrence years after initial presentation because of medication overuse, new medical conditions, and new life stressors. In light of the challenge that CDH presents to patients and providers alike, further research and provider and patient education are certainly highly valued.

In testimony to the US Senate regarding the challenges of headache pain, Shapiro aptly noted: "As our best treatments have only become available in the last decade, hopefully the pace of development will continue to accelerate for this disabling, poorly understood, under-recognized, undertreated, and underfunded disorder."[46]

REFERENCES

1. Rapoport A, Stang P, Gutterman DL, et al. Analgesic rebound headache in clinical practice: data from a physician survey. Headache 1996;36(1):14–9.
2. Mathew N. Medication misuse headache. Cephalalgia 1998;18(21 Suppl):34–6.
3. Gladstone J. From psychoneurosis to ICHD-2: an overview of the state of the art in post-traumatic headache. Headache 2009;49(7):1097–111.

4. Willis T. De anima brutorum quae hominis vitalis ac sensitive est exercitationes duae. London, 1672. English version. Two discourses concerning the Soul of Brutes, which is that of the vital and Sensitive of Man. The Remaining Medical Works of that Famous and Renowned Physician Dr Thomas Willis, London. 1683:121–2.
5. Evans RW. An update on the management of chronic migraine. Headache: The Journal of Head and Face Pain 2013;53(1):168–76.
6. Bigal ME, Lipton RB. Modifiable risk factors for migraine progression. Headache 2006;46(9):1334–43.
7. Halker RB, Hastriter EV, Dodick DW. Chronic daily headache an evidence-based and systematic approach to a challenging problem. Neurology 2011;76(7 Suppl 2):S37–43.
8. Diener H-C, Dodick DW, Goadsby PJ, et al. Chronic migraine—classification, characteristics and treatment. Nat Rev Neurol 2012;8(3):162–71.
9. Post RM, Silberstein SD. Shared mechanisms in affective illness, epilepsy, and migraine. Neurology 1994;44:S37–47.
10. Silberstein SD. Migraine and medication overuse. In: Schoenen J, Dodick DW, Sandor PS, editors. Comorbidity in migraine. Oxford (UK): Wiley-Blackwell; 2011. p. 96.
11. Mercante JP, Peres MF, Guendler V, et al. Depression in chronic migraine: severity and clinical features. Arq Neuropsiquiatr 2005;63(2A):217–20.
12. Evans RW. A rational approach to the management of chronic migraine. Headache 2013;53(1):168–76.
13. Headache Classification Committee of the International Headache Society (IHS). The international classification of headache disorders, (beta version). Cephalalgia 2013;33(9):629–808.
14. Dodick DW. Chronic daily headache. N Engl J Med 2006;354(2):158–65.
15. Diener H, Dodick D, Aurora S, et al. Onabotulinumtoxin A for treatment of chronic migraine: results from the double-blind, randomized, placebo-controlled phase of the PREEMPT 2 trial. Cephalalgia 2010;30(7):804–14.
16. Diener HC, Holle D, Dodick D. Treatment of chronic migraine. Curr Pain Headache Rep 2011;15(1):64–9.
17. Saper JR, Lake AE, Cantrell DT, et al. Chronic daily headache prophylaxis with tizanidine: a double-blind, placebo-controlled, multicenter outcome study. Headache 2002;42(6):470–82.
18. Spira PJ, Beran RG. Gabapentin in the prophylaxis of chronic daily headache. A randomized, placebo-controlled study. Neurology 2003;61(12):1753–9.
19. Blumenfeld AM, Schim JD, Chippendale TJ. Botulinum toxin type A and divalproex sodium for prophylactic treatment of episodic or chronic migraine. Headache 2008;48(2):210–20.
20. D'Amico D. Pharmacological prophylaxis of chronic migraine: a review of double-blind placebo-controlled trials. Neurol Sci 2010;31(1):23–8.
21. Silberstein SD, Lipton RB, Dodick DW, et al. Efficacy and safety of topiramate for the treatment of chronic migraine: a randomized, double-blind, placebo-controlled trial. Headache 2007;47(2):170–80.
22. Magalhães E, Menezes C, Cardeal M, et al. Botulinum toxin type A versus amitriptyline for the treatment of chronic daily migraine. Clin Neurol Neurosurg 2010; 112(6):463–6.
23. Saper JR, Silberstein SD, Lake AE, et al. Double-blind trial of fluoxetine: chronic daily headache and migraine. Headache 1994;34(9):497–502.
24. Calandre EP, Garcia-Leiva JM, Rico-Villademoros F, et al. Pregabalin in the treatment of chronic migraine: an open-label study. Clin Neuropharmacol 2010;33(1):35–9.

25. Drake ME Jr, Greathouse NI, Renner JB, et al. Open-label zonisamide for refractory migraine. Clin Neuropharmacol 2004;27(6):278–80.
26. Silberstein SD, Peres MF, Hopkins MM, et al. Olanzapine in the treatment of refractory migraine and chronic daily headache. Headache 2002;42(6):515–8.
27. Spengos K, Theleritis C, Paparrigopoulos T. Memantine and NMDA antagonism for chronic migraine: a potentially novel therapeutic approach? Headache 2008;48(2):284–6.
28. Yang C, Chang M, Liu P, et al. Acupuncture versus topiramate in chronic migraine prophylaxis: a randomized clinical trial. Cephalalgia 2011;31(15):1510–21.
29. Grazzi L, Andrasik F, D'Amico D, et al. Behavioral and pharmacologic treatment of transformed migraine with analgesic overuse: outcome at 3 years. Headache 2002;42(6):483–90.
30. Varkey E, Cider Å, Carlsson J, et al. Exercise as migraine prophylaxis: a randomized study using relaxation and topiramate as controls. Cephalalgia 2011;31(14):1428–38.
31. Queiroz L, Peres M, Kowacs F, et al. Chronic daily headache in Brazil: a nationwide population-based study. Cephalalgia 2008;28(12):1264–9.
32. Peres M, Rozen T. Melatonin in the preventive treatment of chronic cluster headache. Cephalalgia 2001;21(10):993–5.
33. Bigal ME, Serrano D, Reed M, et al. Chronic migraine in the population: burden, diagnosis, and satisfaction with treatment. Neurology 2008;71(8):559–66.
34. Silberstein S, Dodick D, Lindblad A, et al. Randomized, placebo-controlled trial of propranolol added to topiramate in chronic migraine. Neurology 2012;78(13):976–84.
35. Weibelt S, Andress-Rothrock D, King W, et al. Suboccipital nerve blocks for suppression of chronic migraine: safety, efficacy, and predictors of outcome. Headache 2010;50(6):1041–4.
36. Ashkenazi A, Matro R, Shaw JW, et al. Greater occipital nerve block using local anaesthetics alone or with triamcinolone for transformed migraine: a randomised comparative study. J Neurol Neurosurg Psychiatry 2008;79(4):415–7.
37. Bond D, Vithiananthan S, Nash J, et al. Improvement of migraine headaches in severely obese patients after bariatric surgery. Neurology 2011;76(13):1135–8.
38. Novack V, Fuchs L, Lantsberg L, et al. Changes in headache frequency in premenopausal obese women with migraine after bariatric surgery: a case series. Cephalalgia 2011;31(13):1336–42.
39. Guyuron B, Kriegler JS, Davis J, et al. Five-year outcome of surgical treatment of migraine headaches. Plast Reconstr Surg 2011;127(2):603–8.
40. Saper JR, Dodick DW, Silberstein SD, et al. Occipital nerve stimulation for the treatment of intractable chronic migraine headache: ONSTIM feasibility study. Cephalalgia 2011;31(3):271–85.
41. Zhao, Yang, et al. Comparison of medication adherence and healthcare costs between duloxetine and pregabalin initiators among patients with fibromyalgia. Pain Practice 2011;11(3):204–16.
42. Gaul C, Van Doorn C, Webering N, et al. Clinical outcome of a headache-specific multidisciplinary treatment program and adherence to treatment recommendations in a tertiary headache center: an observational study. The journal of headache and pain 2011;12(4):475–83.
43. Lipton R, Silberstein S, Saper J, et al. Why headache treatment fails. Neurology 2003;60(7):1064–70.
44. Manack A, Buse D, Serrano D, et al. Rates, predictors, and consequences of remission from chronic migraine to episodic migraine. Neurology 2011;76(8):711–8.

45. Seok JI, Cho HI, Chung CS. From transformed migraine to episodic migraine: reversion factors. Headache 2006;46(7):1186–90.
46. Shapiro R. Headache disorders. Pain in America: exploring challenges to relief. Testimony submitted to the United States Senate. Health, Education, Labor, and Pension Committee. Washington, DC. 2012;2(14):12.

Pain and the Injured Worker

James P. Robinson, MD, PhD[a],*, Lee S. Glass, MD[b]

KEYWORDS

- Claims manager • Disability • Maximal medical improvement
- Independent medical examination • Functional capacities evaluation
- Vocational rehabilitation counselor • Objective findings

KEY POINTS

- Physicians who treat injured workers with painful conditions face complex challenges that require skills beyond those of a clinician.
- In order to address these challenges effectively, physicians need to understand the logic of workers' compensation systems and the interests of the various participants in the systems.
- They must be prepared to interface constructively between their patients and the workers' compensation carrier and to accept the fact that, in order to help their patients, they must attend to a multitude of administrative issues.
- In the present article, the authors provide an extended case history with commentary to illustrate the challenges that physicians face and the ways they can respond to these challenges.

INTRODUCTION

Many physicians avoid treating injured workers (IWs) with complaints of acute or chronic pain. Various reasons are offered for such avoidance, ranging from concerns of excessive administrative burden, to patients not recovering as expected, to inadequate reimbursement. It is the authors' view that an understanding of the practical and philosophic underpinnings of our nation's workers' compensation systems will assist physicians in dealing more efficiently with the agencies that provide workers' compensation insurance. The authors also think that IWs' safe and efficient return to health, function, and employment is central to the survival of the tens of thousands of small businesses that power much of the nation's economy and the larger employers that to survive and continue to keep workers employed must compete on the national and international levels.

[a] Department of Physical Medicine and Rehabilitation, University of Washington, Seattle, WA, USA; [b] Department of Labor and Industries, Olympia, WA, USA
* Corresponding author.
E-mail address: jimrob@uw.edu

Phys Med Rehabil Clin N Am 26 (2015) 391–411
http://dx.doi.org/10.1016/j.pmr.2014.12.004
1047-9651/15/$ – see front matter © 2015 Elsevier Inc. All rights reserved.

The present article uses an extended case history to illustrate challenges that physicians face when they manage painful conditions in IWs. The case history assumes that the reader regularly treats patients with musculoskeletal conditions. The comments accompanying the case history are written from 2 perspectives:

- That of a physiatrist (JPR) who works in Washington State, where workers' compensation benefits are available only through a monopolistic state fund and through self-insured employers that by law must adhere to the state fund's regulations and policies
- That of an associate medical director (LSG) of the same state's department that provides workers' compensation insurance and who regularly meets with the state's IWs, physicians, attorneys, and employers

The author of the entries in the several comments sections is indicated.

SOCIETAL BACKGROUND

There was a time before workers' compensation, a time when there was not sufficient societal wealth to support a system that replaced the wages of those whose injuries prevented them from working. People were injured in the course of employment; but absent some voluntary contribution by their employers, IWs had to look to the courts for any money they might seek. The laws that governed the resolution of disputes among the colonials were largely derived from the laws of England, laws that had been developed by the church and state to preserve order in a societal structure in which some were masters and many were servants. Should a servant be injured in the course of employment, the servant would have to prove the master negligent. If the master showed the servant to be culpably negligent to even the slightest degree, then the servant would take nothing. Such was the concept of fairness before and during the industrial revolution.

The industrial revolution generated great wealth. Between the early 1800s and the early 1900s, the industrialization of the United States proceeded at a pace never before witnessed in history. Coal mines provided the energy to turn iron ore into steel. Steel became railroads that punched their way across a continent, providing the means for transporting raw materials to commercial centers and goods to far-flung communities. Steel became derricks that allowed the extraction of oil. Oil further fueled the economy, allowing the efficiency of production that came with mass production to accelerate at a geometric speed. Steel supported the construction of skyscrapers that became the highly visible, upward-pointing metaphor for progress and wealth.

For industrial growth, workers were needed. They came to these shores by the shipload. They came, sometimes prompted by famine and sometimes prompted by visions of wealth, to work. It was their labor—in factories, in the sweatshops of the garment industry, blasting rights of way for rails and crossties—that made the pace of industrialization possible. That labor was performed largely under the same rules that had governed the resolution of disputes in a distant time in a distant land, and the result was that those who were injured in the course of employment had no real ability to obtain either medical care or monetary compensation for their injuries.

The wealth created by the country's industrialization was far greater than had ever been possible in the preceding agrarian economy. With the obvious concentration of much of that wealth—in families with names such as Carnegie, Rockefeller, and Mellon and in corporations and trusts—came clamors for change.

From approximately the last years of the nineteenth century to World War I, the country saw social change at a rate and in a scope that was unprecedented. Those years, the Progressive Era, as historians refer it to, saw change institutionalized in almost every aspect of life. Women got the right to vote. Alcohol was outlawed. Senators were directly elected. And nowhere was change more profound than in the arena of labor relations. Judges, in an era of ever-increasing wealth, were finding reasons to erode the traditional defenses asserted by industry when faced with claims for damages caused by on-the-job injures. For its part, industry was seeing more and more value in having a stable workforce and a quick and efficient means of resolving issues related to industrial injuries.

The ability of business and labor to find shared interests of a magnitude sufficient to form the basis for an agreement was nowhere more evident than in the legislation that created the country's first workers' compensation systems in 1911. However, nothing in the past 100 years has been sufficient to allow business and labor to consistently focus only on those shared interests. For a century, the laws governing workers' compensation have as much reflected turmoil in the relations between business and labor as they may have reflected what is most helpful in returning IWs to health and function.

The fundamental compromise between business and labor that is reflected in all workers' compensation systems in this country is labor giving up the right to sue in exchange for business providing no-fault payments for health care, time-loss payments, and vocational benefits when they are necessitated by industrial injuries. What makes today's workers' compensation systems fundamentally different from the forms of group medical insurance with which physicians routinely interact is the manner and extent to which business and labor, legally and by design, remain directly or indirectly involved in the health care of IWs.

In most private health insurance models, a funding source (often but not always an employer) enters into a contract with an insurer. The contract specifies the beneficiaries of the policy and the scope of the policy's benefits. If a dispute arises, it is virtually always between the beneficiary and the insurer; the funding source is only rarely involved. In workers' compensation, however, the funding source and/or the employer in most states are by law parties in the beneficiary's workers' compensation claim. Therefore, the employer and/or the insurer may intercede as a party in any such proceeding. In this manner, the business interests of an employer can become entangled in the health care of an IW. Although such involvement may actually be in the best interests of a worker (for example, when an employer correctly asserts that a proposed surgery carries far more risk of harm than of benefit), it is generally perceived as being adverse to the interests of the IW.

A full understanding of the diagnosis and treatment of pain in a workers' compensation case is benefited by an understanding that a physician's health care services are to be provided to a specific individual but within a complex system that, ultimately, has a role that goes far beyond the provision of health care to a specific IW. A principal goal of workers' compensation as a system remains what it was in 1911: a means of helping to ensure the economic well-being of the economic backbone of the state through the delivery of affordable, necessary health care services to IWs. It should, therefore, come as no surprise to a physician treating the pain complaints of an IW that his or her health care decisions may be called into question when, if the same patient's care was funded by a group medical insurer, no such issue would, or could, be raised.

Viewed from the aforementioned perspective, it can be seen that the physician treating the pain complaints of an IW has responsibilities that may not be intuitively obvious to the worker. The right to treat an IW carries with it, in virtually all workers' compensation systems, the responsibility of responding to queries that go far beyond the specific health care services that have been or may be provided. For example, a physician may be asked whether an event was a proximate cause of a condition, which is a question that raises both medical and legal issues. A physician may be asked to apportion the responsibility for a condition among multiple employers, which is an exercise requiring skills that are likely not a part of the curriculum of any accredited medical school. For better or for worse, society has a need for such questions to be answered; treating an IW may lay that responsibility on the shoulders of the treating physician.

Many IWs, and many physicians, do not intuitively grasp the layered responsibilities of health care providers who offer services to IWs. When those responsibilities require that a physician voice an opinion that is at odds with the way in which an IW perceives his or her best interests, conflicts can arise. Central to the successful treatment of IWs, especially those in pain, is the setting of clear understandings and expectations as to the role of the physician in providing health care services.

In summary, the physician treating an IW is doing so as a participant in a much larger system. That system imposes responsibilities on physicians that would not be present in other health care funding models. Understanding by both the IW and the physician of the needs of the workers' compensation system for information is critical. The failure of the workers' compensation system to obtain needed information in a timely fashion generally results in an inefficiency that is costly both in terms of time and dollars. Such inefficiency harms workers, employers, health care providers, and society as a whole.

CASE HISTORY

June 1, 2012: Mr Smith, a 40-year-old auto mechanic, calls your office. He seeks an urgent evaluation because he sustained a low back injury yesterday in the course of his work. He was bent over the hood of a car and was lifting out a battery when he felt a pop in his low back and abrupt onset of severe low back pain. He denies pain, sensory loss, or motor loss in the lower extremities. He reports that he has not noticed any problems with bowel or bladder control.

Past medical history is noteworthy in that the patient filed a workers' compensation claim a year ago because of a low back injury that he sustained at work. He underwent an L5-S1 discectomy and was out of work for 6 months. He was eventually able to return to work as a mechanic, and his claim was closed. Although his low back pain never fully resolved after the injury a year ago, he is very definite that his symptoms during the past 24 hours have been much worse than any he has had since the day of his injury a year ago. His employer now is different from the one he had when he was injured a year ago. The rest of his past medical history is unremarkable.

Social history indicates that the patient is a high school graduate. All of his work experience has been in the area of automobile repair. He is married and has 2 children aged 10 and 7 years.

Physical examination is noteworthy in that he stands leaning forward, with complete flattening of the lumbar lordotic curve. He walks very slowly. Palpation reveals diffuse spasms in the lumbar paraspinal muscles, along with significant soft tissue tenderness. The patient demonstrates virtually zero range of motion of the lumbar spine in all planes. Straight leg raising is limited by back pain rather than radicular symptoms. The neurologic examination reveals diffuse, bilateral lower extremity weakness that seems to reflect pain inhibition. The only focal sign is a diminished right ankle jerk, which the patient says has been present since his original back injury. He is positive on 3 of the 5 Waddell signs.

He says he is in too much pain to work.

The patient asks you to fill out an industrial insurance accident form (**Fig. 1**). You indicate the following:

No. 41: Diagnosis: lumbosacral strain (847.2)

No. 45: Objective findings: muscle spasms, severely restricted lumbar range of motion in all planes, diminished right ankle jerk

No. 47: Was the diagnosed condition caused by this injury or exposure? Probably

No. 48: Will the condition cause the patient to miss work? YES, 10 days

No. 49: Is there any preexisting impairment of the injured area? YES

No. 50: Has patient ever been treated for the same or similar condition? YES

You agree to become the attending physician for Mr Smith's claim, and you outline a conservative treatment plan for him. It consists of a referral to physical therapy and prescription of diclofenac 75 mg twice a day.

Comments

1. JPR: The patient's presentation is a typical one: acute onset of nonradicular low back pain.
2. JPR: In filling out the required accident report, you are forced to make several judgments about impairment and disability:
   a. You must decide whether to conceptualize the patient's problem as a new injury or as an aggravation of the lumbar spine problem he developed a year earlier. If the problem is conceptualized as a new injury, claim opening is fairly easy. If it is conceptualized as an aggravation, the question will be whether his claim from a year ago should be reopened. To determine the answer to this, workers' compensation claim managers will probably ask you to review past records on the patient and indicate whether there is objective evidence that his condition has worsened.
      i. The diagnosis of lumbosacral strain embodies the concept that you are conceptualizing the patient's problem as a new injury.
   b. LSG: Administrative agencies often require that a physician buttress his or her conclusions with objective findings. This requirement may serve as a source of conflict: On the one hand, the physician may think that there is no uniformly accepted definition of objective findings[1]; on the other hand, the insurer and employer may be unwilling to pay significant sums of money in response to a claim that lacks objective findings of injury. In this example
      i. JPR: Most physicians would accept the objectivity of a depressed ankle jerk reflex. In this patient, it is quite likely that the depressed right ankle jerk reflex stems from the back injury a year ago. But if an insurer insists on the identification of objective findings, you should strongly consider listing the abnormal reflex in answer to item No. 45.
      ii. JPR: The status of muscle spasms and restricted lumbar range of motion is less clear. They are not completely objective because patients have some control over the tightness of muscles in their backs and over how much they move when a physician assesses active range of motion.
      iii. LSG: What *is* clear is that an answer to item No. 45 is needed in some way. As a practical matter, the claims managers who review accident reports are likely to have only the medical information on the report and perhaps that which appears in a contemporaneously prepared clinic note. For that reason, and because the information in the report will serve as the medical foundation on which the remainder of the claim will be built, it is important

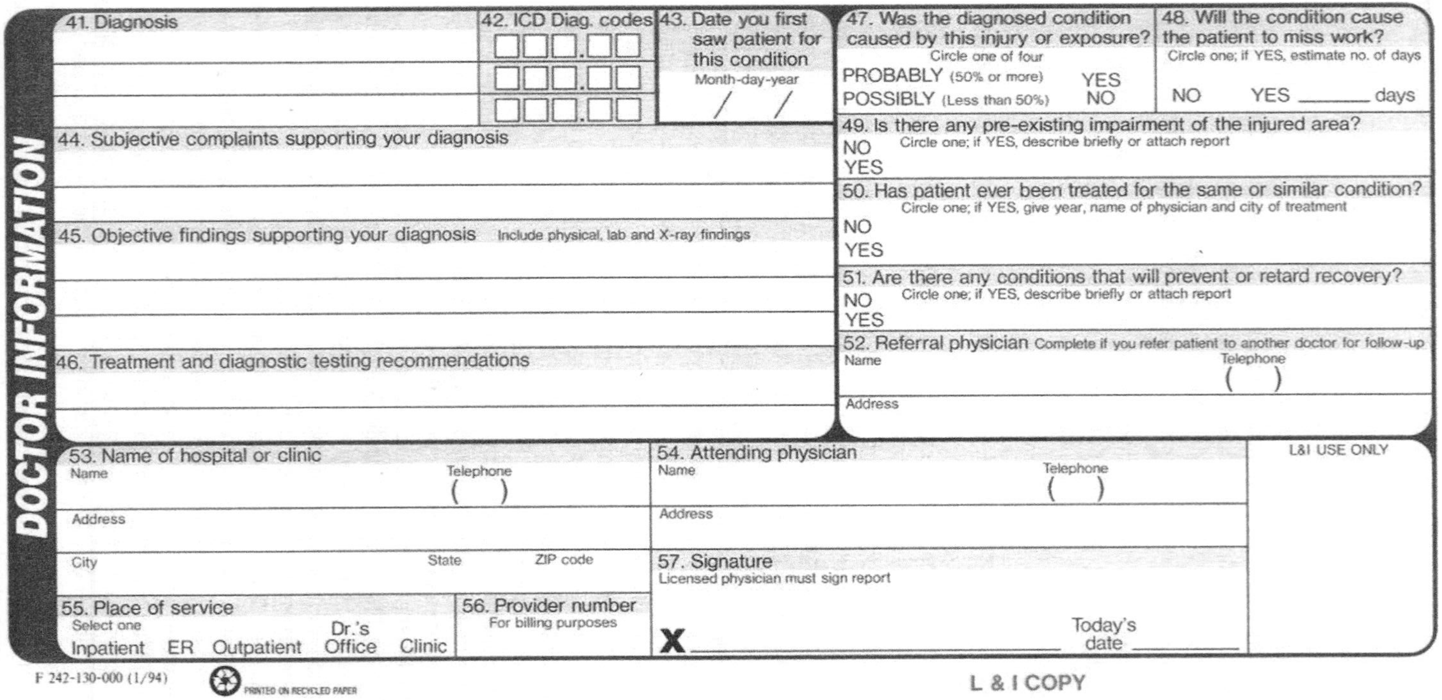
DOCTOR INFORMATION

41. Diagnosis

42. ICD Diag. codes

43. Date you first saw patient for this condition
Month-day-year
/ /

44. Subjective complaints supporting your diagnosis

45. Objective findings supporting your diagnosis Include physical, lab and X-ray findings

46. Treatment and diagnostic testing recommendations

47. Was the diagnosed condition caused by this injury or exposure?
Circle one of four
PROBABLY (50% or more) YES
POSSIBLY (Less than 50%) NO

48. Will the condition cause the patient to miss work?
Circle one; if YES, estimate no. of days
NO YES ______ days

49. Is there any pre-existing impairment of the injured area?
Circle one; if YES, describe briefly or attach report
NO
YES

50. Has patient ever been treated for the same or similar condition?
Circle one; if YES, give year, name of physician and city of treatment
NO
YES

51. Are there any conditions that will prevent or retard recovery?
Circle one; if YES, describe briefly or attach report
NO
YES

52. Referral physician Complete if you refer patient to another doctor for follow-up
Name Telephone ( )
Address

53. Name of hospital or clinic
Name Telephone ( )
Address
City State ZIP code

54. Attending physician
Name Telephone ( )
Address

L&I USE ONLY

55. Place of service
Select one
Inpatient ER Outpatient Dr.'s Office Clinic

56. Provider number
For billing purposes

57. Signature
Licensed physician must sign report
X ______ Today's date ______

F 242-130-000 (1/94) PRINTED ON RECYCLED PAPER
L & I COPY

Fig. 1. Example of a portion of a report of industrial injury or occupational disease: selected questions. *From* Washington State Department of Labor and Injuries, Olympia, WA.

that it be as accurate as possible. Most states, through regulation, judicial determination, or general practice, expect that claim managers will, in the absence of a clear reason to do otherwise, accept the information on the accident report form and make claim allowance determinations accordingly.

c. JPR: When a physician gives a diagnosis (No. 41), states objective findings that support the diagnosis (No. 45), and reports that the diagnosed condition was probably caused by the patients' work (No. 47), he or she is in effect urging the insurer to accept the patients' condition as work related. This step is necessary on the way to medical or disability benefits, that is, a worker must have a valid workers' compensation claim before he or she can get workers' compensation benefits.

d. JPR: The indication that Mr Smith's condition will cause him to lose 10 days of work (No. 48) supports the contention that he is work disabled and, therefore, entitled to disability benefits (ie, cash payments to substitute for his inability to work). In the language of workers' compensation law, Mr Smith deserves benefits if he is judged to be temporarily, totally disabled from work.

e. LSG: Items No. 49 and No. 50 address the issue of previous problems that Mr Smith has had with his lumbar spine. As noted earlier, his new symptoms can be construed as either an aggravation of an old lumbar spine condition or as a new injury. The issue aggravation of an old injury vs. occurrence of a new injury can have significant economic consequences for an employer; as a result, the issue of employer liability is often the source of litigation.

f. LSG: In a general way, it is important to note that in filling out the required accident report, you have made important judgments regarding Mr Smith. There are now contentions that he has a musculoskeletal injury, that the injury was likely caused by his employment, and that he is disabled by virtue of his injury. Such judgments are typically made primarily by what patients say; it is rare to have completely objective indices of the severity of patients' incapacitation from low back pain; often physicians do not have independent confirmation that patients became symptomatic because of their work.

g. LSG: Unless a physician has caused an insurer to doubt the veracity of his or her documentation, the workers' compensation system tends to be permissive when it processes accident reports in that the accuracy of the reporting physician's statements is rarely questioned.

3. LSG: A decision to become attending physician for Mr Smith's claim carries with it significant responsibilities. In part, it means that you will be required to not only orchestrate his treatment but also to address a multitude of administrative issues that may come up regarding the claim.

a. The attending physician's treatment plan should reflect his or her multiple responsibilities and, to the extent possible, take into consideration the needs of all the participants in a workers' compensation claim. For example, a claim manager will react positively to a time-limited, goal-oriented, global treatment plan that incorporates a branching algorithm of treatment possibilities, all of which end with the worker at maximum medical improvement. Claim manager agreement with such an approach will likely be heightened if the plan includes the following elements:

   i. The overall duration of the plan is specified. In a case such as the one here, it might be reasonable to conclude early on that all likely approaches to this patient's low back pain, including surgery, if that was to become an option, could be concluded in 1 year. The maximum length of such a plan, therefore, might be 1 year.

ii. The goals of the treatment plan should be clearly articulated. A physician might phrase such a goal as follows: return to work in employment that does not require lifting more than 15 pounds or frequent bending

iii. The frequency at which progress toward the plan goals will be measured should be included. This frequency may vary depending on the specifics of the plan at any one time. Monthly measurements of progress might be appropriate at some points, and every 2 weeks might be more appropriate at others.

iv. The objective criteria by which the physician will determine whether progress toward the plan's goals is being made should be included. The statement, *patient has less pain today*, may be accurate but it will not likely meet the needs of an insurer that reads such comments daily in the claim files of workers who are not progressing in any meaningful health care direction.

v. The agreement of the IW and, if appropriate, the IW's spouse or significant other that the plan is one to which the worker will give his or her best efforts to help it succeed should be included.

August 1, 2012: Mr Smith seems to have improved modestly from his conservative treatment program but continues to complain of persistent, localized low back pain that is severe enough to prevent him from returning to his auto mechanic job. His employer contacts you and requests a conference to discuss Mr Smith's ongoing symptoms and prospects for returning to work.

Comment

LSG: Many experts in workers' compensation emphasize that treating physicians who communicate with employers regarding return-to-work issues can be highly effective in minimizing disability by, for example, helping an employer see the benefits of a return to restricted employment during the recovery phase of an injury.[2] Ironically, patients may perceive their doctors' communication with an employer as a suspicious activity, whereas an employer may conclude that a doctor whose knowledge of the work site comes solely from an injured employee is not getting accurate job-related information. Such problems can be minimized if the treating physician on the first visit sets his or her patients' expectations, one of which should be that the doctor will be taking all appropriate steps to having patients back to a wage-earning position as quickly as possible. Communication regarding the return-to-work job requirements should be accurately understood by all concerned. This understanding can generally be arrived at most efficiently through an in-person or teleconference that involves the physician, the worker, and an employer representative.

October 1, 2012: You receive a letter from the workers' compensation insurer. It asks whether Mr Smith has reached maximal medical improvement and whether he continues to have impairments that prevent him from working. It requests that you present the objective findings on which your conclusions are based. You respond that Mr Smith's functional capacities as measured by his physical therapist continue to increase, so that he is not yet at maximal medical improvement. Also, you express the view that he needs further evaluation, specifically, a lumbar MRI scan and surgical consultation. You offer your opinion that he is not currently able to return to his job as an auto mechanic. You cite his limited lumbar range of motion and his diminished right ankle jerk reflex as objective findings buttressing your conclusion.

Comments
1. JPR, LSG: The issue of maximal medical improvement is closely linked to disability issues for an individual with a workers' compensation claim. Specifically, compensation law generally requires that some decision be made about a worker's employment capabilities when he or she is judged to have achieved maximal medical improvement. Typically, compensation systems are more willing to accept at face value the opinions of treating physicians during the first few weeks after an injury, principally because such opinions relate mostly to purely medical issues. But later in the course of a claim, when an opinion may more directly relate to the continuation of time loss or other payments, claims managers may be more likely to challenge the opinions of the attending physician, for example, by commissioning an independent medical examination. The issue of maximum medical improvement embodies substantial monetary issues and is a frequent source of litigation in workers' compensation cases.
2. LSG: At its roots, the need for objective findings is economic, not medical. Somebody has to pay the bills generated by workplace injuries. In workers' compensation cases, that somebody is generally the employer or its insurer (which will spend the employer's premium dollars). To assure that the workers' compensation system comes as close as possible to providing needed benefits to IWs without burdening employers with payments to people who could be gainfully employed, workers' compensation systems seek objective evidence on which to base their payment decisions.
3. JPR: In this case, your conclusion that Mr Smith cannot work as an auto mechanic is based largely on the following considerations: (1) He has a complex lumbar spine problem that can produce intolerance of physically demanding work. (2) He has repeatedly stated that he cannot handle the physical demands of work as an auto mechanic. (3) Having treated him for 6 months, you have formed the clinical judgment that his reports regarding his physical capacities are credible. The following is an example of the fundamental dilemma of assessing disability based on pain: The patient reports severe activity restrictions because of his pain; but there is nothing you can do in your office to confirm or disconfirm his statements about his activity restrictions. To a large extent, your decision about whether to support his assertions rests on whether you find the assertions credible. The compensation system, however, seeks objective evidence to verify your subjective opinions. As suggested in the case history, probably the best way to address this mismatch is simply to state the patient's physical findings, regardless of whether they lead inevitably to a conclusion about the patient's work capacity.

November 15, 2012: Mr Smith has now undergone an MRI scan and has had a surgical consultation. The MRI showed severe degenerative disk changes at L5-S1, with loss of disk height and Modic changes. But there is no evidence of compromise of neural elements. The surgeon whom Mr Smith saw concluded that lumbar spine surgery was unlikely to be helpful.

Comment
JPR: As a general rule, lumbar spine surgery is much more likely to be helpful when treating symptoms of radiculopathy rather than when treating mechanical low back pain. Some spine surgeons think that patients who have low back pain but no evidence of radiculopathy can benefit from spinal fusions. However, at least among IWs, spinal fusions for low back pain have produced very disappointing results.[3] Thus, the assessment of the surgeon seems to be appropriate.

12/1/12: You refer Mr Smith to a pain specialist for opinions regarding therapeutic options to facilitate his recovery. She concludes that Mr Smith might benefit from a modest dose of opioids and prescribes oxycodone/acetaminophen (Percocet) (5/325) tablets for him, with instructions that he can take up to 4 tablets per day. By the time you see Mr Smith 4 weeks later, he is taking Percocet and is emphatic that it permits him to function better. His physical therapist corroborates Mr Smith's assessment; she indicates that his performance in physical therapy has improved substantially since he started Percocet. Because there is credible evidence that initiation of Percocet therapy has allowed Mr Smith to function better, you elect to keep him on the medication and take over prescribing it.

Comment

JPR: In this case history, there is credible evidence from the IW and from his physical therapist that he has been able to function better after starting Percocet. But this positive outcome from an opioid is by no means guaranteed. In fact, the efficacy of opioid therapy in the context of work injuries is questionable. Although short-term randomized controlled trials on patients who are not IWs provide reasonably persuasive evidence that opioids may reduce pain, evidence for functional improvement from opioid therapy is much less impressive. Evidence from workers' compensation agencies should also give the clinician pause about the efficacy of opioids for IWs. Several recent studies have shown that IWs who receive opioids are likely to remain disabled for longer time periods than ones who do not receive opioids.[4–7] Thus, in these studies, opioid therapy could be viewed as a risk factor for prolonged disability. It should be noted that research based on large workers' compensation databases can be misleading. In particular, one could argue that IWs with more severe problems may be more likely to receive opioids than those with less severe injuries. Thus, severity of injury could be the driving force behind both use of opioids and delayed recovery. For example, Gross and colleagues[5] state: "As expected, claimants with more severe injuries were more likely to receive opioids. An association was observed between early opioid prescription and delayed recovery, however, this is likely explained by pain severity or other unmeasured confounders."[5(p525)] In summary, though the findings from some workers' compensation database studies are not conclusive, at a minimum they certainly challenge the hypothesis that opioids have a role in facilitating functional recovery for IWs with noncancer pain.

In applying these data to individual IWs, it is crucial that a physician who prescribes an opioid makes sure that the worker receiving the medication demonstrates improved function. Mr Smith did in fact demonstrate such improvement, so it was reasonable for him to be continued on a modest dose of opioids.

February 1, 2013: Mr Smith has now been assigned a vocational rehabilitation counselor by the insurer. The vocational rehabilitation counselor has filled out a job analysis for the position that Mr Smith held at the time of his injury. You review the job analysis with Mr Smith at his next scheduled visit. He complains that it is grossly inaccurate. For example, although the job analysis says that his job requires no lifting more than 35 pounds, Mr Smith insists that before his injury he frequently had to lift objects weighing up to 80 pounds. He also asserts that he is unable to spend long periods of time bent over the hood of a car. You request a formal physical capacities evaluation to determine his lifting capacity and his ability to work in the postures required by his auto mechanic job. Based on Mr Smith's statements, your physical examination findings, and the results of the physical capacities evaluation, you indicate that in your opinion Mr Smith is not able to do the work described in the job analysis.

Comments
1. JPR: It is common for IWs to complain that job analyses provide a distorted picture of what their work actually requires. It is important for you to discuss a job analysis with an IW so that you learn whether there is a significant difference between the job as described in the job analysis and the worker's perception of what the job requires. If there is a significant gap between the employer's description of the job and the perception offered by the worker, the differences need to be resolved without unnecessary delay. A physician seeking to remain objective in his or her assessment of job requirements might choose to request that the employer allow the physician a tour of the workplace with an emphasis on the patient's work station and duties.
2. LSG: It should be noted that physicians often place themselves into positions of conflict that could easily have been avoided. The communication of the conclusion that Mr Smith is not able to do the work that is described in the job analysis will likely cause unnecessary conflict: One party takes one position and the other the opposite, and the physician is in the hot seat. The way for the physician to avoid such conflict is not to become a party to it. As a neutral in such disputes, the physician can offer a statement to the following effect: If the job is as described by the employer, my patient can safely return to that work. If, however, the job is as described by my patient, he cannot. I will leave it to others to come to a decision as to the requirements that the job entails.

   Apart from the potential for introducing otherwise avoidable conflict, a physician's statement that an IW cannot perform a particular job may not turn out to be in the best interests of the patient. It is likely that the statement to the employer will result in litigation, which will delay the patient's progress through the workers' compensation system. Another possibility is that it will result in the worker losing a job that was being held for him. At some point in the future, the patient will likely be seeking employment; a potential employer, although never admitting the real reason, may be disinclined to hire somebody whose prior employment ended in a workers' compensation claim. In the long run, the patient may be better served by a prompt return to safe employment; both the employer and the insurer may be open to discussions that have such a focus.

   Patients, employers, and insurers can become equally invested emotionally in disparate beliefs regarding any given issue in a workers' compensation case. In the end, patients, employers, and insures will all benefit from a process that leads to an accurate assessment of, and planned response to, an issue that generates such conflict. By virtue of their knowledge and training, attending physicians can facilitate the analysis and resolution of such issues. Physicians can facilitate the effectiveness of the workers' compensation process by establishing at the outset that the role of the physician in a workers' compensation case is to assist the worker in safely returning to employment at the earliest reasonable date. They can also help workers understand that although the role of lawyers is to get their clients what their clients want, the role of doctors is to get their patients what the patients need to return to health and function as safely and as efficiently as possible.

3. LSG: Should there remain unresolved differences between the stated demands of the job and the demands perceived by a patient, the physician should explain via a letter to the employer what the patients' working restrictions are and notify the employer that the patients is not being released to work that is beyond those restrictions.

4. JPR: It is often difficult for a physician to determine how restricted an IW is in work activities from office examinations. In this setting, functional capacities evaluations (typically performed by physical therapists) can provide objective data about what an IW actually does in a test situation (eg, how much he or she lifts, how long he or she sits continuously, and so forth). A functional capacities evaluation is by no means a foolproof solution to the problem of determining activity limitations in patients with a chronic pain problem or the ability of patients to do various kinds of work.[8–10] But at least it provides some performance data, which is more than a physician can glean simply by doing an office examination on a patient.

March 1, 2013: Mr Smith brings 2 forms to his scheduled office visit. The first is from a company that has financed the purchase of the car he owns. When he arranged financing, he purchased an insurance option; it stipulates that his car payments will be deferred if his treating physician asserts that he is totally disabled from any kind of work and that the disability is likely to continue for more than a year. You agree to support his request for deferment. The second form is from the Department of Motor Vehicles. It is an application for a disabled parking sticker. The patient says he needs to have a disabled parking sticker because his back pain becomes intolerable if he has to walk more than 200 yards. You tell him that you will not support his application for a disabled parking sticker.

Comments
1. JPR, LSG: These 2 requests have no inherent relation to Mr Smith's workers' compensation claim. But they give a flavor of the types of disability decisions a treating physician is called on to make. These extraneous disability requests can create stress for the treating physician and may well have an impact on patients' perceptions regarding their work disability. Also, they may undercut the physician's message that return to work in the near future is an achievable and desirable goal. Although a physician's acquiescence to a request that he or she knows is not in the patients' best interests may provide short-term relief of the physician's stress from the encounter, it will not really help patients and in the long run and it will not help the physician either. If the physician thinks that what is being requested is not in the patients' best interests, the most helpful approach the physician can offer patients is a caring encounter that is focused on a return to an able-bodied life.
2. LSG: The auto financing insurance form creates a potential legal problem for the physician because to be effective it requires the physician to characterize Mr Smith has having long-term, total disability when the physician presumably knows that such is not inevitably the case. Chronic low back pain is not necessarily disabling; if it is, the disability is not necessary lengthy. Wounded soldiers have returned from battlefields with far worse conditions and have returned to gainful employment. If the message to the auto financer is incongruent with messages regarding disability that are being given to Mr Smith in relation to his workers' compensation claim, the question of fraud may be raised by the insurer.
3. JPR: A disabled parking sticker raises similar issues, though likely of a lesser nature. At a minimum, the physician's assistance in the acquisition of the sticker may also affect Mr Smith's perception of himself as a permanently disabled person. Although there is no logical incompatibility between Mr Smith's having a disabled parking sticker and his returning to work, there may well be a psychological inconsistency.

April 1, 2013: Mr Smith indicates that his workers' compensation claims manager has strongly urged him to apply for Social Security Disability Insurance (SSDI). He indicates that he has started the SSDI application process and has been told that disability adjudicators for the Social Security Administration (SSA) will soon be asking you to provide information about his medical condition. You urge him to delay the SSDI application process until he has gotten definitive information about whether his workers' compensation insurance carrier will provide vocational rehabilitation services for him.

Comments

1. LSG: Although nominally the interests of the IW, his or her employer, and the workers' compensation insurance carrier would seem to be aligned around a single, common interest, the safe and efficient return of the worker to health, function, and employment, in reality their interests may be quite divergent. Communication with the various participants in a workers' compensation claim will likely be most efficient if it is interest focused.

   In this case, the insurer's effort to transfer the burden of disability costs to SSDI is contrary to the purpose of workers' compensation insurance and it is contrary to the purpose of the SSDI program. In all likelihood, the claims manager is well aware that what is being requested is not in keeping with the purpose of either form of insurance.

   One possible explanation for the claims manager's reaction is that it is a response to the push by the IW and his doctor for permanent total disability status as the result of an industrial injury that created symptoms that are experienced on a regular basis by a significant percentage of the working population and does not require surgery. The claims manager's interest may be to limit the insurer's liability for a permanent, total disability claim that does not, to the insurer, seem valid.

2. LSG: At this point, the employer's interest in the outcome of the workers' compensation claim is unknown. If an IW has been a good employee, many employers will do what they can to help the worker return to his or her job. Still the bottom line for private sector employers is that they must either make a profit or go out of business, and that reality may force an otherwise willing employer to cut its losses by permanently replacing the IW and seeking to minimize the costs of the existing claim.

   Thus, for 2, possibly 3, of the parties to the worker's claim, the SSDI application is not in their best interests. This undesirable turn of events is likely frustrating for all concerned. It does, however, offer the engaged physician the opportunity to engage in communication that may better align the direction of the claim with the parties' respective interests.

3. JPR: In terms of perceptions of disability by an IW, an SSDI application represents a kiss of death. An individual can obtain an SSDI award only if he or she can convince adjudicators that he or she is totally and permanently disabled. Long-term studies show that only about 12% of individuals who are awarded SSDI benefits ever return to the work force on a sustained basis.[11] Although it is theoretically possible for a person to continue to seek employment while he or she is applying for SSDI, informal observation and the limited data available[12] strongly suggest that an individual's probability of vocational rehabilitation is low once he or she starts the SSDI application process.

4. JPR: The treating physician is often in an uncomfortable position when an individual on workers' compensation starts an SSDI application. On the one hand, the

physician will appropriately anticipate that the worker will be more refractory to vocational rehabilitation once he or she starts the SSDI application process. On the other hand, he or she may well be concerned about timelines and backup plans for the worker. One issue is that individuals who apply for SSDI because of painful conditions like low back pain often have their initial claims denied.[13] Their claims may be accepted on appeal, but the process of going through multiple levels of the SSA appeals process can easily take more than a year. In the mean time, the worker faces the risk of having his or her time-loss benefits abruptly terminated by his workers' compensation carrier. From this perspective, an early application for SSDI might be viewed as an insurance policy for a worker who is having difficulty returning to work, even if he or she has not totally given up the goal of returning to work. In an ideal world, workers' compensation agencies would work cooperatively with other agencies to make sure that IWs do not get caught in the middle between different benefit programs. In fact, this kind of cooperation rarely occurs.

May 1, 2013: Mr Smith's claims manager schedules him for an independent medical examination. The examination is performed by an orthopedist, a physiatrist, and a psychiatrist. The orthopedist and physiatrist collaborate to generate a medical/surgical report; the psychiatrist submits a separate report. The medical/surgical report states that the patient has reached maximal medical improvement from his lumbar strain of June 1, 2012. He is thought to have no permanent partial impairment over and above the 10% impairment that was awarded when his earlier lumbar spine claim was closed. The report states that are no objective findings that would prevent Mr Smith from working on a full time basis in a job with medium physical requirements." The psychiatrist diagnoses pain disorder associated with psychological factors and a general medical condition (*Diagnostic and Statistical Manual of Mental Disorders* [Fourth Edition] 307.89).[14] Both the medical/surgical and the psychiatric reports indicate that Mr Smith's claim is ready for closure. A copy of the independent medical examination report is sent to you, and you are asked: (1) to indicate your agreement or disagreement with it and (2) if you disagree with the report, to state the objective findings on which your opinions are based. You respond that Mr Smith probably has reached maximal medical improvement but that you do not think that he can work on a full-time basis as an auto mechanic. You note that he has shown consistent activity limitations and that his reported activity limitations are credible. You indicate that he needs a careful vocational assessment and identification of specific job options before his claim is closed.

Comments

1. LSG: There are 2 principal means of resolving medical issues in workers' compensation cases: consultations and independent medical examinations. The attending physician typically seeks consultations. When they occur with the agreement of the insurer, they usually promptly provide either resolution of a medical issue or a recommendation for further exploration of the issue. Independent medical examinations are typically sought by insurers to resolve medical or medical-legal issues. They usually occur without the agreement of the attending physician, and they often polarize rather than resolve matters of concern. Rightly or wrongly, such evaluations are a source of considerable stress for many IWs; they often do more to impair collaborative discussion among the parties than further such conversations.

2. JPR: Independent medical examinations routinely perpetuate the assumption that physicians can objectively measure impairments and associated work restrictions. The statement that "There are no objective findings that would prevent Mr Smith

from working on a full-time basis in a job with medium physical requirements" could be made about virtually every patient with low back pain. But the reality is that back pain is one of the most common causes of disability in working-aged people.[15] To paraphrase Osterweis and colleagues,[13] back pain disables people not because their backs fail mechanically but because back problems can create unbearable sensations that limit activities. Treating physicians need to avoid falling into the conceptual trap of concluding that disability can be supported only if there are objective findings that make the disability inevitable.

3. JPR: Nonpsychiatric physicians may well feel intimidated by psychiatric evaluations that purport to say what is really underlying an IW's pain complaints. It is important to realize that, although psychiatric disorders may well be major factors underlying the pain complaints of some patients, this is by no means universal. Even if patients with chronic low back pain have a psychiatric condition, the role that this plays in their ongoing pain complaints is often uncertain. Also, although diagnostic criteria for some psychiatric disorders, such as major depressive disorder, are well established, the diagnoses given to many patients with chronic pain are much less well validated. In particular, you should look with some skepticism on a diagnosis of pain disorder.[16]

4. LSG: An attending physician might well feel overwhelmed by a strongly worded independent medical examination report signed by 3 physicians. Regardless, the attending physician will best serve the interests of his or her patients if he or she responds articulately and unemotionally to whatever opinions the independent medical examiners may have offered. The attending physician should understand that the workers' compensation process has well-defined rules for giving weight to the evidence with which it is presented. Medical issues are generally resolved by lawyers or judges who have no training in medicine by applying rules that may be equally distant from a medical nexus. The process and its rules are reflective of the system's shared ownership by business and labor. In this system, medicine plays a supporting, not a leading, role in the resolution of workers' compensation disputes.

July 1, 2013: The workers's compensation insurer's claims manager indicates that the insurer has accepted your assessment that Mr Smith is not able to return to the job of auto mechanic and that his claim is not ready for closure. She retains a new vocational rehabilitation counselor to do an employability assessment on Mr Smith (ie, to see whether Mr Smith's physical capabilities and past work history permit him to work in any field other than auto repair). The vocational rehabilitation counselor notes that, at 18 years of age, Mr Smith worked for 3 months as a dishwasher and asks you to sign a job analysis for this kind of work. You meet with Mr Smith to discuss the job analysis. He protests that dishwashing requires more bending, lifting, and standing than he can do. He also notes that he and his family will be impoverished if he is left with no choice other than doing entry-level work. You refuse to sign the job analysis on the ground that the physical demands of dishwashing exceed Mr Smith's capabilities.

Comments
1. LSG: Vocational rehabilitation services in the various states' workers' compensation systems reflect the differing degrees to which legislatures have been willing to fund, or mandate funding, to retrain IWs. The deliberations of legislators, and the compromises they make, usually occur far from the offices of the physicians who will be involved in workers' rehabilitation processes. Although such a process may be a formula for disappointment, it generally establishes a fairly clear process for the assessment and resolution of vocational rehabilitation issues.

In most states' systems, through compromise and release, an IW may settle a workers' compensation claim through an agreement with the insurer. In many states, such settlements may resolve all vocational rehabilitation issues as well as other issues, such as medical care, time-loss payments, and the like. Some states, however, are far more restrictive; such settlements are either not allowed at all or are allowed only in very narrowly defined circumstances.

In the example case, the claim manager may or may not be acting within the scope of a governing law or administrative regulation in seeking a declaration that Mr Smith is employable as a dishwasher. Regardless, the vocational issue raises a medical issue: disregarding for a moment Mr Smith's statements regarding his level of pain, does he have the physical ability to engage in the occupation of dishwasher? The attending physician might find it productive to request that the insurer fund another physical capacities assessment by a person or entity that is agreeable to both the physician and the insurer. Such evaluations can add a degree of objectivity that otherwise would be absent in a discussion of vocational rehabilitation issues.

Ultimately, it will be the responsibility of the workers' compensation system to determine whether the IW is capable of successfully returning to some form of gainful employment. The discussions that occur in this regard rarely address a fundamental irony that is an inherent part of the system: the cross-purposes at which the workers' compensation systems and the Americans with Disabilities Act work.

Most vocational rehabilitation disputes place the attending physician in the position of the physician in the example case: The physician must state whether a patient can or cannot return to some specified form of employment. Physicians generally think that they face a difficult choice: They can agree that patients can safely return to work in the specified form of employment and thereby risk alienating the patients or they can offer the opposite opinion and in the process alienate the insurer with all of the potential administrative complications that such alienation could cause.

There is a different way to approach resolution of such disputes, and it is one that places the resolution more in alignment with all (not just some) of our laws: Rather than ask whether the worker can return to work in the named job, the question can be framed as follows: If the worker seeks employment in the named job, could I, as a physician, in good faith support the worker's efforts? Phrased in that manner, both the interests of the workers' compensation system and the Americans with Disabilities Act are advanced.

In our country, if an IW was refused a job because of an actual or perceived disability, if the worker could perform the essential functions of the job with or without a reasonable accommodation, the refusal of employment would be illegal. Phrasing the issue as just suggested changes the focus from the results of a physical capacity assessment with which the worker might disagree to what the workers' compensation system really needs to know: If the worker wanted to, could he or she succeed in the job? A second benefit from framing the issue as just suggested is that by being phrased hypothetically, it is less likely to directly conflict with the position of a worker who does not want to return to employment as a dishwasher.

2. JPR: When an IW is judged not to be able to return to the job he or she had at the time of injury, at least some workers' compensation systems ask a vocational rehabilitation counselor to review his or her entire work history and to determine whether, based on his or her skills and physical capabilities, the worker can

perform any kind of work. Most workers who go through this kind of vocational assessment are placed in one of 3 categories:

a. They are judged to be employable based on work they have done at some earlier time in their lives. (Workers in this category typically have their time-loss benefits terminated.)

b. They are judged to need vocational retraining in order to be employable. (Workers in this category are typically authorized for vocational rehabilitation services.)

c. They are judged to be unemployable under any circumstances. (Workers in this category typically receive a pension.)

IWs and treating physicians often look at category No. 1 with some skepticism. One issue is that workers may be judged employable by the entry-level work that they did when they first entered the labor force. Even if a worker is physically able to do such entry-level work (eg, a job at a fast food restaurant), the remuneration from the work is often very low. Also, some of the jobs that are proposed by vocational rehabilitation counselors seem contrived. For example, a person with a severe lumbar spine condition might be judged to be employable as a telephone solicitor.

September 1, 2013: Mr Smith is accepted for vocational rehabilitation services. He and his vocational rehabilitation counselor develop a plan for him to work in an auto parts store. It is determined that Mr Smith will need 6 months of training in order to have the skills needed for this kind of work. The workers' compensation insurer requests that you review the physical requirements of a salesman in an auto parts store. You review the appropriate job analysis with Mr Smith and sign it. Mr Smith goes through the 6-month training program.

Comments

1. JPR: A formal vocational rehabilitation plan represents the last step in most insurers' procedures for assisting IWs in their return to the work force. A vocational rehabilitation counselor assigned by the insurer typically first works with an IW to develop a vocational rehabilitation plan. Most insurers provide only modest funding for retraining and generally insist that the attending physician indicate that the job for which patients will be trained is within their physical capacities.

May 15, 2014: Mr Smith has finished his vocational training and has applied for jobs in several auto parts stores. All of his applications have been rejected. He expresses the view that employers are discriminating against him because he continues to use Percocet.

Comments

1. JPR: Even if an IW on opioid therapy reports pain relief, improves functionally, and seems to be ready to return to work, continued opioid therapy may act as a barrier to his or her successful return to work. Issues related to the ability of IWs on opioids to return to work divide into 2 groups: impairment in work activities secondary to opioid use and unwillingness of employers to hire IWs on opioids. It is beyond the scope of this article to review the voluminous research that has been done on cognitive impairment from opioids that might adversely affect the ability of an individual to work.[17]

2. JPR: The authors are unaware of systematic data on the frequency with which employers reject job applicants because of their use of prescription opioids. Clearly, though, efforts by IWs on opioids to return to work may run afoul of programs established by private industry and governments at the federal and state level to create drug-free workplaces.[18] For example, the Drug Free Workplace Act of

1988 required organizations that contract with the federal government to establish programs to reduce drug abuse by employees.[19] As one component of programs to reduce inappropriate use of illicit drugs and alcohol, many companies have required employees to undergo urine drug tests.[20,21]

Discussions about drug-free workplaces are routinely framed in terms of the need to prevent workers from using illicit substances, psychoactive substances that have not been prescribed for them, or excessive alcohol. The status of prescription opioids is ambiguous. For example, in a recent publication entitled "What Employees Need to Know About [Department of Transportation] DOT Drug and Alcohol Testing," the DOT[22] stated: "Prescription medicine and [over-the-counter] OTC drugs may be allowed."[22(p3)] The document then listed requirements that must be met in order for patients on prescription medications to engage in safety-sensitive work for the DOT. One requirement is that prescribing physicians indicate that the medication "is consistent with the safe performance of your duties."[22] But the DOT makes clear that meeting the stated requirements may not be sufficient because subsidiary organizations within the DOT might establish different standards regarding opioids. As an example of this, the Federal Aviation Administration, a subsidiary of the DOT, does not permit pilots to use any prescription opioid.[23]

3. JPR: Given the multiple policies used by governmental organizations and private companies, it is difficult to know how likely it is that patients' job applications will be compromised by their use of prescription opioids. To make matters more complicated, cases regarding the rights of opioid users in the workplace are currently being litigated.[24] The balance between an employer's right to maintain a safe, drug-free work environment and an employee's privacy rights and right to work while using medications sanctioned by a physician has not been determined.

In theory, at least according to the Equal Employment Opportunity Administration, applicants for jobs do not need to provide information about their prescription medications.[25] But the practicality of this protection of privacy is vitiated by the fact that employers have the right to demand urine drug testing before an applicant is accepted for a job.[26] Thus, prospective employers can learn that a job candidate is using opioids. Although urine drug testing is supposed to be deferred until after an applicant has been assured of a job, this safeguard can easily be circumvented.

In summary, although the implications of prescription opioids for reintegration into the workforce are not entirely clear, physicians need to be aware that when they treat IWs with long-term opioids, they may well be prejudicing the chances of the IWs to reenter the work force. In the present case example, Mr Smith was rejected by many employers for unknown reasons. His use of Percocet may have prejudiced employers against him, but there is no way to be certain of this.

August 1, 2014: Mr Smith is finally hired for a full-time position as a salesman in an auto parts store. Although he continues to complain of back pain, he is able to carry out his job responsibilities consistently, with no time lost from work because of back pain. His workers' compensation claim is closed 4 months after his successful return to work.

Comment

JPR: This case history has a happy ending. Mr Smith makes a successful reentry into the work force, and his claim is closed. In real-life situations, the likelihood of the outcome described in the example is low for a person who has been disabled for the past 2 years. Moreover, an outcome that is successful from the standpoint of an *individual claim* may not be successful from the standpoint of the *person* with a chronic low back problem.[27–29] Long-term follow-up data indicate that an individual like Mr Smith is at high risk to have still another back injury and file another compensation claim before the time when he reaches retirement age.

GENERAL COMMENTS

The aforementioned example highlights the kinds of challenges that a physician treating an IW often confronts. A few general points deserve emphasis:

1. The dates given for various events in this hypothetical case cover the interval between June 1, 2012 and August 1, 2014 (ie, more than 2 years). To some extent, the slow evolution of Mr Smith's claim reflects the complexity of the workers' compensation and the multiple decisions and interventions that must be made before the claim is resolved. But regardless of why the claim is so prolonged, the fact that it is prolonged increases the risk of a poor outcome. The unfortunate reality is that individuals who have been out of work for extended periods of time often have difficulty reentering the work force. This circumstance is true both for IWs[25] and for people who have no medical problems but have been laid off from their jobs.[30]

2. The treating physician's role is not just one of providing medical care for an IW. In fact, judgments about Mr Smith's disability status required an enormous amount of time and effort on the part of the physician.

3. Judgments about disability in the workers' compensation system are multilayered and interwoven. It is rarely the case that a treating physician renders a single judgment about the ability of patients to work. Instead, as the example shows, the physician is repeatedly asked or required to make judgments that bear on the disability status of his or her patients. Also, the physician may end up interfacing between the patients and several organizations (eg, the workers' compensation insurer, the SSA, the Department of Motor Vehicles, and Mr Smith's automobile credit company. As the example shows, the contradictory needs of different agencies make the difficult task of disability evaluation even more taxing.

4. The questions posed to the physician in the aforementioned example were not explicitly about pain. Pain was central to the entire problem because Mr Smith's medical condition was one in which activity limitations are created primarily by pain. But the role of pain was by itself insufficient to allow the system to make necessary decisions. Facing patients who perceive their life to be limited by pain, it can be frustrating for a physician who is asked to corroborate such elements of the patients' history with objective findings that for whatever reason may not be obtainable. The physician should understand that what seems to make no sense medically may make abundantly good sense to a system charged with consistently and appropriately redistributing societal wealth. In short, physicians should recognize that others fund the system, and it is, therefore, others who own it.

5. The treating physician in this example included Mr Smith in crucial decisions and generally paid a great deal of attention to Mr Smith's concerns. Some physicians might take a very different approach to this kind of patient. For example, a physician might focus on the fact that Mr Smith lacked unequivocally objective findings and support early closure of the claim. The authors are of the opinion that the right

approach is the one that most safely and efficiently assists the IW to a return to health, function, and employment.

REFERENCES

1. Robinson JP, Turk DC, Loeser JD. Pain, impairment, and disability in the AMA guides. J Law Med Ethics 2004;32(2):315–26.
2. Attending doctor's handbook. Olympia, Washington: Department of Labor and Industries. Publication F252-004-000. 2012.
3. Maghout Juratli S, Franklin GM, Mirza SK, et al. Lumbar fusion outcomes in Washington State workers' compensation. Spine (Phila Pa 1976) 2006;31(23):2715–23.
4. Volinn E, Jamison DF, Fine PG. Opioid therapy for nonspecific low back pain and the outcome of chronic work loss. Pain 2009;142(3):194–201.
5. Gross DP, Stephens B, Bhambhani Y, et al. Opioid prescriptions in Canadian workers' compensation claimants: prescription trends and associations between early prescription and future recovery. Spine 2009;34(5):525–31.
6. Franklin GM, Stover BD, Turner JA, et al. Early opioid prescription and subsequent disability among workers with back injuries: the Disability Risk Identification Study Cohort. Spine 2008;33(2):199–204.
7. Webster BS, Verma SK, Gatchel RJ. Relationship between early opioid prescribing for acute occupational low back pain and disability duration, medical costs, subsequent surgery and late opioid use. Spine 2007;32(19):2127–32.
8. Trippolini MA, Dijkstra PU, Côté P, et al. Can functional capacity tests predict future work capacity in patients with whiplash-associated disorders? Arch Phys Med Rehabil 2014;95 [pii:S0003-9993(14) 00934–4].
9. Gross DP, Asante AK, Miciak M, et al. Are performance-based functional assessments superior to semistructured interviews for enhancing return-to-work outcomes? Arch Phys Med Rehabil 2014;95(5):807–15.
10. Reneman MF, Soer R, Gross DP. Developing research on performance-based functional work assessment: report on the first international functional capacity evaluation research meeting. J Occup Rehabil 2013;23(4):513–5. http://dx.doi.org/10.1007/s10926-013-9425-1.
11. Mamun A, O'Leary P, Wittenburg DC, et al. Employment among Social Security disability program beneficiaries, 1996-2007. Soc Secur Bull 2011;71(3):11–34.
12. Rucker KS, Metzler HM. Predicting subsequent employment status of SSA disability applicants with chronic pain. Clin J Pain 1995;11:22–35.
13. Osterweis M, Kleinman A, Mechanic D, editors. Pain and disability. Washington, DC: National Academy Press; 1987.
14. Diagnostic and statistical manual of mental disorders. 4th edition. Washington, DC: American Psychiatric Association; 1994.
15. Franklin GM, Wickizer TM, Coe NB, et al. Workers' compensation: poor quality health care and the growing disability problem in the United States. Am J Ind Med 2014. http://dx.doi.org/10.1002/ajim.22399.
16. King SA. Review: DSM-IV and pain. Clin J Pain 1995;11:171–6.
17. Robinson JP. Workers' compensation and disability. In: Ballantyne J, Tauben D, editors. Expert decision making on opioid treatment. New York: Oxford University Press; 2013. p. 103–14.
18. Available at: www.drugfreeworkplace.org. Accessed February 20, 2012.
19. United States Department of Labor. Drug-Free Workplace Act of 1988. Available at: http://www.dol.gov/elaws/asp/drugfree/screen4.htm. Accessed February 19, 2012.

20. Bush DM. The U.S. mandatory guidelines for federal workplace drug testing programs: current status and future considerations. Forensic Sci Int 2008;174:111–9.
21. Walsh JM. New technology and new initiatives in U.S. workplace testing. Forensic Sci Int 2008;174:120–4.
22. What employees need to know about DOT drug and alcohol testing. Washington, DC: U.S. Department of Transportation, Office of the Secretary; 2005.
23. FAA accepted medications. Available at: http://www.leftseat.com/medcat1.htm. Accessed February 20, 2012.
24. Drug testing poses quandary for employers. New York Times 2010.
25. Cheadle A, Franklin G, Wolfhagen C, et al. Factors influencing the duration of work-related disability: a population-based study of Washington State workers' compensation. Am J Public Health 1994;84(2):190–6.
26. EEOC NOTICE number 915.002 Date 10/10/95. Available at: http://www.eeoc. gov/policy/docs/preemp.html. Accessed February 20, 2012.
27. Robinson JP. Disability in low back pain: what do the numbers mean? American Pain Society Bulletin 1998;8(2):9–13.
28. Butler RJ, Johnson WG, Baldwin ML. Managing work disability: why first return to work is not a measure of success. Ind Labor Relat Rev 1995;48(3):452–69.
29. Johnson WG, Baldwin M. Returns to work by Ontario workers with permanent partial disabilities. (Report to the Workers' Compensation Board of Ontario). Ottawa (Canada): Workers' Compensation Board of Ontario; 1993.
30. It's still bad for the long-term unemployed. New York Times 2014.

Index

Note: Page numbers of article titles are in **boldface** type.

Phys Med Rehabil Clin N Am 26 (2015) 413–426
http://dx.doi.org/10.1016/S1047-9651(15)00019-4
1047-9651/15/$ – see front matter © 2015 Elsevier Inc. All rights reserved.

pmr.theclinics.com

Printed and bound by CPI Group (UK) Ltd, Croydon, CR0 4YY

03/10/2024

01040496-0008